Yoga For Freedom

John P. Vourlis

Yoga For Freedom

~

How twenty yoga students from America
traveled to Nepal to raise awareness about
child slavery and came home forever changed

~

John P. Vourlis

Hometown Media Productions

Cleveland, Ohio

Hometown Media Productions
Cleveland, Ohio

www.hometownmediaproductions.com
info@hometownmediaproductions.com

ISBN: 978-0-615-93719-9

Library of Congress Control Number: 2014904964

Library of Congress subject headings:
Vourlis, John P. -- Travel – Nepal.
Travel writing.
Nepal -- Social conditions -- 21st century.
Yoga-Philosophy

Back Cover author photo by Melissa Lynn Holt

Photos are ©2014 by photographer as noted in book. All other photos ©2014 John Vourlis.

Book Cover & Design by Jaime Lombardo, Eriepro Ltd., www.eriepro.com

1.1

This book is dedicated, with love, to my parents:

Rose Vourlis & Pete Vourlis

Prologue
The Writer's Perspective

I make no pretext that this book will somehow define or explain Nepal to you, nor do I claim that it will give you a complete understanding of the individuals who went on this amazing Yoga For Freedom journey with me. I can't say that it will make you want to go to Nepal, or even make you want to try downward dog or chaturanga. What this book will do, I hope, is tell the remarkable story of a group of people who, for their own particular reasons, traveled together halfway around the world to Nepal and then throughout that country for fifteen days in the summer of 2010.

Much of this book will be told in my fellow travelers' own words, through journals we all kept, so you will get more than my view of things. The voices at times may contradict each other, dispute each other, condemn or affirm each other. I won't try to give you a "definitive truth" or take sides too often. The noise level of twenty voices all speaking on the same subject might get a bit confusing, argumentative, and even cacophonous at times. To which I can only say this: that is how it was.

Wrapping one's mind around a place like Nepal could take an outsider like me a lifetime. For those of us who went on the Yoga For Freedom trip, just being able to take in all that happened, all that we saw and heard, touched, smelled, tasted and felt in two short weeks, and then make some sense of it all when we got back wasn't that much less of a challenge. To say we were overwhelmed by it all at times would be an understatement. This amazing journey pushed us all to our breaking points, emotionally as well as physically. All I can tell you with certainty is that this trip was, for me and I think most of the others as well, the trip of a lifetime. I also know with certainty that I would do it all again tomorrow. And someday, I probably will.

John Vourlis
May, 2014

Part 1
Before the Journey

*"We don't receive wisdom; we must discover it for ourselves
after a journey that no one can take for us or spare us."*
~ Marcel Proust

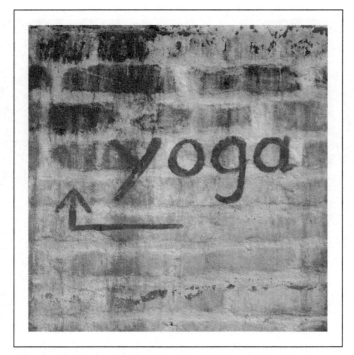

A hand painted sign on the wall of a building in Kathmandu, Nepal.

Everything Begins With An Idea

Be the change you want to see in the world.
~ Mahatma Gandhi

In the summer of 2009, Jesse Bach was volunteering in Kathmandu with Nepal Orphans Home (NOH), walking the children to school with Michael Hess, founder of NOH. It must have been quite a sight for any Nepali watching these two very different looking men strolling up the street like pied pipers followed by a gaggle of happy kids.

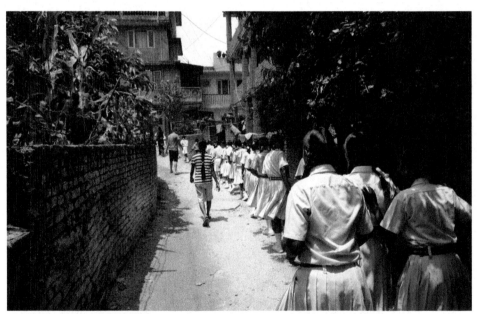

The children of Nepal Orphans Home walking to school. Photo courtesy of Candace Koslen.

Jesse Bach is a big dude. Bigger than life. He's in his 30's, about 6'2" and 300 pounds. He grew up in Parma, Ohio, a working class suburb of Cleveland, where he played high school football until his senior year, when he blew out a knee. He attended Kent State University as an undergrad, earned his Master's Degree in Education from Ursuline College and, at the time of this trip, was a shop teacher at his home town high school. He has an enormous shaved head, an impressive goatee, tattoos and earrings, all of which give the effect of a circus strongman. He was a devoted student of yoga and active member of the Cleveland yoga community. Jesse laughs loudly at times, and at other times he withdraws completely.

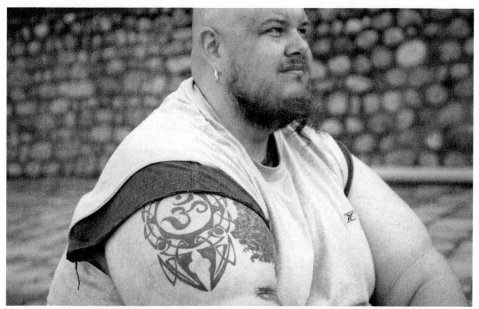

Jesse Bach. Photo courtesy of Candace Koslen

Jesse was no traveling naïf; on previous trips to Nepal, he had gone off on his own into the back country to places where few, if any, outsiders had ever ventured. On one such solo adventure, he had to perform immediate surgery on his own big toe using only a Swiss Army knife. Jesse was well aware of Nepal's many serious problems. He knew all the statistics about poverty, life expectancy, infant mortality, and child trafficking. In 2007, he had spent a month in western Nepal working with girls rescued from the Kamlari system, a kind of indentured servitude of children that has a long tradition in Nepal. During that time, he had an agonizing revelation, one of those moments of epiphany that can strike a person without warning and change their lives forever. These children aren't statistics, he realized. They are people, and they need help. When he returned to Cleveland, he promptly founded the Imagine Foundation to bring awareness to the problem of child slavery and human trafficking in the world, a cause for which he remains both passionate and committed to this day. Not knowing a single thing about charity work, but hoping to help these kids in any way he could, in 2009 and 2010 Jesse held benefits to raise money for the Nepal Orphans Home. These benefits drew the attention of Michael Hess and NOH.

Michael Hess is a thin, wiry, quiet man in his late 50's, a shade under 6' tall and 150 pounds soaking wet. He often wears a Cleveland Indians baseball cap, a gift from a volunteer, the bill pulled down to shade his eyes. His voice is soft, his demeanor gentle. He's also very steady and pragmatic. A carpenter from Florida, Michael had never traveled outside of the United States, until he went to Nepal for a month in early 2004 as a volunteer with a nongovernmental organization restoring a school building outside of Kathmandu. He found the experience so fulfilling that he returned again in March of 2005.

They walked several miles to the outskirts of the city, and as they crested a hill at the edge of the valley, Michael spotted an abandoned-looking building. His friend told him that this house was the orphanage she had wanted him to see. When

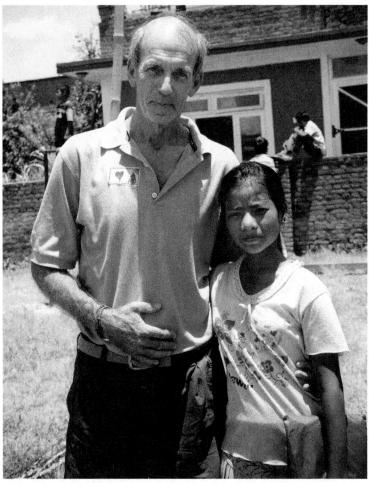

Michael Hess and one of the girls at NOH. It is the policy of Nepal Orphans Home not to identify by name the children living there to the media, a policy we have respected. Photo by Candace Koslen.

they approached, Michael's friend called out, "Namaste!" and a group of young children emerged from the run-down house. The conditions in and around this home were deplorable. There was no running water, and just one outhouse with no door. A wide broken gate in front of the building tilted on one hinge, useless and ignored, in the middle of a wall with broken glass embedded into the top. A sign on the gate read "Humanity Concern Center"; the irony of that name did not escape Michael. He found the children in a horrible state, malnourished, in poor health and not attending school. These kids were being forced by the orphanage owners to beg in the streets, his friend told him, a crude and commonplace money-making strategy. At the time, the vast majority of orphanages in Nepal were run by unscrupulous people, smooth-talking operators who used children for their own gain. These people would pocket whatever money the children could separate from unsuspecting tourists, and then abandon the children. Such was the case with this orphanage. It was at this moment, standing before this house and these children, that Michael had his own epiphany.

He returned to Kathmandu that evening, bought new clothes, shampoo and medicine, along with enough vegetables and rice for a full meal for all the kids, and came back the next day. The owners of the orphanage showed up and begrudgingly allowed Michael to supply the children there with the basic medical care and food they had been lacking for a very long time. These sham operators thought that Michael would eventually give up caring for the kids and leave. It took them months to realize he wasn't going anywhere. Once they did figure it out, they left in the middle of the night, taking supplies and children to set up operations elsewhere. Some of the children were found and eventually brought back. Over the next year, Michael sold his home and business in the United States, assumed control of this orphanage, renovated the building and began caring for the children. That was the beginning of Nepal Orphans Home.

That Jesse and Michael, such outwardly different men, could see the world in the same way, see the need to help those far less fortunate than themselves as a calling, is as much a testament to basic human goodness probably as anything else. This particular day, as the two men walked with the children to Skylark Academy where the kids of NOH now attended school, Jesse began talking to Michael about the loving nature of the yoga community that he was a part of in Cleveland, and how it would be amazing to bring people like that to Nepal to see firsthand the work that Michael was doing at the Nepal Orphans Home and to let them experience this amazing country for which they both shared a deep love. Over the next few weeks and months Jesse and Michael continued talking and from those long conversations, Yoga For Freedom was born.

Yoga For Freedom was not meant to be a relaxing spa holiday. The purpose of the Yoga for Freedom trip, Jesse and Michael decided, would be not only to educate people and raise their awareness of Nepal, but to allow outsiders to experience Nepal fully. The good (of which they knew there was plenty), the bad, and the ugly. Experiences usually reserved for the pages of National Geographic are what Jesse and Michael wanted to make available to those unfamiliar with Nepal. Traveling halfway around the globe to a poor, developing country, they both realized, would be a test of anyone's physical, spiritual and emotional limits. Their hope was that Yoga For Freedom would unite the spirit of yoga with the beauty of Nepal's natural landscape, to help effect change and improve the lives of the children of NOH.

From a practical standpoint, the trip would also serve as a platform to raise funds for the children of NOH. Though the cost of living in Nepal is unbelievably low, running an orphanage, feeding, clothing, educating and housing 120 children, does require money. So the two men decided that $850 of each traveler's cost of the Yoga For Freedom journey would be donated to NOH. This modest amount would be enough to support one child completely for an entire year. This combination of idealism and pragmatism is the perfect reflection of what Jesse and Michael represent. That's essentially why I wanted to be a part of this journey. I wanted my trip to be about more than just fulfilling my own need for adventure. The idea of helping a child, an orphan, to be taken care of for a whole year seemed a pretty special opportunity to me. So, in June of 2010, I joined a group of 19 other yoga teachers and students from the Cleveland area, and one from Hong Kong, on a two-week trip to Nepal, for the inaugural Yoga For Freedom journey.

The idea for this book came from one of our fellow travelers, Minling Chuang, who was in her late twenties with a degree from USC and an MBA from Indiana University. Minling's idea was to have the trip make even more of a long term difference. She wanted the trip to live on within the pages of a book that would help provide support for NOH, and she and Jesse also thought the book could shed some light on the Kamlari system in Nepal. All of us hope the book will inspire concrete action, whether through donations or volunteerism, to help children everywhere limited by circumstances, as well as to help raise funds for the children of NOH. In that vein, the majority of proceeds from this book will be donated to NOH to help feed, clothe, shelter and educate these remarkable kids. Every child deserves at least that.

Why Nepal?

You see things, and you say, 'Why?'
But I dream things that never were,
and I say, "Why not?"
~George Bernard Shaw

Going to Nepal isn't like traveling to Disneyworld or hiking the Grand Canyon. It's not like going on a tropical vacation or a ski trip to Aspen. Things we take for granted in the United States, like electricity, refrigerators, and air conditioning, are extreme rarities in Nepal. Garbage collection, traffic lights, and street signs are almost non-existent, as is healthcare. It takes an entire day of flying, dealing with luggage and airports and all the hassles of modern travel, just to get there.

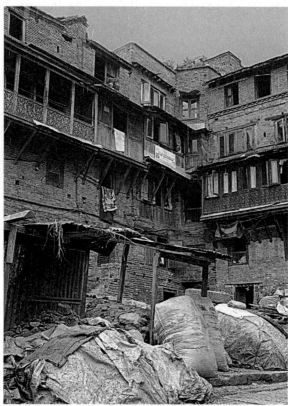

Garbage collection is sporadic at best in Nepal. More often than not it's burned, or just dumped. Photo by Candace Koslen.

When you do finally arrive, your sleep patterns are completely disrupted. What you feel should be night time is actually the middle of the day because your body clock has been turned upside down. The food looks and tastes different from what many Westerners are used to, and the language is quite foreign to most Americans.

So why go to a small, third world country like Nepal, then? If it's volunteer work you want to do, why not go somewhere closer to home, somewhere in the United States to help out? If it's charity you're interested in, why not just write a check to NOH and be done with it? What kind of vacation would it be anyway, going to an impoverished nation that lacks so many of the creature comforts of home? These questions, and many more, were being asked of us often as we prepared to head off on the Yoga For Freedom adventure. To answer them, you first have to know a little about Nepal.

For those who aren't familiar with Nepal, the country is located just about halfway around the world from the United States, where the Indian subcontinent collides with Asia, the result of this collision being the world's tallest mountain range, the Himalayas. Nepal is bordered to the north by the People's Republic of China and the Chinese occupied nation of Tibet, and to the south, east, and west by the Republic of India.

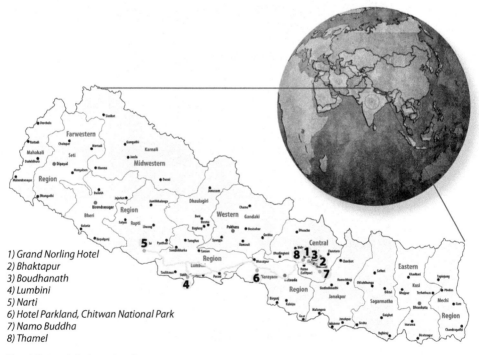

1) Grand Norling Hotel
2) Bhaktapur
3) Boudhanath
4) Lumbini
5) Narti
6) Hotel Parkland, Chitwan National Park
7) Namo Buddha
8) Thamel

Nepal. Our route is shown in yellow.

Nepal has a rich geography. The mountainous north has eight of the world's ten tallest mountains, including the highest point on Earth, Mount Everest, called Sagarmatha in Nepali. It contains more than 240 peaks over 20,000 ft. (6,096 m) above sea level. As a contrast, North America has one mountain taller than 20,000 feet - Mt. McKinley in Alaska. The fertile and humid south is heavily urbanized. With an area of 147,181 square kilometers (56,827 sq. mi.) and a population of approximately 30 million, Nepal is the world's 93rd largest country by land mass and the 41st most populous country. Kathmandu is the capital and the country's largest city.

Nepal may be a small country, but it is one of the most beautiful places on the planet. You can take in spectacular vistas of the highest mountains on Earth one day, and the next day join an elephant safari through lowland jungles where you can see rhinos and tigers in the wild. This is an untamed land, a world where rice farming, one of the most labor intensive forms of agriculture, is critical to the lives of not only vast numbers of peasant farmers, but the whole nation. The views throughout the country of hillsides terraced with rice paddies, peasants tending the fields, are serene and often-times stunning.

Nepal is also one of the most spiritual places in the world. Monks are as common in Nepal as teenagers in a western shopping mall. Hinduism is practiced by a large majority of the people. Buddhism, though in the minority, is also linked historically to the country since it is the birthplace of the Buddha, founder of Buddhism, one of the world's major spiritual philosophies. Many Nepali, in fact, do not distinguish between the two religious practices, and follow both traditions. Nepal is also one of the centers of that other great eastern philosophical export, yoga, the practice of which is closely related to both Buddhism and Hinduism. The landscape of Nepal is dotted with some of the most beautiful Buddhist art in the entire world, too. There are breathtaking monasteries and wondrous temples and stupas everywhere.

Nepali's are also some of the sweetest, most gentle people you will meet, people who would gladly share their meal with you or go hours out of their way to direct you to where you are going. But despite all the natural beauty and Buddhist serenity, Kathmandu, the capital, is intensely hectic. Though crime doesn't seem rampant, the people generally seem to govern themselves. Just take a ride through Kathmandu, where you can watch a lone traffic cop stand on a raised concrete platform in the middle of one of the capital's busiest boulevards, valiantly, futilely attempting to do his job, a job that requires him to wear a dust mask to save himself from the pollution of thousands of vehicles hurtling past him - cars, trucks, vans, buses, motorcycles and gas powered rickshaws.

Throughout most of its history, Nepal was a monarchy ruled by various royal factions, some allied with the British, who ruled neighboring India from the early 1800's to the mid-1900's. A recent decade-long Civil War between royalists, the military, and Maoist insurgents led to the murder of the Nepali king by his nephew. The war and the assassination culminated in mass protests by all major political parties, until the conflict was finally resolved in November 2005. The ensuing elections for a new Parliament in 2008 abolished the monarchy and established a federal multiparty representative democratic republic whose first President was sworn in on July 23, 2008.

Despite having resolved some major political issues, Nepal still grapples with a host of other troublesome problems. Population growth and poverty are two of the biggest ones. The population in the Kathmandu Valley has doubled between the 1990's and 2000's and is rising at an unsustainable rate. Much of the population lives in poverty, and the majority of the people live as subsistence farmers. Life expectancy is just sixty-three years, and one in twenty children die before the age of five. In addition, an estimated 1 in 3 Nepali children fall victim to child slavery.

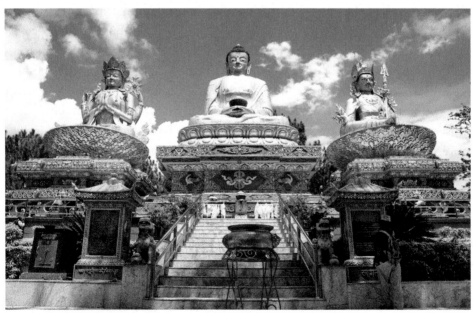

Exquisite statues like the ones at Swayambhunath in Kathmandu are not uncommon in Nepal. Also known as the Monkey Temple because the monkeys living there are considered holy by both Buddhists and Hindus, this 1500 year-old temple area is among the oldest religious sites in Nepal. Photo by Candace Koslen.

Child slavery has a long, reprehensible tradition in Nepal. Widespread poverty leaves children vulnerable to a form of indentured servitude known as the Kamlari system. In rural areas, poor families are pressured by financial hardship into taking money in exchange for sending children, as young as six years old, to work in the homes of wealthy people as indentured laborers, because such an exchange can help the remainder of the family buy things like food and medicine that are necessary for survival. In the local language of Western Nepal, Kamlari literally means "slave."

Here is a brief account of what that experience was like for one of the young girls at NOH named Sarita.[1]

> My mother died when I was ten and my father sold me to home owners. They did not work, I did it all. I would wake up at 4 am and start to work, and I would finish my work at 11 or 12 at night. The family never let me go [to] sleep, they would always give me more work to do; if they found me sleeping they would scold and then beat me.
>
> My sister Sapana talked to Papa [what the children of NOH call Michael] about where I was and what was happening to me. Papa sent Vinod [a young Nepali man who worked at NOH]... to the village where I was [to] take me. When they got to me the family refused to let me go; one man in the house was always beating me and I was scared, but Vinod... told the house owner I was going with them and took me.
>
> If not being rescued I would never escape the Kamlari system, I don't know what would have happened with not good food, little sleep, all the time work, all the time beaten what would happen to me.

Over half of the 120 children in Nepal Orphans Home are former Kamlaris like Sarita. As Sarita says, she did not know what would have happened to her if she had not been rescued. Often sent far from their homes, Kamlari girls are terribly isolated and vulnerable to physical violence and sexual abuse. However Dickensian it sounds to the average westerner, the simple fact remains that such horrors still exist in the modern world, which in itself was reason enough to draw like-minded, conscientious individuals like ourselves to Nepal to see if we could somehow make a difference. As idealistic, perhaps even naïve, as that might seem, that is exactly what Michael and Jesse had done. They had gone to Nepal, had seen the problems firsthand, and then decided to do something about them. And as a result, both ended up making a very real difference.

So, why Nepal, then? Well, to paraphrase George Bernard Shaw - "Why not?" This amazing little country is where we chose to go, full of noble intentions and

---

[1] Children's names used here by permission of Nepal Orphans Home.

good will. We were a smart, motivated group of spirited and caring individuals, and we were going to make a difference there, of course. How could we not? Blissfully unaware of the challenges to come, we jumped right in to the adventure, and discovered that it's one thing to want to effect change, and quite another to get twenty people to all pull in the same direction to make it happen.

The Travelers

"You are three people:
The one you think you are - the body.
The one others think you are - the mind.
The one you really are - the divine."
~ Sai Baba

Below are all the people who would eventually go on the Yoga For Freedom trip:

Jesse Bach

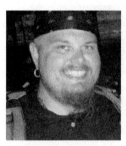

Minling Chuang

Terri Bahr

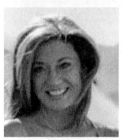

Eve Ennis

Robb Blain

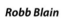
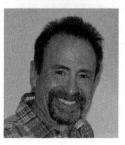

Joyce Fijalkovich

Jaime Furda 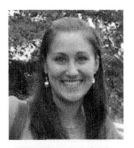 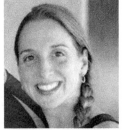 *Candace Koslen*

Kathy Hayes 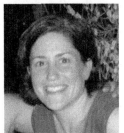 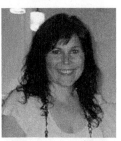 *Deanna Lee*

Christina Jankus 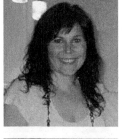 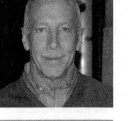 *Marc Nathanson*

David Kampinsky 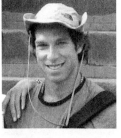 *Tingting Peng*

Gabrielle Stickley-Klein 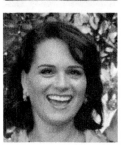 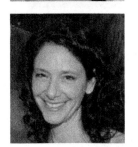 *Marni Task*

Rachel Vincent

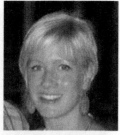

Jennette Zimmerman

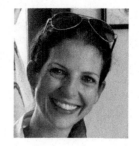

John Vourlis

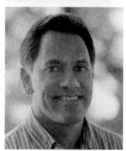

There were twenty members of the group traveling to Nepal, including Carola Drosdeck, our spiritual den mother and contact at NOH. Eleven of the travelers were yoga teachers, and the others were yoga students from the Cleveland area, except for Tingting Peng, who lived in Hong Kong. There were five men and fifteen women, ranging between nineteen and sixty years of age. We represented a wide variety of occupations, as well as a mix of religious, spiritual and cultural backgrounds. Each one of us held an appreciation for Buddhism, and some of the members were daily practitioners. Four of the travelers were parents, and the youngest member was a college student. Most of us were college graduates, from places as varied as MIT and Cleveland State University. Several people, myself included, had advanced degrees from universities such as Case Western Reserve, Indiana and USC.

This little band of yoga brothers and sisters was accompanied by four exceptional Nepali's. **Basu Panday** of Nepal Social Treks was our group's guide and a longtime friend of Jesse and Michael. Jesse also brought along **Subash Adhikari**, a Nepali yoga instructor to teach yoga classes to us every day of the trip. We were, after all, yoga students, and what better place to practice yoga than in the heartland of that philosophy? Two important additions were **Buddha Saktia**, our bus driver extraordinaire, and **Sun Tze**, his always smiling assistant. These four men provided invaluable help, knowledge, instruction and friendship along our journey.

Basu Panday

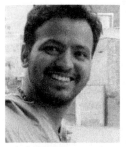

Subash Adhikari

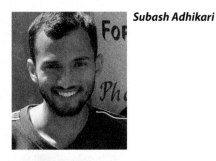

Buddha Saktia

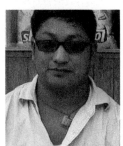

Sun Tze

This is a snapshot of who we were. From a philosophical viewpoint, it's not always 'Who' that is most interesting, but more often 'How' and 'Why'. Why this group of people? Why this journey? And why now? Was everyone on this trip like me, just looking for an adventure? Or were they seeking something deeper, more profound? Why were we brought together at this time, for this trip? Was it meant to be? Or was it just coincidence, a random series of events leading up to this point in time? Even more important questions, perhaps, were these: Were we naïve enough to think we could actually make a difference in these children's lives in the short time we would be in Nepal? And how would this trip affect us, both as individuals and as a group? Only time, and the journey, would tell.

Discovery

"Adventure is just bad planning."
~ Roald Amundsen

I found out about the Yoga For Freedom trip in a yoga class at Cleveland Yoga, in Beachwood, Ohio, where many of the travelers practiced. It was around Christmas of 2009, and one of the teachers there mentioned a trip to Nepal that would be taking place the following summer. That was a part of the world I had always wanted to see, so I filed that little bit of information away in the back of my brain as something I might want to do.

When I had first heard about the trip, I was working as a freelance writer, splitting my time between Los Angeles and Cleveland. Not long after that class, I headed back to LA for business and soon forgot about the trip, until one day an ad for it popped up on my Facebook page. I clicked on the Facebook ad, and soon realized that this must be the trip the yoga instructor in Cleveland had mentioned. I quickly sent an email to Jesse Bach, the trip organizer, asking him if there were still spots available. He wrote back:

From: <Jesse Bach>

To: <John Vourlis>

Date: Sun, Jan 24, 2010 9:00 am

Well this might sound like it was planned, but it totally wasn't. I just opened my e-mail this morning [and] the first message was an unfortunate cancellation; a member of Yoga for Freedom had to drop out. The second e-mail was you...

Attached to this e-mail is our brochure and description letter; ... fill out the Application and send it to me... so I can hold [a spot] for you...

- Jesse Bach

I read the attached introductory letter and brochure. "**Yoga for Freedom: One traveler, two lives forever changed**… This trip is life changing for all people involved; the traveler as well as the child who this trip will support." A vacation with an altruistic twist; very intriguing. I looked over the itinerary: Grand Norling Resort Hotel, Mt. Everest flight, Lumbini - the birthplace of the Buddha, Chitwan National Park - home to elephants, rhinos and tigers! Not one, but two Buddhist Monasteries. Yoga twice a day, morning and evening. This trip sounded amazing. I wanted in.

We had four months to prepare for our trip, and I wasn't in any rush to get started. I do procrastinate, especially where money or travel commitments are concerned. Here there were both, so I was really dragging my feet. Planning for a trip like this is as much about mental preparation as it is about the physical logistics. Of course, you need to buy tickets, procure visas, and get immunizations, as well as decide what to pack and how much money to bring. But you also have to deal with all the issues in your life that a trip like this forces you to confront. And that can prove a far bigger challenge than deciding on a backpack.

Travel can act as a backlight for the problems you're already dealing with in your day-to-day life, and sometimes casts a spotlight on all the dark corners of your psyche, where your deepest fears reside. Once those fears are brought to light, like a wild animal cornered, they tend to lash out. On this trip, fear was going to play an important role, like Iago in Othello, a catalyst for the drama, driving the action forward. What none of us realized at the time, myself included, was just how very important a role this fear would play.

February 25, 2010 _____

My head is spinning. It's easy to get caught up in your story… A lot is going through my mind right now, and it's all about me. New house is a mess. Have to sell this house. Have to move. Have no money. Ayla's going to a new school.

Right when we get settled…I am off to Nepal for two weeks. I am trusting the universe that it just knows – what's best – that everything will work out. Have to admit… I am overwhelmed. I am scared. I am having second thoughts. Am I strong enough to leave my own children?

But have made the commitment.

_____ *Candy Koslen*

March 1, 2010 _____

Today I was reminded that my layover is in Abu Dhabi in the Arab Emirates… My layover is 12 hours. Great fear shot through my body when I realized that no one [from YFF] is on the same flight as me. The fear went through me leaving me in state of panic. I don't know why I was so overcome. I guess its fear of the unknown. What do I do with that amount of time? Should I get a hotel? Should I wait to see how my flight schedule pans out, and maybe I won't need a hotel? Should I view this as an opportunity to see another part of the world that I had not anticipated seeing?

As always, I allay my fears with research. Research and knowledge is a good cure for fear of the unknown.

_____ *Christina Jankus*

When it comes to dealing with your fears, to some extent Christina was right. Knowledge is power. Fear used well can lead you to knowledge, understanding, even wisdom. It can push you to learn about the world around you, and the world within you. The more you know and understand, the more manageable are your fear. Regardless, it doesn't hurt to have the support of others. After all, we weren't traveling alone. There would be twenty of us on this journey, walking into the unknown together. Ideally, we'd be able to lean on each other when necessary.

It never hurts to maintain a sense of humor, either, to be able to laugh and to understand, as Rick says in Casablanca, that our own individual problems don't amount to a hill of beans in this crazy world. I think that Robb, among all of us, had the best sense of humor about things. It probably helped that he was one of the older members in our group, and that he'd served in Vietnam. He had the kind of life experience that many of us lacked, the kind that prepares you for venturing into the unknown, and this gave him a healthy perspective on things, including journaling…

March 13, 2010 _____

I'm sorry I have not been better with my journaling, but I refuse to write every day that I'm excited about my journey to Nepal for which I truly am. But I'm not going to waste trees and ink with that redundancy.

_____ *Robb Blain*

Goals and perspectives aside, the size and composition of the group continued to grow and change through the early months of 2012. Jaime Furda joined the trip in late March. She brought an air of youthfulness and wonder to our mix that was refreshing. Everything on this trip was new to her. A talented musician with a terrific singing voice, which we all were able to enjoy at various times on the trip, Jaime also had some of the same issues as the rest of us. Like me, she wasn't sure if she had the means to go on this trip. But where there's a will, there turns out to be a way.

March 30, 2010 _____

[Jaime] contacted me in December, right after I got back from celebrating Christmas in Nepal with the kids. Out of the blue, she decided she wanted to go to Nepal. I met with her over coffee, said she just loved the stories I would tell and now that she was older, wanted to experience them for herself. She's a [college] student now, around 20 years old. She planned a benefit concert for herself, to raise the funds to get herself there. I was extremely impressed, I really like people who make things happen, and she was making things happen. Then the venue fell through about a week before the concert, and her trip dreams were extinguished. She had given up all hope. I received a phone call the night the concert was supposed to go on, a friend who chose to remain anonymous wondered if it was possible to sponsor someone on the trip. A person, with a simple signature on a check changed someone's life forever; no, she changed multiple lives forever. She will be home this weekend, I'll tell her the good news. The universe works in amazing ways.

_____ *Jesse Bach*

On April 3rd Jesse sent out an email to the group to announce a fundraising event, a scholarship party to raise funds to help send another person on the trip. This was attached to his email…

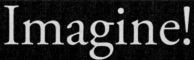

Imagine!

What's possible if we just try!

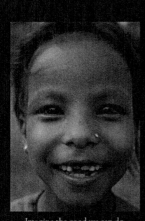

Imagine the good we can do.
Imagine the wrongs we can right.
Imagine what's possible if we just try.

Her name is Sita, she is six years old.

Imagine a world where you can be a super-hero to children.

I'm pleased to tell you it's possible. On Friday April 16th from 6:30-10:00pm Imagine will be hosting a "Yoga for Freedom scholarship party", to raise funds and awareness to send a volunteer to Nepal to help in the work of Nepal Orphans Home.

You can join us at:

The Murray Hill Galleries
The Yoga Room
2026 Murray Hill Rd
Cleveland, Oh 44106

Join us for a Yoga practice at 6:30pm followed by Kirtan and party at 8pm. There will be food and drinks, silent auction items and performances.

There is a suggested $20.00 donation, however no-one will be turned away. Please direct any questions Jesse Bach at theimaginebenefit@gmail.com facebook.com/imaginebenefit facebook.com/yogaforfreedom

The party went off without a hitch, and Jesse raised enough to fund the scholarship. Now he just had to get people to apply for it. The application process involved three questions, which Jesse borrowed from the movie "Bucket List". He loved the theme of that movie: two people living it up before they die. The questions were:

1. Have you lived a joyful life?

2. What have you done to bring joy to others?

3. How will this experience change things?

He hoped that the recipient of the scholarship would answer the questions honestly, without fluff or insincerity. He really wanted the recipient to be the right person.

The day after the party, there was a gathering for everyone going on the trip at Jennette Zimmerman's home. I was a bit nervous. Meeting a bunch of new people all at once can sometimes be overwhelming. At least I would know the yoga instructor who had first mentioned the trip, I thought to myself, but as soon as I arrived, I found out she wasn't there, and that she wouldn't be going on the trip after all. Yikes. I didn't know a single person who would be traveling with me. I had only communicated with Jesse via email, and hadn't met any of the others. No matter. I wanted an adventure, and now the adventure was beginning.

At the meeting, I introduced myself to Jesse. My first impression was confirmed—a happy, sincere, circus strongman. Jesse introduced me to Jennette and the others. Everyone was exceedingly nice. They all seemed to know each other, and I felt a little bit like an outsider to the group, but I was okay with that. All part of the adventure - that was my mantra. We 'noshed' awhile on pizza, hummus and veggies, and sipped some wine and other beverages before gathering in the living room. We sat on pillows, and Jesse led a discussion on the book Sold, about the plight of children who have fallen victim to the horrible practice of child enslavement, told through the eyes of Lakshmi, a young Nepali girl who is sold into slavery in India. He had asked us to read the book before our trip, and it had a powerful effect on all of us who read it.

March 19, 2010 _____

Il was haunted by Lakshmi in my sleep last night. I am jarred awake several times with the frustration and desperation of not being able to save her. Right before I jolt awake I am dreaming that I have Lakshmi in my arms running and a very cruel man takes her from me.

It was horrible! I was sweating, and breathing shallow. I went downstairs to the kitchen to get myself a cold drink of water to try to calm myself down since it seemed so real to me.

_____ *Christina Jankus*

Following the book discussion, we watched a short documentary on the Nepal Orphans Home and its founder, Michael Hess, by the Canadian filmmaker Toni Thomson. (You can learn more about Toni, her documentary and the works she's doing in Nepal on her website at www.possibleworlds.ca). It was the first time most of us had actually seen or heard Michael or the kids of NOH. This short film was a trailer for a longer project Thomson was working on, yet it was powerful and poignant. Suddenly, the trip was becoming less abstract, more real. My fanciful thoughts of seeing Mt. Everest and the land of Buddha began taking on darker shading. Nepal wasn't going to be all fun and adventure. Our trip was also going to raise awareness about the disturbing real world of child trafficking. I wondered what kind of man Michael Hess must be to undertake a noble cause like this – was he a saint or just plain crazy? Perhaps a little of both.

After the movie, Jesse handed a flyer to everyone inviting us to journal about our experiences leading up to, during, and after the trip, and informing us that, if we chose to participate in this unique group exercise, what we wrote in our journals would be compiled into a book to be published and sold to benefit the children we would be meeting on the trip.[2] I read the flyer and was a bit trepidatious. Even though I am a writer and a published author, I don't like journaling. I like to keep all those thoughts and emotions swirling in my head like a primordial soup, out of which I draw inspiration for my writing. Or at least that's what I told myself then.

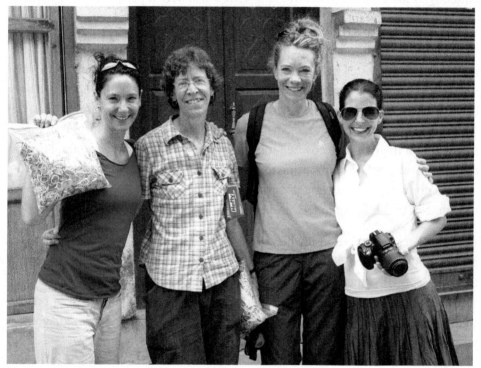

Marni, Carola, volunteer Tamara Chante, and Jennette. Photo by Candace Koslen.

Carola Drosdeck, a member of the NOH Board of Directors, then spoke to the group about Nepal, NOH, our journey and its purpose. A school teacher living in Cleveland, Carola came across as warm and kind, with the unpretentious demeanor of a caring "earth mother". She didn't try to sugarcoat the trip, or the plight of the children. You could see in her eyes and hear in her voice that she was totally committed to NOH.

---

[2] *Several people were already journaling on their own about the trip even before Jesse handed out the flyer.*

Carola was going to be in Nepal while we were there, working full-time as a volunteer at the orphanage, which she had been doing for several years. It turned out that three members of the group, Jennette, Candace and Marni would also be going as volunteers. They were yoga instructors in the Cleveland area who wanted to give something back to the world through NOH and the Yoga For Freedom trip. We would only meet up with these volunteers at a few stages along our journey, since the rest of us would be trekking around the country most of the time. Ours would be a separate experience from theirs, but we planned to come together intermittently to share a few adventures and relate our different perspectives of Nepal.

Hearing her speak, I liked Carola right away, and as she talked about the journal-to-book idea, I began to soften my attitude about a practice that as a writer, up until this trip at least, I had not warmly embraced, perhaps because, along with my disdain for it, I also feared journaling a little too. Words as thoughts are one thing, but words on paper are something else entirely. They are a commitment, on the record, of your feelings. A journal is a snapshot, or series of snapshots of those feelings in all their raw uncensored form. I'm one whose mind likes to mull things over a long time before committing thoughts to words on paper, but when journaling, you don't always have time to think. I came to learn that that's part of the point, though. Not to think, but to feel, and express those feelings. In words. On paper.

A little scary, yes, but in my life, I've learned a few things, and one is you have to confront your fears if you want to grow. Maybe I would give journaling a try I thought, especially since it had a goal. Maybe it would help me grow, if not as a person, then as a writer. A book constructed from the journals of twenty or so people sounded pretty cool to me, too. Whoever writes that book, though, is in for a really big challenge. On that count, I turned out to be absolutely correct.

Anxiety & Anticipation

"If pleasures are greatest in anticipation,
just remember that this is also true of troubles"
~Elbert Hubbard

I went back to LA a few days later with a lot to think about. I began to research possible flights and the necessary immunizations. I had been overseas before, and I knew that Kaiser in LA had a travel office with a list of all the immunizations you needed to travel anywhere in the world. Since the internet has pretty much made the travel agent obsolete, I went online to search for flights, and found dozens of options on dozens of carriers. I asked around for advice, but quickly realized I'd have to figure it out for myself. Everyone else was going through similar logistical trials and tribulations:

April 18, 2010 _____

I am a bit freaked about the bus trip through the mountain ranges, the cliffs, and the airplane trip over the Himalayas. I hope I can be okay with my fear of heights, and not have an anxiety attack get in the way....

_____ *Marc Nathanson*

Once again, knowledge took the edge off our anxieties and fears. Jesse sent everyone an email with links to many of the places where we would be staying. It got everyone, myself included, pumped up with anticipation for the adventure that lay ahead of us.

April 23, 2010 _____

Yesterday Jesse sent us the websites for most of our accommodations. They looked awesome. It also took away a bit of the unknown of how we were going to live for two weeks. I was thinking a dorm-like setting and tents, but the pictures were of nice hotels with an Eastern culture look and feel.

_____ *Marc Nathanson*

You can't really fear the unknown if there is no unknown to fear. Like Marc, I was truly impressed with the accommodations Jesse had arranged for us. So, on April 26, I finally 'bit the bullet' and wrote Jesse a check for payment in full for the trip. Doing that made me feel like there was no turning back. For me, it was no small chunk of change. Then I remembered some advice a friend had once given me: When in doubt, go! And I really did want to go, so… the check was in the mail.

Meanwhile, Jesse was stressed about the scholarship:

April 29, 2010 _____

Tomorrow the scholarship application is due and no one has applied. That's a little frustrating but understandable. It's a huge commitment and scary to head to the other side of the world. I learned a lot from it though. I don't know if we will do it again next year. We spent all this time, money and energy and not one person applied…

I'm depositing everyone's money and getting horribly nervous about it. It's a big number growing in that account, the biggest number I've ever seen. I now understand what Michael said about Nepal Orphans Home. When it was his money, it was no big deal; once outsiders involve their money it's a completely different story. With my money I just don't care, with their money I do.

_____ *Jesse Bach*

It was eventually decided that the scholarship money would be granted to a traveler whose tuition fee was paid by an anonymous donor, and who had little resources for airfare. Everyone who attended the event had donated specifically to help someone without the financial means to go to Nepal on Yoga For Freedom, so this decision appeared to be the best solution.

On May 7, Jesse sent an email with a checklist and the arrival and departure schedule. I downloaded the checklist and began reading it over. The trip was now 'official', so naturally, some people were getting the pre-trip jitters. Others were just plain excited to get going. I fell in the jittery camp. As I said in the beginning, traveling to Nepal, halfway around the world, is not like going to Disneyworld, no matter how enticing the accommodations.

I started thinking about practical things like packing for the trip. Do I need a backpack? I have a regular sized one, I'll use that. Can I fit everything on the checklist in a duffle bag? Travel guru Rick Steves recommends a 12 x 24 one, so I'll buy a cheapie. At Big 5 Sporting Goods on Wilshire, I was lucky to find a collapsible duffle bag for a mere $19. If it got ruined, lost, or stolen, I wouldn't be too upset. Last big question: how many pairs of underwear do I bring for a two week trip? 5? 7? 10? I decided to bring 14.

As the day of departure drew near, people were doing their best to get prepared:

May 9, 2010 _____

...this week I went to a hypnotherapist to try and deal with my fear of heights. I am scared and worried about the bus trip into the Himalayas. So I went to this session, hoping to be able to focus on something other than my fear. We will see if it really works.

_____ *Marc Nathanson*

Around this time, things in Nepal started to become a bit squirrely, politically speaking. The country had just come out of a long civil war between those loyal to the King and Royal family, and Maoist insurgents mainly drawn from the peasants in the countryside. The civil war had taken many lives, and badly divided the country. After several years of armed struggle, a tentative peace took hold, and the competing factions attempted to create a new democratic state and a new constitution. The writing of that constitution, however, proved to be very difficult. Despite the dysfunctional government, Nepal and its people simply carried on. We weren't Nepali's though, and some members of our group were becoming seriously concerned about traveling to such an apparently unstable country.

May, 2010 _____

...we started receiving information about the travel warnings issued by the Department of State about the safety of travel to Nepal. There was a lot going on politically before we left and there were frequent instances of violent riots. Reports were also stating that there were several instances of people being robbed, sometimes by groups of armed men, while asleep in hotels or traveling popular tourist trails, even in daylight. It was advised not to travel in public transportation, especially in tourist buses day or night, or with large groups of foreign women. We were doing all of the above so a few of us began to become afraid for our safety. The news began reporting the story of the yoga teacher who had recently disappeared while in Nepal and this raised our eyebrows even further; we knew this trip would be intense on certain levels but intentionally putting ourselves in harm's way seemed a foolish idea. Upon hearing affirmation from volunteers at the Nepal Orphan's Home that everything was okay and we would be safe we were set at ease but still a little hesitant. After much consideration and reassurance that we didn't have to take part in anything that made us feel unsafe we packed up and began our journey.

Deanna Lee

I wasn't immune to the anxieties myself. Around May 22nd, I read an article on the internet about a missing backpacker, the same story Deanna was referencing.

Nepal police search for missing U.S. hiker[3]

KATMANDU, Nepal (AP) — Police are scouring a remote region in northern Nepal, searching for a Colorado woman who has been missing since last month when she failed to check in after a solo hike in the Himalayan mountains, an official said Wednesday.

Aubrey Sacco, 23, of Greeley, was reported missing by her family. She had arrived in the Langtang area in the northern region of Nepal in April for a trek that was to last just over a week.

Her mother, Connie Sacco, said Aubrey had promised to check in by e-mail around April 29 but did not.

The young woman was hiking alone without a guide or porter. There were not many other backpackers in the area because it was end of the trekking season.

The police chief in the Rasuwa area, Om Bahadur Rana, said police teams were searching the trekking route and interviewing inn owners and villagers. Word has been sent to local monasteries, which are often visited by foreign trekkers....

The search was unable to begin sooner because mass protests on May 1 and a general strike imposed by the Maoist former rebels shut down all transport in Nepal until May 7.

It was a very sad story, one that still has not been resolved, unfortunately (as of November 2013, Aubrey was still missing). I emailed Jesse about the article. He said that when trekking in a third world country, especially one that has undergone recent political turmoil, even an experienced traveler should have a guide, and stay in contact with someone there. We will have twenty or so people with us, as well as a Nepali guide, so this should not be a problem, I thought.

The past week has been filled with uncertainty about the trip; whether or not to drop out due to fear. I was so blind to it before, I was ignoring any possibility of danger because I didn't want to believe it. Then, I allowed the fear to penetrate... eventually consuming and controlling me. It was awful. Up and down with: "Yes, I'm going, I need to," to "No, I have to cancel"...after all of the "what ifs" blanketed my busy mind. Today was beautiful. I sat on the back patio with Kristal in the early morning after Alex's graduation. We talked, relaxed. Then went home and had lunch with Mom. We talked at LENGTH of my fears, paranoia. I spent hours alone allowing thoughts in... I knew I had to allow the decision to just come to me without trying to force it. Mom went to yoga with me, her first class ever. It was incredible to share my love of yoga with her. Upon arriving, I saw Terri. She hugged me and asked if I was going. I said "YES." I knew it that moment. 'Yes' was the right answer. Great practice. Held Mom's hand in savasana and cried. Then I got to tell her, "Yep...I'm going." She was so glad to hear my decision. I shared it with everyone. It felt like real relief. Sometimes you have to face your fears to grow. I can't wait to grow on this journey....

_____ *Rachel Vincent*

Less than a week later, however, I read some more unsettling news on the web. An Air India plane had crashed. It was reported online in the New York Times:

Scores Feared Dead in Southern India Plane Crash[4]

by LYDIA POLGREEN   *published: May 22, 2010*

NEW DELHI — An Air India flight from Dubai carrying 166 people crashed into a heavily wooded valley moments after landing at an airport in southern India on Saturday morning, killing almost everyone on board...

Yikes. Even though it happened quite far from where I'd be traveling, it was close enough to rattle the nerves a bit. I have a dark sense of humor though, and almost immediately I thought of the immortal words of TS Garp, from John Irving's great book, The World According to Garp. When a plane crashes into the house Garp wants to buy, instead of abandoning the deal, he closes the purchase, because in his mind, everything will be fine now. "What are the odds of another accident like this hitting the house?" he says. "It's been pre-disastered." Now this trip has been pre-disastered too, I thought.

---

[4] http://www.nytimes.com/2010/05/23/world/asia/23india.html?_r=0

When people travel to faraway lands, the trip doesn't just affect them. It has an effect on the people around them. Mothers worry. Fathers worry. Girlfriends and boyfriends, husbands and wives, they all worry. Sometimes travelers like myself grow tired of continually reassuring friends and family that we will be alright, and having to explain why we're still going. Some people can accept that…

May 2, 2010 _____

I talked with my mom on the phone. My mom told me that my aunt asked why she would let me go to Nepal when it is so dangerous. My mom's answer was

(a) Christina is 45 years old. What am I going to tell her?

(b) When has anyone been able to tell Christina what to do?

Thanks Mom!!!

_____ *Christina Jankus*

And some people can't…

June 13, 2010 _____

[X] is attempting to put some guilt on me for [going to Nepal]. So I am trying to keep detached with love. Sometimes it's a challenging goal, but I am trying.

_____ *Marc Nathanson*

Whether we believe it or not, and even if we have no way of knowing the future, travelers like me are always confident that everything will be fine, and that we will all return safely home. The truth is that there is some risk involved in this kind of travel. If you go into it with your eyes closed and your head in the sand, you are doing yourself a disservice. If you know the risks and plan for them, keeping safety of paramount concern, you will usually be okay. Despite all the reassurances from the travelers to family and friends, some folks were having more difficulty than others in convincing their loved ones.

June 10, 2010 _____

My mom has been experiencing panic attacks…. My concern is that she is more worried about my going to Nepal than she is letting on. I don't want to upset her so that she has a heart attack!

_____ *Christina Jankus*

They worked through their issues, and no one ended up cancelling their trip. I have no doubt that each family understood why we weren't letting their fears, or our own, deter us from doing something about which we all felt so passionate. They gave us their support, and for that, we love them.

June 11, 2010 _____

Now I had to ask my mom if she is fearful of me going to Nepal. Her reply was no, she isn't fearful of me going. She is concerned for my safety and hopes I stay with the rest of the group as I have a tendency to wander. I promised her I will not wander from the group.

_____ *Christina Jankus*

Another thing that happens with a big trip like this one is that it often causes travelers to reassess their lives up to that point. Perhaps it's a subconscious fear that we may actually not come back, or maybe these trips just act as some kind of milestone in our lives. Our group was certainly no different, and Jesse's entry at that time is a perfect example:

May 19, 2010 _____

I often wonder what life would be like if I had chosen a different path; if I didn't become a teacher, if I didn't go to Nepal, if I didn't give a damn.

I used to be different; I used to not care. I was happier then. I only had myself to worry about and that was nice, it was really nice. I didn't know things, only had superficial contact with people and only regarded them for what they could do to benefit me.

I wouldn't change anything though. Even though my days are no longer mine and at times I feel completely overwhelmed, utterly alone and like I'm fighting losing battles at every turn, I wouldn't change anything. I can't Imagine going back, not having seen, not having met, not having experienced my current life.

I need to be around the kids for the summer, to see that my life actually means something.

My biggest fear is to waste what little time I have on this amazing planet, to not have meant anything to anyone, to not have made a difference; to leave this life having only taken and not given.

_____ *Jesse Bach*

Momentum was building; the kind of momentum that propels you to the finish line, or in our case the starting line, despite whatever last minute issues may pop up. I, for one, couldn't wait for this amazing adventure to begin.

Last Minute Details

"If it weren't for the last minute, nothing would ever get done."
~ Anonymous

I used to have this habit in college of making calendars on the back of notebooks. The calendar would cover all the days of the semester, and I'd cross off each day as it came and went. I must have been bored, or anxious to get the semester over with, or worried about finals. Whatever the reason, I dropped that habit once I was in the real world. Instead, I just ignored the fact that deadlines were fast approaching. In the case of the YFF trip, I did a lot of ignoring. I was focused on writing a script at the time, and I tried to squeeze in travel plans around that. The end result was that I raced around doing a lot of last minute preparations.

As June approached, I still had some items to cross off the checklist, so I decided to cram it all into the last week before the trip, once I was back in Cleveland. At the same time, Carola sent out an email to us with a last minute request:

From: Carola Drosdeck

Sent: Sat, May 8, 2010 6:41 am

I currently have about 75 pounds worth of paperback books collected, with probably more to come. Is anyone willing to take some of them in their luggage?

I wrote her back, telling her I'd be happy to carry some of the items with me to Nepal. I was planning on traveling as light as possible, but I was sure I'd be buying souvenirs and things, so having an empty bag for the trip back would be a good thing.

In addition, I was having some trouble with my travel visa for India. Apparently, the San Francisco consulate had lost my paperwork. I had already made arrangements to stay overnight at the Hotel Lohmod, near the airport in Delhi. I would shower and sleep there, and have breakfast in the morning before heading on to

Nepal. However, I wouldn't be able to leave the Delhi airport without that visa. Worse yet, I had included my passport with the visa application, so I wouldn't even be able to leave the United States unless my visa application was resolved.

The irony is that the Indian consulate in San Francisco had outsourced their visa application process to a San Francisco based company, which had no record of my application. After several phone calls, in which I disguised my panic with a calm, cool, Ghandi-like demeanor, they found my paperwork. One month before my departure, I was notified that my visa had been processed, and my passport was on its way back to me. I breathed a little sigh of relief.

I was trying to finish the script I'd been working on before leaving LA for Cleveland, and ended up having to postpone my flight twice. I flew to Cleveland just one week before I jumped on the plane for the real beginning of my Nepali adventure. I was stressed, certainly, but I was also psyched. I could almost taste the adventure now.

Just after I arrived in Cleveland, I received a call from American Greetings, the card company based there. I had applied for a job with them months ago. I had been thinking of making a change for a long time, especially moving out of LA, but I had lost track of all the resumes I had sent out. I wasn't sure I wanted this kind of job, writing greeting card aphorisms, but it paid well, and it was in Cleveland, where my family and many of my longtime friends were living. The HR person asked if I would be available for an interview the following week. I said of course. What day did they have in mind? They said how about June 17th? I stifled a laugh. Or more of a panicked yelp. That was the day before I was to leave for Nepal, and they wanted me to come in for a job interview? What the hell, I thought. Maybe I'd have a real job when I returned.

The day of the interview was a crazy one. I raced to get a haircut, and did some last minute trip shopping (bug repellent, hand sanitizer, soap, shampoo, toothpaste), and then showered, shaved and threw on a suit and tie, and rushed across town for my job interview. The interview was pleasant enough, but one moment stood out. I had told the HR person that if they had to reschedule for any reason, it would have to be for after the Fourth of July, because I was about to leave the country on vacation. During the interview, the main recruiter asked me where I was going.

"Nepal," I said.

"Really?" she replied. "I have a friend who's going to Nepal. When are you leaving?"

"Tomorrow," I said.

"So is she!" said the recruiter.

I was flabbergasted. What are the odds of that? I wondered. Then I asked her if she could tell me her friend's name...

"Sure," she replied. "Kathy Hayes."

I just shook my head. That cliché about it being a small world? Apparently it's true. I met Kathy the next day, on the flight from Newark to Delhi. She got a huge kick out of it when I recounted the incident to her. And me? I didn't get the job, but I got a heck of a good story out of the whole deal.

Up, Up, and Away...

"No flying machine will ever fly from New York to Paris ...
[because] no known motor can run at the requisite speed for
four days without stopping."
~ Orville Wright

On June 16th, the first people in our group began their trip. Terri, Eve and David were flying through Dubai, staying there a couple of nights, and then heading to Kathmandu. Rachel, Jesse, and Jaime were leaving together from New York City for Kathmandu on the 17th.

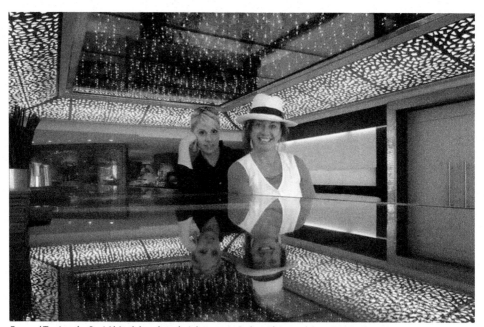

Eve and Terri at the Burj Al Arab hotel on their layover in Dubai. Photo courtesy Eve Ennis.

Most of us were going to depart on the 18th of June. My flight was scheduled to leave Cleveland at 4:55 p.m. When I arrived at the airport, I looked around for the travelers who would be on the same flight. I first found Robb Blain. Robb and I had talked on the phone two days earlier and had made plans to meet at the gate. We knew from the trip schedule emails that Gabby would be joining us on this flight as well. We also found out that Deanna would be on our flight too. We made quick introductions as we waited to board. I liked this group already.

Before we left, Marc, Kathy, and Minling showed up at our gate. Their original flight had been scheduled to go through Chicago, but it was cancelled due to bad weather. Luckily, there were still three seats left on our flight to Newark. They would be joining us all the way to Delhi and Kathmandu. Now we had nearly half the group traveling together. This was going to be fun. We all grabbed a quick bite of food at the airport in Newark, our last American food for two weeks. As soon as we finished eating, we boarded our flight for Delhi. The real beginning of the trip was finally here!

I quickly found my seat and settled in for the 13 hour flight to India. I was sitting next to a couple of young folks whose final destination was India. I started telling them about Nepal, NOH, and the kids we were going to help. It was at least a half hour before I realized that I had turned into that guy -- the one who sits down next to you on a plane and doesn't shut up for the entire trip. To their credit, they were polite, and nodded and smiled often as I continued on about my noble quest. Having exhausted some of my pre-flight energy, I finally gave my seat mates a break from my yakking so they could get some sleep. The trip was overnight, but I'm not much for sleeping on planes myself. The seats are fairly comfortable for the average person on an average flight, unless you're trying to get some significant shut-eye and like me, you have to be horizontal to really zonk out. I'd been on long flights before, and I knew that the signature feeling I was going to experience for the next twelve hours was boredom. Looking out the window revealed only darkness. I had my iPod with me, and the newer planes do have video screens in the back of the seat right in front of you, which can help with the tedium a bit. But thirteen hours confined to a plane, even a big one, is an exercise in patience. I watched movies, listened to some music, got up a few times to stretch and use the bathroom, and then shut my eyes to rest as best I could.

The remainder of the flight was uneventful. One "dinner" and one "breakfast" were the bookends of the trip. There was hardly any turbulence to shake things up and get the heart pumping. Trans-Atlantic jets are so huge that the ride feels even smoother than a bus trip on the turnpike. The whole experience is like being locked in a cramped living room watching your own little TV or listening to your own music, while dozens, or in this case hundreds of others like you, are doing the same thing. There's a weird combination of community and isolation on these long plane trips. You hardly know anyone, but you feel like you all have a common goal – landing safely.

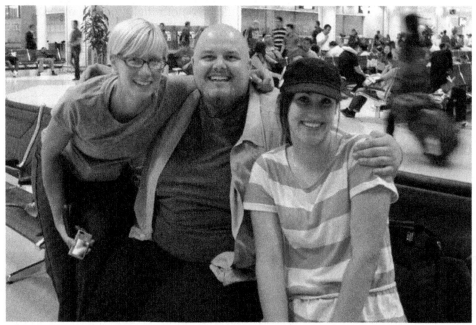

Rachel, Jesse, and Jaime on their layover in Qatar. Photo courtesy of Jaime Furda.

For me, the most interesting thing to do was watch the triptych on the video screen. It would tell you how far you'd flown, how far you had to go, the plane's altitude, the outside temperature, and the local time at your destination. There was a little visual of the plane as it flew over the earth. First, you're over the North Atlantic for about six hours, then over Europe and Asia for another six hours. At one point, I saw on the trip screen that we were flying over Afghanistan and Pakistan. At 40,000 feet, you can't see much of the landscape below, especially since it was still dark, but I felt oddly unnerved. Forty thousand feet is nearly eight miles, but that put me closer to a war zone than I think I've ever been in my life. Below us were American and NATO troops in armed conflict with Taliban and al Qaeda fighters. Somewhere down there, Osama bin Laden was probably just waking up. It all made me think of that John Carpenter movie, Escape From New York, where the president's plane crashes in a hostile futuristic Manhattan, and Kurt Russell is sent in to save him. I just hoped I wouldn't have to experience anything like that on this flight.

I slept maybe a total of two or three hours on the flight. When we arrived in Delhi, it was about 10 p.m. local time, and I was remarkably awake. Those of our group who were on the flight all congregated at the bottom of the jet way. Everyone seemed fine. Deanna had a friend who worked for the airline, and had arranged for the group to be taken to an overnight airport lounge where they could drop their backpacks and relax somewhat comfortably. But, once in Delhi, there was no one there to meet the group. Deanna considered staying downstairs in the transfer lounge that night to save some money, but Kathy and Minling convinced her to go with them to the regular airport lounge, which had food, internet access, and some comfortable chairs for sleeping. It was quiet too, which was nice since there was a lot of noise and commotion in the transfer lounge area with people coming and going.

I had made other arrangements. I had received my Indian visa and would be staying at a nearby hotel overnight. I said my temporary goodbyes, and told the group I'd see them all in Kathmandu. I checked through immigration, picked up my baggage, and exchanged some currency. Then I went out to look for a cab to take me the ½ mile from the airport to my hotel.

Stepping outside, I immediately felt the heat. Of course, I had been anticipating it being hot in India, as this was late June, but it's one thing to anticipate it, and another to feel it. Your body, all your senses are hit with stimulus overload, and your brain races to make sense of it all. The temperature was over 100 degrees at ten o'clock at night. The air was thick and dusty, and the pickup area was loud and noisy. Hundreds of people were jostling for cabs, and you could smell them, perspiring in the humid night air. None of the cabbies spoke English, but I somehow managed to find a driver who seemed to understand where I wanted to go. He took my luggage and tossed it in his trunk, and off we went. I was hoping that this pleasant, smiling man understood me when I told him the name of my hotel.

As soon as we left the airport, I got a second shock to the system. We pulled out of the airport roundabout onto a main boulevard, and the traffic was insane. Bikes, cars, cabs, mini-buses, motorcycles with three and even four people on them, all raced down the boulevard, weaving amongst each other, like some sort of crazy race. My cabbie merged quickly but carefully into the stream of vehicles. That no one hit anyone seemed to me a small miracle. Horns constantly blared, warning other drivers of impending doom, which they seemed to ignore until the last possible moment, when they would swerve quickly, effortlessly, almost nonchalantly out of the way. These folks had obviously driven these roads many times before. I hoped my cabbie had too.

I knew my hotel was only a half-mile away, but that drive was still a little unnerving. In a few moments, I actually spotted the hotel coming up quickly across the road on our left, but then we drove right past it. I got the driver's attention and

47

pointed back to the Hotel Lohmod where I was staying. He nodded and smiled, and pointed down the road in the other direction. "Traffic very bad," he said. "We go round." You're the boss, I thought to myself. Just don't get me killed. When we reached the end of the boulevard, I realized the driver had to go all this way because there was nowhere else to make a safe u-turn. Trying to do so earlier would have meant certain death for both of us. He made a gentle, smooth loop under a bridge and came back up on the other side of the street, then merged easily into the traffic heading back toward the airport and my hotel. In a few short moments, we arrived. I paid him, and thanked him for getting me to my hotel safely. I think he understood my sentiments, if not my words.

I checked in, got the key, and arranged for a wakeup call for 7 a.m. My flight was around eleven, and the hotel concierge said it would be early enough to check out and reach the airport in time to catch my flight to Nepal. When I got to my room, I found a modest little sleeping area, a couch and TV, and a bathroom and shower. It reminded me of the small hotel rooms I'd stayed in in Paris and Athens. Clean, simple, and inexpensive. My first order of business was to take a shower. After fourteen hours on a plane, the water washing over me felt nice. Cool, but not cold. Refreshing.

As I was soaping up my hair, I heard the strangest sound; an enormous whooomp combined with a long, low rumble. And then the power went out. I stood there in complete darkness, soap dripping into my eyes, and realized that this was a brownout. I'd experienced one or two of these mini power failures during exceptionally long heat waves in LA, but never at night, in the shower, covered with soap. I laughed, and then worked my way under the nozzle and rinsed myself clean. I fumbled out of the shower like a blind man, and searched with my hands for a towel. In a few minutes, there was another whooomp, this time softer, and the lights flickered on, at perhaps 25% power. Good enough I thought.

I went back into the sleeping area and tried the TV. No luck. Not enough power. It was late, so I thought I'd just turn in. I was feeling tired now, and though the AC wasn't working, the fan was steadily whirling. I lay on the bed underneath it and fell fast asleep.

I woke with a start. It felt like I had been sleeping for twelve hours, and I suddenly got panicked that I'd missed my flight to Nepal. I jumped out of bed and looked for the clock, but couldn't find it. Of course, I'd forgotten to bring a watch. Ever since cell phones started keeping time, I had quit wearing a watch. Want to know what time it is? Just check your cell phone. But now I was in India, and my cell phone didn't work there. I fumbled around until I found the TV remote and turned it on. This time it came on. There was a little clock on the TV. It read 2:30 a.m. Shit, I cursed. I was wide awake, and I had almost five hours to kill before I had to get up. What to do? Well, the TV was on, so I started watching. Half the shows were in Hindi, the other half English. I watched CNN World News for a while, then some other news programs, and a sports program. The World Cup had started, but I couldn't find any news on it. Soccer is a huge sport worldwide, but India to my knowledge had never had a team in the World Cup. The big sport here is cricket. It's like baseball, but looks more like lacrosse. And if you don't know the rules, forget about trying to understand it.

After an hour or so of television, I rolled over and tried to go back to sleep. Then I got up again, and read a book. At 6 a.m., I finally gave up and rose out of bed for good. I took another shower, this time with the lights on, and packed up and headed down to the lobby for breakfast. When I found out the restaurant wasn't serving until 7 a.m., the hotel manager offered me a seat outside the restaurant and the day's newspaper to read. I wanted to thank him, so I asked him how you say "thank you" in India. He smiled and said, "Thank you." I realized he was joking, and we had a good laugh. But I was serious too, and asked again. He said there are several ways, but the most common is the Sanskrit word, "dhanyabad." Sanskrit is one of the most common languages in the region that includes India and Nepal. I repeated it, and he corrected my pronunciation. "Dah-nee-ah-bod," I said. He smiled and nodded, very pleased that I got it right. I asked if there was a business center in the hotel, and he pointed me to his office, which consisted of one computer at his desk. "Dhanyabad," I said, winking and smiling, and went in to check my email. At 7 o'clock sharp, the restaurant doors opened, and I went in for breakfast. Toast, a boiled egg, and tea. Lots of tea. Then I checked out. The hotel manager arranged for a cab for me. We were old friends by now. "Dhanyabad," I said to him for the tenth time at least that morning. He laughed, and waved goodbye to me as I left.

When I stepped outside to wait for the cab, I noticed two things. First it wasn't quite as hot as last night, and second, the hotel was no more than 10 feet from the busy boulevard we'd driven to get here the night before. And there was no curb or sidewalk, just stairs leading straight down to the street. A small parking area for cabs was just in front of the hotel, and cars were already whizzing by at this early hour on a Saturday. I could only imagine how busy it was on a weekday. I thought about taking a walk, but decided it was better not to risk it. I went back in the lobby and waited for the cab. A taxi soon arrived, and I headed to the airport to take the noon flight on Jet Air to Kathmandu.

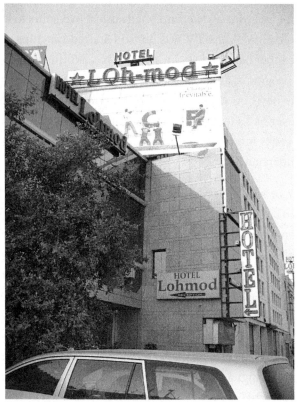

Outside the Hotel Lohmod in Delhi.

As we flew over India to Nepal, I looked out the window of the plane. India has a population of nearly a billion people, and I somehow expected to see every square inch of land covered by human dwellings. But that was not the case. From the time we left the airport until we arrived over Kathmandu, there was nothing below me but large tracts of open green land. The world really is a big place, I thought.

Part 2

The Real (Third) World: Nepal

"I prepared excitedly for my departure,
as if this journey had a mysterious significance....
"'Til now," I told myself, "you have only seen the shadow
and been well content with it; now, I am going to lead you
into the substance."
~ Nikos Kazantzakis, Zorba the Greek

"The world out there is a school.
Life is the only real teacher."
~ Socrates

"Everybody's got plans... until they get hit."
~ Mike Tyson

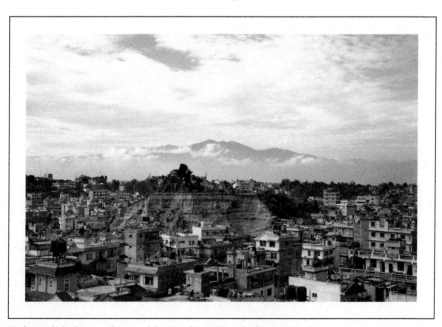

Kathmandu looking north toward the Himalayas. Photo by Candace Koslen.

June 21, 2010

Day 2 of the trip

Kathmandu

Stepping off the plane in Kathmandu, I found myself in a rather small airport that reminded me of the ones I had been to in Mexico and the Caribbean. There was no jet way to take you from the plane to the airport, just a large metal staircase they rolled up to the plane's door so passengers could disembark. I climbed down the stairs, walked across the tarmac and into the main building. It felt cooler here than in Delhi, and the air was cleaner, less dusty. I pulled out my YFF checklist and remembered I had to fill out some paperwork to get my Nepali entrance visa. I made it quickly through immigration, and decided to change some of my money before heading out to look for Jesse.

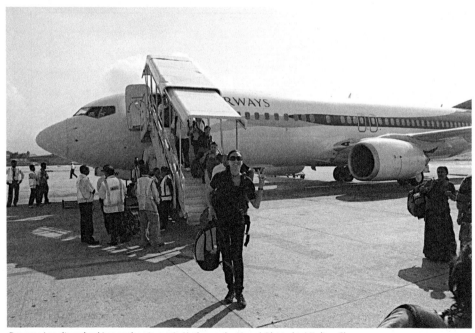

Deanna Lee disembarking at the airport in Kathmandu, Nepal. Photo by Minling Chuang.

I walked outside and into a small sea of people. In moments, I heard someone calling my name. But it wasn't Jesse. It was a Nepali man, in his late 20's or early 30's. This must be Basu Panday, I thought to myself. Jesse had told me to look for him. I waved to Basu, and he quickly came over and grabbed one of my bags before I could stop him, and told me to follow him. I introduced myself as we walked. Jesse was waiting for us in the car, and when he saw me he stepped out and gave me a big hug. I was happy to see him. Then he and Basu presented me with a traditional garland of Nepali flowers, not unlike a Hawaiian lei, to welcome me to Nepal.

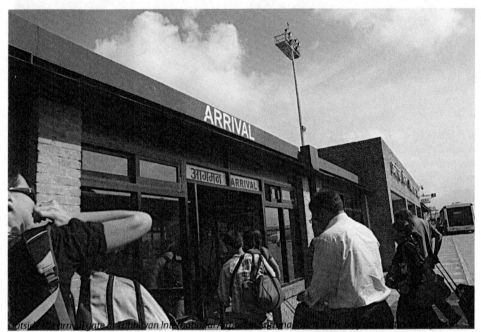

Outside the arrival gate at Tribhuvan International Airport. Kathmandu is the only airport in all of Nepal and has just one domestic and one international terminal. Photo by Minling Chuang.

In no time at all, my luggage was loaded, and we were off to our first destination, The Grand Norling Hotel just outside Kathmandu, where most of the others in our group were already ensconced. The drive from the airport to the hotel was eye-opening. After 24 hours of traveling, most of it spent in a plane, Kathmandu was a shock to the system. Though Delhi was crazy and crowded, it was fairly modern. Kathmandu, despite some trappings of modernity, was something else -- more chaotic, less developed, like a work in progress. The initial experience of it made quite an impact on all of us...

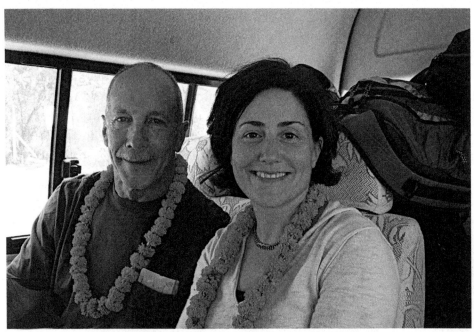

Marc Nathanson and Kathy Hayes wearing traditional greeting garlands on the shuttle from the airport to the Grand Norling Hotel. Photo by Minling Chuang.

June 20, 2010

Kathmandu was packed with people, animals, cars, buses…. What is immediately apparent is that every single building is in some way "under construction." Nothing looks finished. There are people everywhere, walking, talking, and living. And animals – goats, chickens, dogs, cats, and cows. They don't have the happy-go-lucky demeanor of American pets. They are serious here, like residents. There are no wagging tails, nuzzling up to you, just existing in their own animal lives. The sounds are everywhere. Silence is impossible.

Gabrielle Stickley

Chris Jankus, Candy Koslen, Marni Task and Jennette Zimmerman arrived after the rest of us. Christina landed in Kathmandu one day late because of a cancelled flight to Chicago along the way. Candy, Marni and Jennette arrived a couple days later and headed straight for the NOH Volunteer House where they would be working for most of their stay. They all had similar experiences to ours upon seeing Kathmandu for the first time, as Chris and Marni describe…

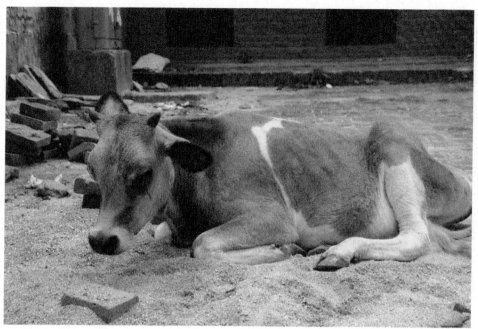

A calf with a bindi marking on its forehead resting outside a building in Kathmandu. Cows are considered sacred by all Hindus. Photo by Candace Koslen.

June 21, 2010

I can't believe I'm here in Nepal! The Kathmandu airport was a crazy scene with men screaming at me to "help me." One man grabbed my packs from my hands and threw them on a cart. He barked his instructions to me through the airport. Somehow because I was with him, I was waved through Customs. I don't know. Maybe his yelling gave him some kind of authority. I tipped him before exiting the airport. I thought once I was outside the scene would change for the better. I was never so wrong!

I was searching the crowd looking for a face I recognized. It seems the crowd consisted of taxi drivers who were yelling to me asking if I needed a taxi. It was so loud it was disorienting.

Finally, I heard my name being called from behind my right side. Thank goodness it was Jesse!

Christina Janku

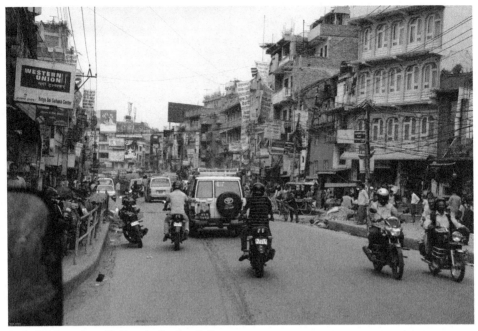

Typical Kathmandu traffic. Photo by Candace Koslen.

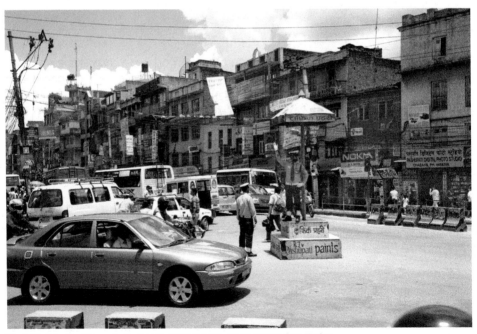

The futile job of traffic cop in the heart of Kathmandu. Photo by Candace Koslen.

Kathmandu… hits you in your senses—in your eyes, you know, there's so much… I guess poverty, but it really also looks like they're just living on the land. It's not all built up, everybody lives literally, simply in these shacks. And so it hit me in my eyes, but really specifically in my nose and in my mouth and in my skin. I could feel the country. So, I was very aware of all the different smells and scents that were completely new for me and somewhat disturbing… the incredible amount of dust and pollution which literally coated my tongue and my skin… I was amazed at how in traffic there, everybody was so calm. There are no traffic lights, and this is what I sort of made up about it: that perhaps because there were no rules—there were no stop signs, there were no lights that said "stop now"— that it was really a free-for-all. And so when there was stopped traffic, it seemed as if everybody knew, "well, of course there's stopped traffic, there's just a lot of it, and when it clears up, it'll clear up." It's not because there's a red light and it's turned green and some pokey guy is checkin' his text messages, and he's not going, where everybody'd start honking their horns. There was no horn-honking, there was no road rage or so it appeared. It seemed like everybody sort of surrendered to this… I dunno… free-for-all, if you will.

_____*Marni Task*

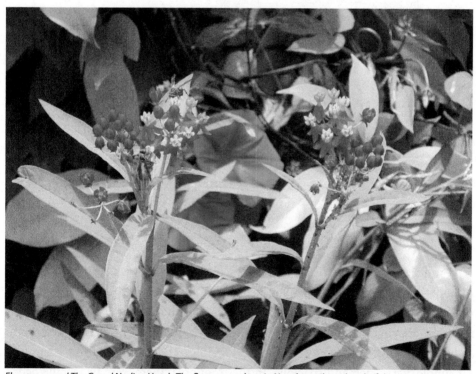

Flowers around The Grand Norling Hotel. The flora everywhere in Nepal are vibrantly colorful.

The Grand Norling Hotel, our first destination, was located on a beautiful hillside overlooking, of all things, a golf course. Who plays golf in Nepal I wondered? Who could afford to? Just the tourists? I had no idea, but no matter, the grounds were beautiful. There were monkeys, deer, flowers of every kind and ample vegetation all around, not to mention all kinds of strange bird sounds filling the air. Behind the hotel was a swimming pool. The noise of the city was now just a far-off thrum. The dragonflies, their wings beating rapidly as they flitted from flower to flower, were louder than the distant traffic.

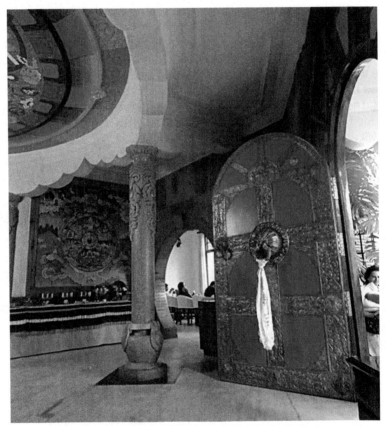

The entrance to the lobby of The Grand Norling Hotel. Photo by Eve Ennis.

I walked into the hotel, and found myself in a small but very charming lobby, with lots of whicker all around. I checked in and took my room key. Jesse told me I would be sharing a room with David Kampinsky. I'd never met Dave, and since he would be arriving a little later in the day with Eve and Terri, I went into the room and picked a bed, and dropped off my belongings. The room itself was beautiful, yet simple, very open and spacious. In the front area, there were two single beds, a couch, a coffee table, air conditioner, a ceiling fan, TV and a small wardrobe. An archway led to another small room with a large wardrobe that contained two robes and some shower sandals, as well as a little desk. Further back was a door that led into the bathroom. I was happy to see a sit-down toilet, a large sink and a bathtub with one of those European style shower nozzles hanging above it.

Jesse had told me to relax and explore the grounds, and that we'd be having dinner around 7 o'clock that evening. Once I had dropped off my things, I went in search of people I knew. At first, I only ran into hotel employees, and like most Westerners, I began greeting them all with the traditional phrase, namaste. Namaste is the customary greeting given when individuals first meet, or when they depart from one another. You hear it all the time at the end of yoga classes. It's sort of like a blessing. The word itself is derived from Sanskrit and is a combination of two words, "Namah" and "te." Namah means 'to bow' and te means 'to you', so namaste literally means "I bow to you." It is, however, a bit formal, as I found out quickly. I felt like a guest in someone's home, so formality seemed like the right approach. My greetings of namaste elicited some big smiles from the young kids who were around, most of whom I learned were not guests, but children of the hotel workers who lived on the grounds. Each time I greeted them with namaste, they returned

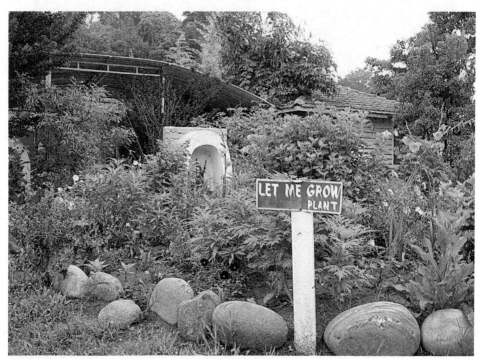

They take their landscaping seriously at The Grand Norling Hotel, not sure about the signage.

the greeting, shyly, politely, but with smiles. As soon as I passed, I could hear titters of repressed laughter and little snippets of conversation. I assumed they were discussing where I was from, and what I was doing here, and wondering why an adult was bowing in greeting to them.

As I walked around the hotel, I met up with Marc and Robb, who were rooming together, and Minling and Kathy, who were also roommates. We found Gabby and Deanna, who were sharing a very interesting room on the top floor:

June 20, 2010_____

I feel like Rapunzel in the top of the castle. The room that has been assigned to us is at the very top of the building. It is completely dome shaped, and every surface is covered in basket-weave lattice. It is like living inside a basket. From the windows we can see out onto the golf course(!) and [watch] the monkeys that come out and play from the woods in the late morning… scampering across the expanse of grass.

_____ ***Gabrielle Stickley***

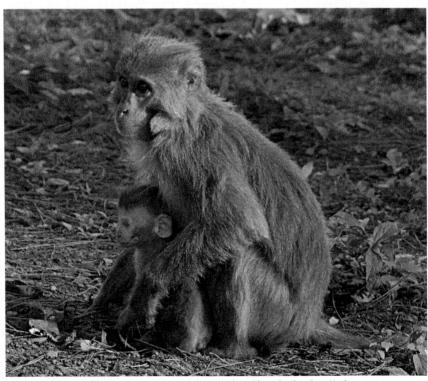

Mama and baby. Monkeys were a common sight at Norling. Photo by Candace Koslen.

Around mid-afternoon, I went back to my room to take a nap. The long flight, the layover in Delhi, and the general lack of sleep had all caught up with me. I stretched out on the small, but comfortable bed and quickly fell asleep. An hour later, around 5:30 p.m., Jesse knocked on the door, and I woke up to find that it was almost dark. He apologized for the early wakeup, but he had been informed that dinner would now be served at 6 p.m., so I roused myself out of bed. Not much later, my roommate David arrived. Standing six feet tall, in his early thirties, with dark wavy hair, Dave is incredibly fit, with what I like to call 'yoga tattoos' on his arms, shoulders and back. Being a yoga instructor back home, he practices yoga virtually every day. He knew all the other teachers on the trip, but he and I had never met. Dave, I quickly came to find out, marches to his own drummer. He is also warm, friendly and very easy-going. I liked him right away.

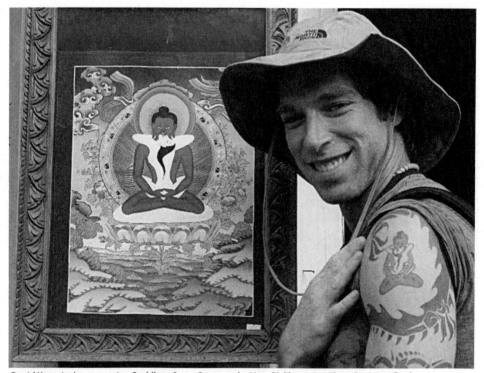

David Kampinsky comparing Buddhas. Same Same as the Nepali's like to say. Photo by Jaime Furda.

I left Dave to wash up, and headed to the dining room to grab dinner which, that first night, turned out to be a little adventure all its own. I love trying different kinds of food from different nationalities, but I had never tasted Nepali food. It's very similar to Indian food in many ways, but in general, it contains less meat and is a little less spicy. The main dish in almost all Nepali meals is dal bhat. It consists of cooked or steamed rice (bhat) and lentil soup (dal), often served with roti or chapati (rounds of unleavened bread). Dal can be cooked with tomatoes, onion, chili, tamarind, garlic and ginger, in addition to lentils or beans. It always contains herbs and spices like coriander, garam masala, cumin and turmeric. A small portion of chutney or pickle (called achar) is usually included. The exact recipe varies by season, locality, ethnic group and family.

The dal bhat at Norling was served with vegetable tarkari - a mix of available seasonal vegetables. Everything tasted incredibly delicious. After the main courses we were served yogurt, which was also exceptionally good. One of the reasons everything tasted so good was because it was so fresh. There is very little refrigeration available in Nepal because the power is so unreliable. The electricity shuts down often and for long periods of time, so people tend to cook and eat the things they've grown or bought at market quickly, before it has a chance to spoil.

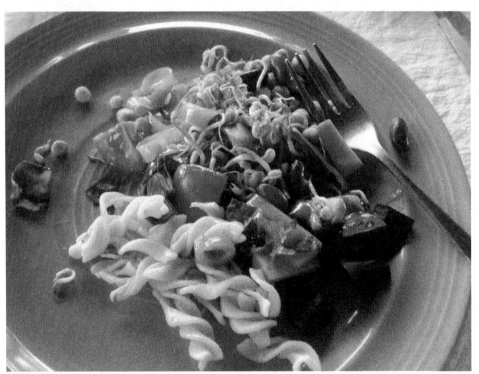

The first of many delicious meals in Nepal. Photo by Tingting Peng.

There was one moment during the meal, though, that gave a jolt to our proceedings. Just as Gabby was about to apply fork to food, a little bug crawled out of the rice she was about to dig into with her fork. Gabby is 40-ish, the proprietor of an estate sale firm, and is quite sharp. At heart, Gabby's a hippie, I think, who you'd just as easily picture at a Grateful Dead show as at an estate sale. Gabby can be intense, but she's also quite practical and pragmatic, and very capable of going with the flow, and she was only momentarily flustered by the appearance of this small unwanted interloper on her plate. Instead of freaking out, she laughed the whole incident off as de rigueur, gently pushing aside the little critter, careful to avoid that bit of food. Like Gabby, we were all soon to find out that in a country like Nepal, you had to develop a certain acceptance of bugs. They weren't intolerable, just unpredictable.

Eve and Terri arrived while we were eating. They had flown in with David, and had stopped by their room to freshen up before joining everyone at dinner. Originally from Kansas, Terri is in her late 40's and a full-time yoga instructor at Cleveland Yoga. Eve is a little younger than Terri, with straight reddish brown hair, and quite tall. She managed an apartment complex near where Terri lived, and the two women often traveled together. Eve also has a great sardonic sense of humor, which I really came to appreciate on the trip.

After dinner, everyone sat around the table drinking coffee and tea and talking, and I got to know Tingting and Rachel a little better. Rachel is in her 30's, and had lived in Columbus and New York before moving back to Cleveland, where she had been raised by her parents who had adopted her as a baby. She had taught yoga, but wasn't teaching currently, instead working fulltime as a bartender and hostess at one of Cleveland's finest Italian restaurants, Michaelangelo's, in the Little Italy section of the city. Tingting, who's in her mid-20's, was born in China, but raised in Boston. She went to MIT where she studied finance, and had once worked on Wall Street. In her free time, she also taught yoga, having gone through teacher training along with the Cleveland Yoga instructor who had first mentioned the Nepal trip to me. Being an only child, Tingting had learned to make friends easily. She also knew how to go with the flow. She had arrived a day earlier from Hong Kong, where she resides, minus one important piece of ladies' travel gear:

June 19, 2010_____

Despite being so prepared, I still managed to forget something – my razor. I laugh a little at this because I've been shaving ever since I was a teenager or something like that and I don't remember the days when everything about me was au natural. Guess I'll find out this week!

_____ *Tingting Peng*

Tingting and Rachel both seemed to have boundless energy, and the three of us talked until fairly late. When Jesse notified us that we'd be waking up at 5:30 a.m. tomorrow for our first yoga practice, I said my goodnights and headed off to bed, all the while wondering how on earth I was going to get up that early, let alone practice yoga at such an ungodly hour. All part of the adventure, I thought to myself, and I wasn't going to miss any of it. Something about starting this adventure here in such a wonderful place, and taking it all in that first day, moved Kathy to write a little poetry in her journal:

> We come together
> Face to face
> From the unknown, creating the known
> Thousands of things came together
> to make this moment possible
> From around the world, so many
> Synchronicities built this
> Hello. Namaste.
>
> We are here now
> In this moment
> You and I
> From here and there
> Through thousands of small
> And millions of large things
> Leading to this
> Why?
> Hello. Namaste.
>
> Why are you, you
> And me, me
> And why do we meet
> Here, now
> Of the places we could be now
> Yet here we are
> Unable to connect through language
> But easily connecting through
> the heart
> You are not you
> Nor me me
> But in our meeting we become we.
> **~Kathy Hayes**

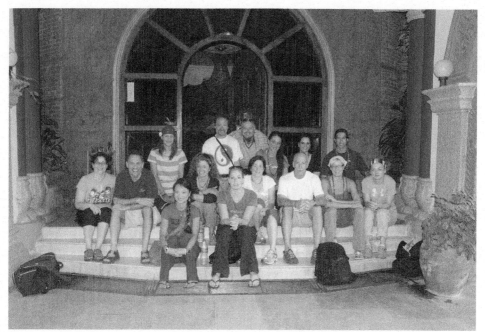

The entire YFF traveling group (minus Minling) outside The Grand Norling Hotel. Photo by Minling Chuang.

I liked Kathy's sentiment -- in our meeting, 'we become we'. The twenty of us on this trip were all meeting for the first time, and on our way, hopefully, to going from me to we. What I'm sure Kathy, or any of us for that matter, didn't realize at the time was just how difficult that was actually going to be.

June 21, 2010

Day 2 of the trip

Grand Norling Hotel & Resort

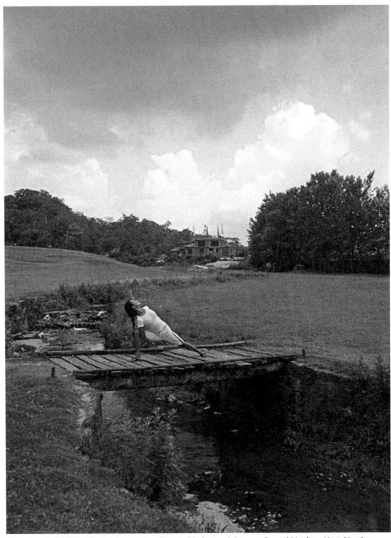

Tingting in Baddha Parsvakonasana (Bound Side Angle) pose. Grand Norling Hotel in the background. Photo by Jaime Furda.

I slept like a happy baby, to borrow a phrase from yoga, and had no trouble getting up at the appointed time of 5:30 a.m. I somehow managed to avoid jet lag in Nepal. Maybe it was the adrenaline, or the fact that I had stayed the first night at that hotel in Delhi. Others, though, were having more difficulty sleeping those first couple of days:

June 21, 2010_____

I was having trouble adjusting to the time change and was over-stimulated by the difference in culture, so I had issues sleeping…. When I finally would settle in for the night my sleep time was spent having lucid, vivid dreams and I would wake up hours before anyone else, but somehow I wouldn't be tired upon waking and got to watch the world awaken around me. One night there was an intense lightning storm that lasted until just before sunrise. For hours I watched as the sky would go from pitch black to brighter than day and back again, and then the storm passed. The sky lightened up to a glowing midnight blue and filled with scarlet and amber clouds, and eventually all the clouds faded and the sun took their place, which got me to thinking of endless spiritual references that warmed my soul. The land beside us was a golf course next to a wooded area, and the hills filled with laughing, playing monkeys. This is how it would go on several occasions, a long, intense storm and then the re-emergence of life and activity.

_____ *Deanna Lee*

Practicing yoga helped me adjust to the 12-hour time change rather quickly. Once I was up and dressed that first morning, I grabbed my mat (each of us had brought a yoga mat donated to the trip by Kulae, which we'd be leaving behind for the kids of NOH) and headed out with David to the lobby. We were all directed to a large pagoda on the grounds behind the hotel. The sun was barely up, and it was cool and pleasant outside. Once together, our mats lined up row after row, four rows deep, Jesse introduced us to Subash Adhikari. Subash was in his 20's, a certified yoga instructor, Reiki healer, and doctor of naturopathy who shared an office and studio with his uncle in nearby Thamel, one of the more developed areas in Kathmandu.

Jesse had met Subash when he was interviewing local yogis for the YFF trip. He had shown up for the interview on his motorcycle, and Jesse, an avid Harley man himself, hired him on the spot. It took us all about 5 minutes to realize that when it came to yoga, Subash was the real deal. He was strong and incredibly flexible. He contorted his body in ways that even the most practiced among us could only imagine. Each morning of the trip, Subash would lead us in a 90-minute practice, starting at 5:30 a.m. When I first heard that we'd be practicing at that hour, I laughed. I am not a morning person. But on this trip, that was part of the adventure, so I dealt with it, and surprised myself. In no time, I was enjoying these peaceful early morning routines. In the evenings, before dinner, one of the yoga instructors from our group would teach another 90-minute class – a sort of cultural exchange we were all looking forward to experiencing, Subash included.

Initially, I had some genuine concerns about how my body would respond to that much yoga. I practice Power Vinyasa Yoga in Cleveland two or three times a week, so I consider myself in decent shape yoga-wise. One of Power Yoga's main proponents is Baron Baptiste, who had taught many of the teachers at Cleveland Yoga. It's a vigorous, physical, and exhausting style of yoga. You sweat a lot, though it's not as dehydrating as Bikram Yoga, which I also practiced regularly, especially when I was in LA. I had taken classes with Bikram Choudury himself, and I enjoyed both styles. To me, the main difference between the two is that while Bikram promotes flexibility, the Baptiste style promotes physical strength.

Much to my pleasant surprise, Subash's style was different from both disciplines. He spent a good 15 minutes at the beginning of each class just warming up the body, especially the joints, from toes to fingertips. In my experience, that's the biggest weakness of the power yoga I practiced in Cleveland -- not enough warm up time. It's probably a reflection of Western vs. Eastern cultures. We in the west tend to want to get to it right away. Subash also liked to spend a fair amount of time at the beginning of his sessions discussing yoga philosophy. He liked to explain why we were doing certain things that day, and how they affected our mental and physical well-being. There was also a greater emphasis on chanting with Subash. As we went through the various Sun A and Sun B poses, he instructed us in the proper verses to chant. These chants weren't just spiritual. They emphasized breathing to a greater extent than I was accustomed. Incorporating laughter as a breathing technique not only made the class a blast, but also really strengthened the core muscles. If you don't believe it, try doing 50 regular sit-ups or bicycle sit-ups while laughing loudly and heartily, and see how it feels. We struggled with the proper pronunciations of the chants and with integrating laughter into our practice, but all the new twists Subash brought to the mat made class a lot of fun.

Another thing that made our yoga enjoyable was practicing it outside. The over-all view of the grounds from the pagoda was beautiful. The sun was just rising, and a haze that hung over the grass and trees gave everything a kind of Shangri-la aura. The morning birds were chirping away, and we saw monkeys roaming near the tree line. It was incredibly relaxing and invigorating at the same time. Eve and Minling's journal entries nicely describe what the yoga practice was like that first morning:

June 21, 2010_____

Jesse knocked on our door at 5:30 a.m. It was cool outside, as we gathered inside a pagoda for our yoga. Very different from Cleveland Yoga (thank God). But, it was great yoga and great fun. We are bicycling and laughing, laughing and bicycling. Quite hysterical.

_____ ***Eve Ennis***

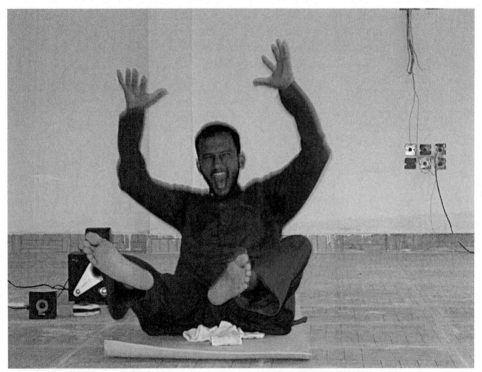

Subash demonstrating Paripurna Navasana (Full Boat) pose with laughing. The laughing makes the pose much tougher. Great for toning the abs. Photo by Kathy Hayes.

June 21, 2010_____

Today we had our first [morning] yoga practice with Subash. His style is so completely different than what I've experienced in Power Yoga, yet it was one of the most powerful, fulfilling, relaxing classes I've ever taken. I'm so used to flow yoga and to going through yoga poses one right after another. It's always an intense workout and I'm always sweaty after class. This one was completely different. We didn't start with the sun salutations, but some warm up exercises. Once our bodies were loose, yoga began. It's funny, I never thought about warming up my body before yoga. I always thought that yoga warmed up my body.

We moved into a series of 12 sun salutations. We did 12 poses 12 different times. Before each pose, we would chant something in Sanskrit. Again, this is not something I've ever done before in a yoga class, but saying these chants made me feel so much more connected to the poses and my body. There was nothing super hard in all the poses that we did. There was no handstand, crow, or anything that exerted a lot of strength. At first it didn't seem as intense as a power yoga class, but my body still seemed to ache after class. In reality it may have been more intense than a power yoga class....

My favorite part about the classes was the fact that Subash would tell us what each pose was good for. "This pose cures indigestion, headaches, and every-thing else." At first I laughed, but then realized that yoga was developed not for the physical fitness, but as a way to naturally heal.... Is this what Eastern Yoga is all about? If so, I love it and want to learn more!

_____ *Minling Chuang*

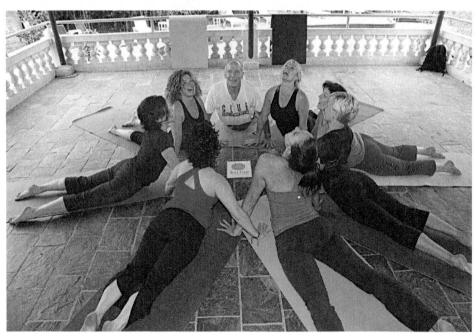

Upward facing dog (Urdhva Mukha Svanasana) pose on the Kulae mats we brought for the kids from the US.
Photo by Minling Chuang.

After morning yoga we all showered and then went to breakfast, which was served buffet style outside in the same pagoda where we had practiced earlier. No dal bhat this morning, but loads of eggs, potatoes and toast with butter and jam. And plenty of tea. Nepalis, like Indians and Brits, love their tea strong, hot, and with sugar and milk if one preferred it sweet. As we ate, Jesse told us that we'd have the rest of the morning free, but we'd meet up at the pagoda at noon for a meditation and journaling exercise. Afterwards, we would be heading out on our first excursion into Kathmandu.

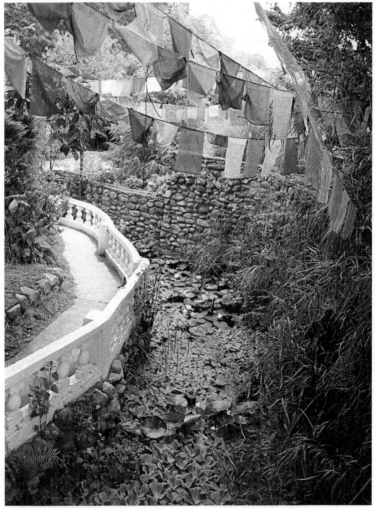

Water lilies and prayer flags adorn the grounds of The Grand Norling Hotel. Traditionally, prayer flags come in sets of five: one in each of five colors. The five colors are arranged from left to right in a specific order: blue, white, red, green, and yellow. They represent the elements, and the different colors are associated with specific traditions. Blue symbolizes the sky and space, white symbolizes the air and wind, red symbolizes fire, green symbolizes water, and yellow symbolizes earth. According to Tibetan tradition, health and harmony are produced through the balance of the five elements (source: http:// en.wikipedia.org/wiki/Prayer_flag).

We finished our meal, and then wandered the hotel grounds for a bit, exploring our new surroundings. As David and I were exploring the scenery, we spotted the biggest spider web either one of us had ever seen. It stretched from a small pine tree just outside our hotel room window, four or five feet across, to the side of the hotel. In the center of the web was what at first looked like a nickel-sized greenish gold arachnid. David nudged the web with a small stick, and in an instant the spider's legs shot out from its body and it grew from nickel size to dollar size. We both jumped back. Whoa! That sucker was huge.

We called the others over to see it, hoping to frighten them, but only managed to mildly scare one or two of the women, who had a fear of bugs. The rest were just as fascinated as we were to check out this eight-legged freak of nature. So much for stereotypes. As we examined the web more closely, we saw dangling from the branches throughout the tree, little sacks of spider silk wrapped around some very unfortunate insects, flies, mosquitoes, and bees that had all been trapped by this huge spider in its enormous web. The little silk sacks were suspended like meat on hooks, for later consumption. Macabre but fascinating.

"No wonder there were no mosquitoes in our room last night," said Dave. "This guy kept them all out."

"Works for me," I said. I love spiders.

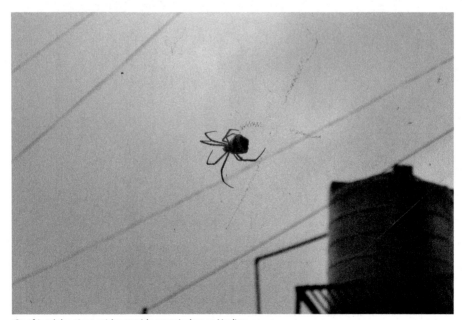

Our friend the giant spider outside our window at Norling.

The day was getting warmer now as the sun burned off the last of the morning haze. We strolled the grounds, and came across a small hut at the back of the resort about a hundred yards behind the pagoda where, we discovered, the resident massage therapist and his family were living. Several of us promptly reserved massages to rid our bodies of the aches and kinks from 14 hours of flying. A Thai massage cost about 1000 rupees, which if memory serves me right was approximately 14 dollars. A pretty good deal, I thought, for a 60 minute massage. I booked one for the next morning, and then resumed wandering the grounds of the hotel, taking pictures and greeting hotel workers and guests alike with a namaste and a smile. The rest of the group had been taking in the new sights and sounds of Norling, as well, and reflected on them in their journals:

June 21, 2010_____

I am really aware of the rhythms of sound today. I heard the clear difference between man-made sound and natural sound. My ears can differentiate that so clearly today. But some sounds are the same, no matter where you go. The sound of children, and of water, these are the universal sounds that we will always have around us, no matter where on Earth we are. We go into town today (yay!). I wonder what sound I will hear there.

_____ ***Gabrielle Stickley***

June 21, 2010_____

As I walked around the landscaped grounds of the hotel, I saw a group of smiling girls coming towards me. When I realized that Jaime was among their group, she asked me to join them in their meandering. "Come walk with us!" one of the girls boldly said. I took my place alongside them and another girl extended her hand, "Let's be friends, what is your name?" I introduced myself to the other girls. They smiled back at me with openness and curiosity.

They danced around me as we strolled through the hotel gardens, always asking "Where should we go?" Was I this carefree and happy when I was 8, 10 or 13 years old? ... Spending time with those girls reconnected me to my own childhood. It's funny to think that I was more confused, more lost in my first few years as an adult than when I was much younger.

... A few of us went for a walk on the golf course adjacent to the hotel. We hopped a wall that was covered in morning glories, and made our way onto the fairway. We were so close to nature here. There were monkeys, dashing across the fairway, and deer trotting through the woods. The air was crisp and the whole view was surreal. We walked up a long staircase made of stone which led us to hole 12 and an opening in the green which was lined with ancient-looking trees and vines stretching far into the distance. Beyond the golf course walls was a city brimming with life – there was life in the bricks that made up the buildings, there was life in the sounds of the streets, there was life in the daily activity of the construction workers, the school children and the house-wives.

Tingting Peng

We gathered again at the pagoda for meditation and journaling at noon. Jesse asked us to keep an open mind about what we were about to do. Now that would be a challenge for me. I had similar feelings about meditation as I had with journaling — skepticism mixed with a dash of cynicism. But I was determined not to give in to those negative feelings, and to see what I could learn from trying new things. Subash gave us some simple breathing exercises to get started, and played some very soothing yoga music, instructing us all to close our eyes and try to clear our minds of any thoughts. Just concentrate on breathing.

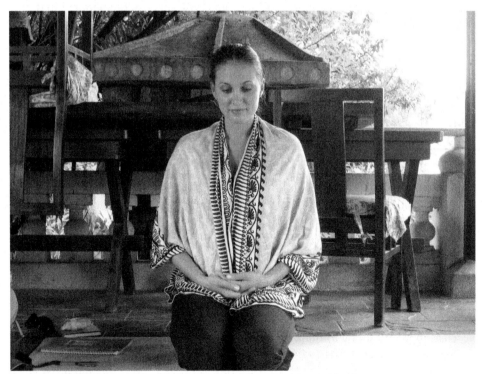

Deanna meditating in the pagoda at Norling. Her journal lies at her right, awaiting the next entry.

Anyone who has tried meditating, especially novices like myself, will tell you that clearing your mind of all thoughts is pretty much impossible. You can do it for a very short time, and then bam! A thought pops up. Subash later explained that instead of resisting the thoughts, the point of meditating was to embrace them, feel them, and then let them go. We did this for about 10 minutes the first day, and afterwards I felt oddly refreshed, like I'd taken a short cat nap. If meditation is like this, I thought, I'm going to be okay with it.

When we finished meditating, Jesse asked us to take out pen and paper and answer the following question in our journals: Why did I come here? I realized right away that my negative thoughts about journaling had not been entirely purged from my subconscious. I'd forgotten to bring paper and pen. I borrowed some and then I sat for a moment thinking, *why did I come here?*

Journaling Exercise: Why did I come here?

Here's what I wrote in my journal:

June 21, 2010 _____

I came not for one reason, but many. First, I've always wanted to come to this part of the world—to see the Himalayas. There is something awe-inspiring about that kind of natural beauty. It is so overwhelming that it puts the daily concerns of life both small and large in perspective. Ironically, you can only see the foothills of the mountains from where we're staying, but their presence, like the future, seems to loom ahead. We have an airplane ride to Everest planned for later in the week that I am really looking forward to.

Second, I've come to see where the Buddha was born and Buddhism began. I have always been fascinated by spirituality in all its forms, read, watched, and listened to Joseph Campbell and Huston Smith, and to go to the center of one of the world's great religions/philosophies is in a small way to connect with that greater spirituality. Someday I hope to also go to Israel and perhaps Mecca in Saudi Arabia to experience where Judaism, Christianity and Islam began. I see the connections between religions, and it saddens me that in the world today all the focus is on the differences. It especially saddens me when those differences are used as excuses to propagate violence against other human beings. Nothing could be further from the truth and spirit of religion.

Third, I've come to Nepal to be around people who are like-minded in their love for yoga. Not "same"-minded, but with the same spirit of exploration into the physical, mental and spiritual aspects of what it means to be a human being alive in the world. For me, that's what yoga is really about.

Another important reason why I came here is for the adventure. Even though much of this trip has been planned for months, traveling halfway around the globe, in a mind-boggling short 15 hours is an amazing adventure. And coming to a place that, at least on the surface, is so different from where I call home, is amazing. It gives you a kind of perspective on yourself and your life that home cannot. It's like changing the lighting in a scene in a movie or a painting—different aspects of the scene become highlighted, different aspects contrast. This kind of change of perspective gives me insight into who I am and what is really important to me. To me, that is the great gift of travel, especially travel to "exotic" places. You come to know yourself better through these adventures.

Perhaps this last one is really the most important reason for me to come to Nepal. It's what makes us human—the sense, the need, to venture out and explore the world. You just never know what you might learn.

_____ *John Vourlis*

Here's what the others wrote in their journals in answer to that most basic question:

June 21, 2010_____

Nepal was not even on my top ten list of places to travel. However, when the opportunity presented itself, I knew I had to make this trip. I wanted to breathe the same air as these people halfway around the world are breathing…

It's funny. I signed up for this trip knowing that it was something I HAD to do – a passion. Then all of a sudden, it was here, and I feel so unprepared. I was afraid of the warnings I was reading about, and of what other people were telling me. Then I realized it was a process I was meant to go through.

It's facing my fears. Now, I really feel like one of the lucky ones. Of all my travels to date, this one trip will affect my life the most. I am here with a group for a purpose. We are all sharing this common mission, but maybe each with our own expectations or agenda…

What is very exciting to me is that this is my first day here, my experience only beginning. That is exciting. The whole journey is waiting to unfold.

_____ ***Terri Bahr***

June 21, 2010_____

Why am I here?

An interesting question… Dynamic answer that is composed of one word "fear." Throughout my 12 year yoga journey, I have been releasing the fear that has been built up over 50 years. A mentally and emotionally abusive father instilled [that] fear [in] me. The fear of accepting myself for who I am. The fear of reaching out for love and getting yelled at. Getting rejected… The fear of not feeling safe within interpersonal relationships. The fear of authority. The fear of doing something wrong… the list goes on and on. Yoga freed me from these fears and helped me replace them with love.

…Fear said to me, "you're not going to go." I agreed. The next two days were a living hell. I had the new liberated Robb on one shoulder saying "you need to go" and I had the fearful Robb on the other saying "you would love this trip, it is just what you need and want, but you will not go." Two days later I allowed love to win. I committed to the trip.

_____***Robb Blain***

…When people asked me why I'm going to Nepal, I told them it was because of the girls we would be helping. The statement is very true for me, I am here because of the girls, but as I look deeper, the answer is not as simple.

Part of why I'm here is to embark on a spiritual journey. For some time now, I've been questioning my life and the purpose of my existence. Am I here to live through life unconsciously? Going to work every day, developing a routine, getting married, having a family, etc., is that it? If it was up to my parents, that's exactly what I would be doing. My parents are fantastic and they love me immensely (and I love them), but I've come to realize that that life is not something I want or crave.

However, I don't exactly know what I want either. I guess you can say that we are all craving happiness and are each figuring out how to get there. Is it the material things or relationships that make us happy? Or is it something much bigger than all of us can imagine?

The universe is so massive and in the big scheme of things, life is so short. Is there ever a right way to live it? I guess I'm still searching for the answer despite the fact that deep down I know that there is no right answer to life and our purpose. …Life is always a constant journey, one that will test our limits and expand our mind and I intend to maximize that journey. It's this expansion of self and learning who I am and what I'm capable of doing that has me be here.

If someone asked me 3 years ago where I would be, would I have said working at a major corporation and beginning my career path towards being a top executive? But that was 3 years ago, before the new path of my life began.

Lately, I've wanted to become more centered – centering on peace from within and being at peace in all situations. Our lives are so full of motion that we can't or won't always stop and appreciate life, the living, the spirit within each person and thing. Wouldn't it be great to have every person appreciate life? If I can't change others, I can at least change myself and be more appreciative, right?

I'm also drawn to this idea of connectedness with people and nature. The idea that everything is one – you are me, I am you, we are all each other. We are one with the earth and its infinite beauty. This connection with each other and earth is not something I've been able to experience in everyday life. So being in Nepal and coming here to connect is a magical experience. I believe this is another reason why I came here…to feel oneness with the earth and other people…to really see the beauty in everything and one…to see the soul of this earth without distractions.

It's funny, after writing all of this and trying to make sense of why I'm here, there are probably more reasons why that I haven't uncovered yet. All I know is that I'm supposed to be here to learn and grow. I was meant to be on this journey and at the end of the trip I'll know why I came here.

Minling Chuang

June 21, 2010_____

What Made Me Come Here?

There's a cat on the patio with us. He's gorgeous, but he doesn't like me very much.

So, what brought me here? To be honest, it was a rather sudden decision, triggered by the pictures I saw posted on Jesse's Facebook—there's a wedding today, and the music has started; it sounds like something you'd hear at a high school football game—of his most recent trip at the time (winter of 2009). I don't mean to sound phony when I say this, but it was mostly the kids that influenced my decision—the music just sped up considerably. There was just something about them… I just knew I had to be here. I mean, I'm not religious or anything, so it's not like Jesus or Buddha or someone called me up and said "Get over there, girl!" The country itself was calling; Nepal was where I needed to be.

Aside from all that, I guess I just needed a change of pace. I've been through a lot since last winter, so—a crowd of about thirty guys watching one man swim laps in the pool… how strange—taking some time off sounded fantastic.

And you know that feeling you get when you do something nice for someone, something that impacts him or her so positively that you just—that is one huge spider; oh! And it jumps. Great—know you've changed his or her life for the better? Yeah, well this is kind of like that, but the extraordinarily brilliant feeling is multiplied by about eighty-four.

I'm just glad to actually be doing something like that. You know, most people might think about doing something like this, but I bet very few actually go out and do it. Change lives, I mean. If you get a chance, I suggest you try it sometime. Right now perhaps—good luck.

_____ *Jaime Furda*

June 21, 2010_____

"why are you here?"

~At first, if you were to ask me why I'd chosen to come here it was difficult for me to put into words. There was a strong feeling, a magnetism that pulled my heart from the moment I became aware of this trip and the Kamlari system. On the surface, yes I wanted to help, but there was something deeper. The more I thought about it the more clear it became – I could have very well been one of the children caught in the system here, any one of us could have. If fate had brought me into the world as one of these children I would hope/pray/dream that someone somewhere would care enough to come and find me and lift me up like the child I was and carry me away to safety. Maybe it's the nurturer in me, the natural maternal instincts of a woman who was once a little girl, or the dreamer in me who brought me here, who believes that if we all gave just a little more we could easily bring peace, healing and light into the darkest places. I am empathetic to these children because I too have suffered at the hands of man… have awakened from the nightmares and carry with me the strength to overcome fear and sorrow, to know that we can make a difference be it in the life of one child or thousands, in our local communities and our global community, if we just try <3

Deanna Lee

June 21, 2010

The last couple of days have been all about figuring out my space, and my comfort level on this trip. I learn about me every day, and this trip is no exception. I have come to know more about the Nepal Orphans Home, and I continue to understand why I am here. It is about suffering. I have been brought here to help me through my suffering, and to help others to support them in their pain.

Today we did yoga and meditation, which is all good, but I want more. I didn't come for a vacation or to have an epiphany. I already had those experiences. So we shall see what happens. Will I find peace? Will I find connection? Will I meet the kids? Will I learn more about Michael? That is why I'm here.

Marc Nathanson

June 21, 2010

How did I end up here? Let me go back approximately a… half year. The moment I knew my life was going to change, I was sitting across from my portfolio manager at Fortress Investment Group, where I had been working as an investment analyst for just a few months. It was a couple days before Christmas and bad news from the financial fall-out that began a year earlier had continued to pour in. The office was doom and gloom, vibrating in fear and anticipation of the biggest shoe yet to drop – the axe was about to swing down from headquarters in New York.

So there I was, sitting with my fingers nervously twiddling on my lap as my PM began his delivery of the bad news – we've all been deemed redundant. Unnecessary. Thank you very much but good-bye.

Rather than feeling the world crashing down around me, I began to feel a weight being lifted from my chest and shoulders. I somehow saw a light at the end of the tunnel. I had been unexpectedly set free from my self-constructed corporate rat cage.

…What is a life worth living? What is a life of success and accomplishments? What do any of these mean if they are not shared with other people? I wanted to come on this trip so I can share what I love, my joys, my energy. I wanted to come on this trip because I wanted to also be on the receiving end of all that.

A journey of challenges, transformation, service and discoveries. So here I am.

_____ ***Tingting Peng***

June 21, 2010_____

"Why are you here?"

I came here to Nepal because I like the sound of the word. Nepal – it's a pretty word to say, to write, and to look at. The opportunity to do something by my-self, while the kids are at camp, is something I didn't want to miss. I am really a full-time mommy. So knowing the kids would be having fun and were safe, and that I had four weeks to fill, made this the perfect opportunity....

The idea of going to Nepal probably took hold (somewhere from 1989-1990), 20 years ago. I was living in Jackson Hole, WY, newly graduated from Ohio State University, and learning to rock climb.

The talk was all about peaks and routs. And, of course, the holy grail of all this was Mt. Everest. At that time, any thoughts of going to Nepal included climb-ing, or at the very least, trekking to Mt. Everest.

As I moved on, and eventually left the Wild West for more civilized locales, the idea of visiting Nepal became a smaller and smaller part of my dreams. It was practically forgotten, until I heard Candy speak a few weeks ago.

_____ ***Gabrielle Stickley***

June 21, 2010_____

Why did I come here?

I knew within 2 1/2 minutes of talking to Jesse about this trip that I needed to do it. The personal reason... I've lived 30 years of my life for myself... needed to fill the void of purpose. Although happy by nature, there is much in my life that is incomplete. I needed to commit to something, to not control everything; to let my guard down and let something in, let something affect me—to change/ better me. I don't have a solid career that I commit to; I resort to the restaurant business...because although I enjoy it and I'm great at it...it's noncommittal. There isn't the possibility that I'll change anything and need to be consistent... there's always an out, always another restaurant/bar. Same with relationships; I've been in many, but since 1 1/2 years ago, I avoid getting in anything too long..."What if it works? What if I'm stuck? What if it's not right and I should've been with _____?"

Living even....I moved back home and won't commit to my own place, al-though it makes sense to stay at home (financially, helping mom, etc...), those are just justifications to avoid the deeper layer...I'm afraid to commit because I don't know where I'm supposed to be, what I'm supposed to be, whom I'm sup-posed to be with, and in addition....not only do I not know the "supposed to's",

I do not know the "wants". I feel this way in most areas in my life and live my life according to these ungrounded aspects of life...that all need grounding, completion, and purpose. God, I sound like a certified "lost soul."

I have the tools... the confidence, the love/support from amazing people, the happiness, the humor... the YOGA!!! I am a complete person, but with an empty purpose. Ironically enough, I do feel absolutely certain that those gaps will be bridged, wants will be know, "supposed to's" will become is/are, empty places will be filled, need to control will be set free. I came on this trip because I feel drawn to it. I believe this is the path... the way... the process that will begin that journey of fulfillment. This experience will form the Rachel that the world already declared me to be.

_____ **Rachel Vincent**

Bakhtapur

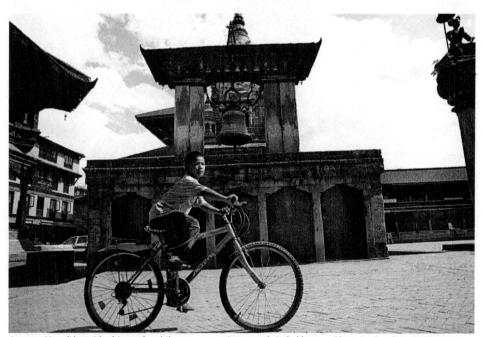

A young Nepali boy rides his modern bike past an ancient temple in Bakhtapur. Photo by Candace Koslen.

June 21, 2010_____

It's difficult to explain in words the sheer craziness of Kathmandu. There are cars, overfilled buses, motorcycles, bikes, and pedestrians. Plus, there is every animal you can imagine in the streets and alleyways. Horns are constantly honking to the point that they have no meaning or effect. Chickens are being slaughtered on the sidewalk, in front of your very eyes. Meat is on the street for sale, infested with flies. Trash and garbage are everywhere. There is no running water. From deep wells, women hoist their buckets down so low it looks like there is hardly any water left.

The heat, dirt, and poverty are overwhelming. There is never a quiet moment, and never an unoccupied space. Every market looks the same. Yet, the countryside is stunningly beautiful. The people of Nepal are amazingly friendly and helpful. They are tough, proud and hard working. Well… the women and girls [at least] are very hard working.

_____ ***Terri Bahr***

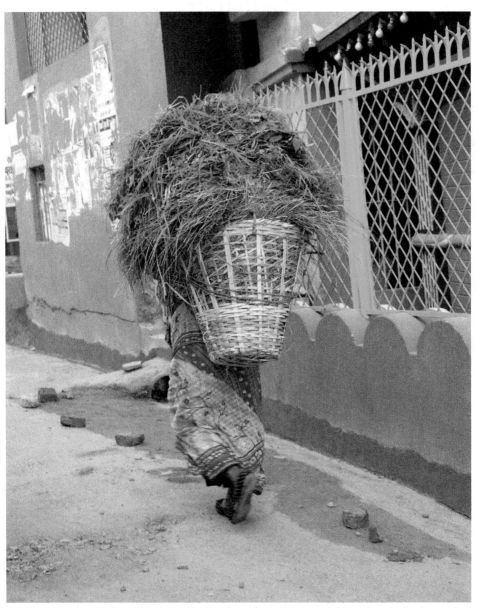

Woman carrying basket of grass fronds to be dried and used for weaving more baskets. Photo by Candace Koslen.

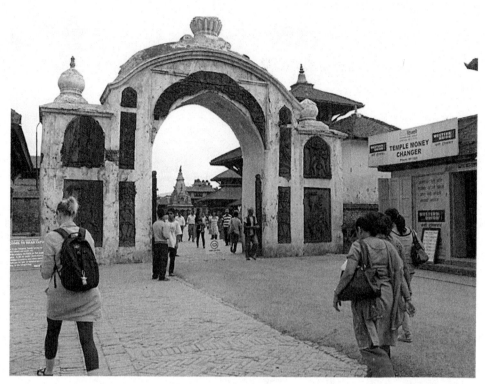

Just outside the gates of the Old City of Bakhtapur. Photo by Terri Bahr.

Arriving at the gates to Durbar Square, we left our bus and bought tourist tickets to enter the Old City; the cost of the tickets helped the Nepalis maintain the site. The first thing you see once you pass through the gates is a series of ancient temples. They look hundreds if not thousands of years old. The stonework and bronze statues that surround them are truly impressive. Then just off the square on the right is the old Royal Palace. It has a large golden door leading inside, where an ancient fountain with a giant bronze cobra on one side once spouted water into a large deep pool. Very cool looking. The other thing we couldn't help noticing was the poverty…

6/21/10 _____

Well, the Old City was something else. Every cliché about a "Third World Country" was on display, right in front of you: the emaciated animals, the begging children, the goat ready for sacrifice at the temple wall, the disfigured, the crazy screaming man, and the woman hauling water from the community well. It was all there, in living color.

The thing that strikes you is – NEED. It is the need for so very much….

_____ *Gabrielle Stickley*

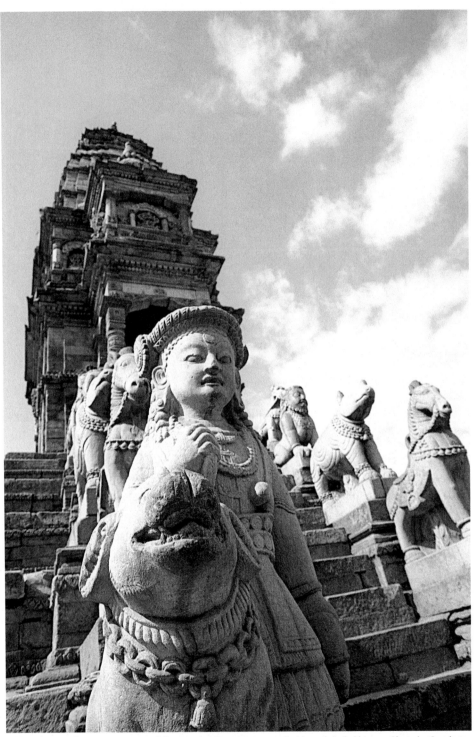

Intricately carved stone statues guard the steps leading up to an ancient temple in Bakhtapur. Photo by Candace Koslen.

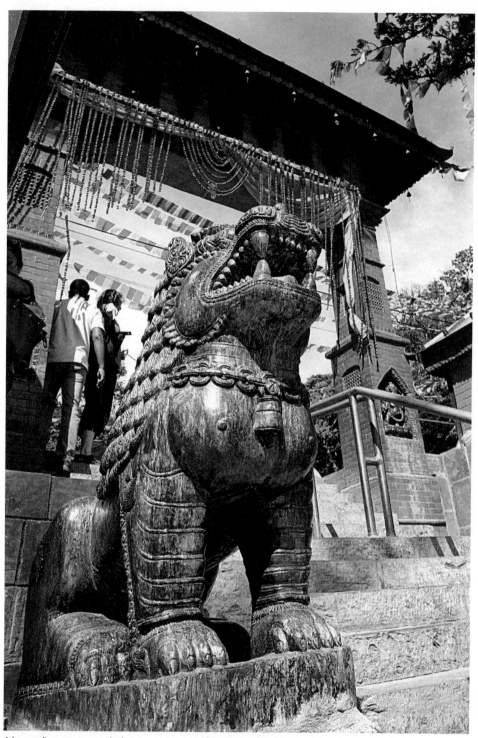

A bronze lion statue guards the entrance to one of the gates of the Old City. Photo by Candace Koslen.

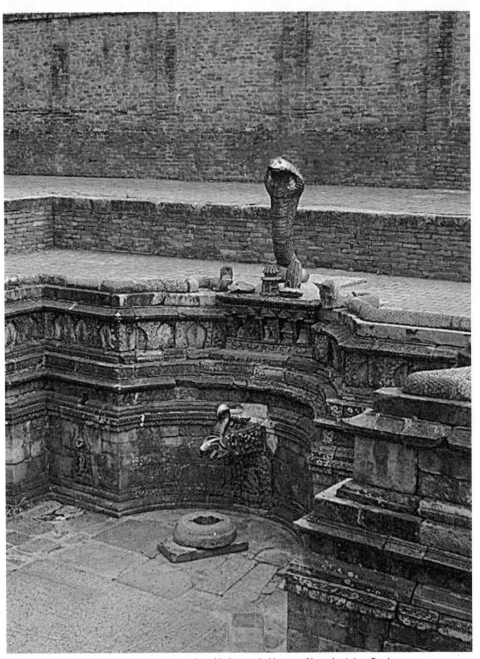

A golden cobra guards the font in the ancient Royal Palace at Bakhtapur. Photo by Jaime Furda.

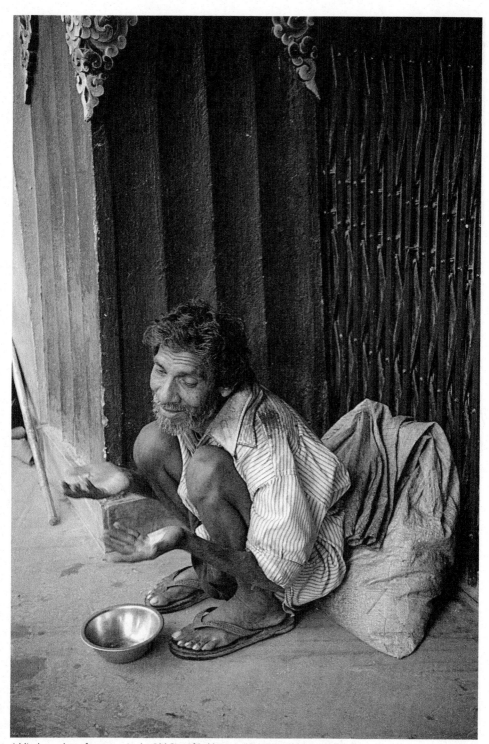

A blind man begs for rupees in the Old City of Bakhtapur. Photo by Candace Koslen.

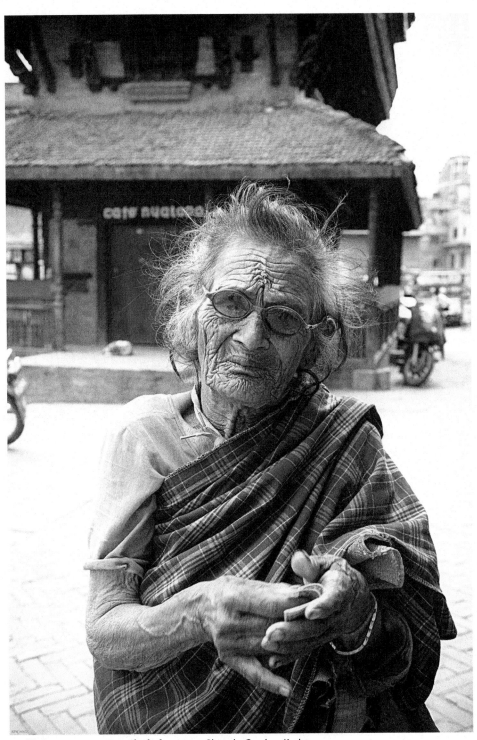

An elderly woman accepts a gift of a few rupees. Photo by Candace Koslen.

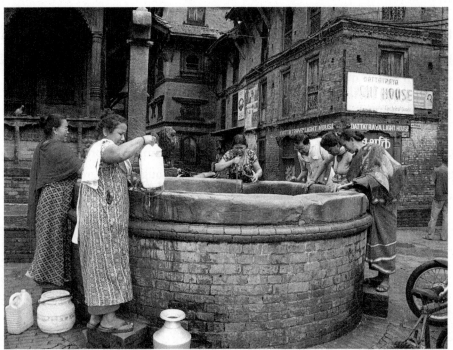

The women of Bakhtapur filling jugs with water from the town well. Running water is only a dream for most Nepalis.

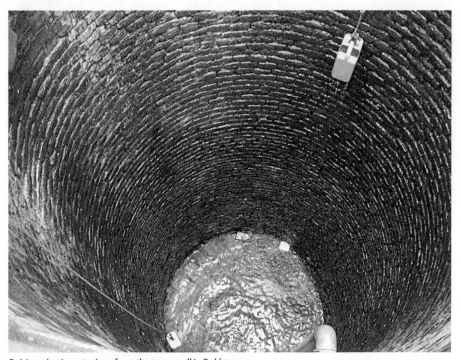

Raising plastic water jugs from the town well in Bakhtapur.

It was overcast this afternoon, and as we toured the old temples and the palace it began to rain. Luckily, Jesse had prepared us for this, and we had brought rain ponchos and umbrellas. The rain turned into a brief deluge and the gutters along the narrow streets quickly turned into rivers of water.

David, wearing his poncho and a hat that made him look like Mel Gibson in Gallipoli, disappeared down an alleyway in the rain (the first of several solo jaunts he would take over the next two weeks), and came back proudly displaying a genuine Gurkha knife in a leather sheath that he'd bought for a great price. David it turned out was an excellent haggler.

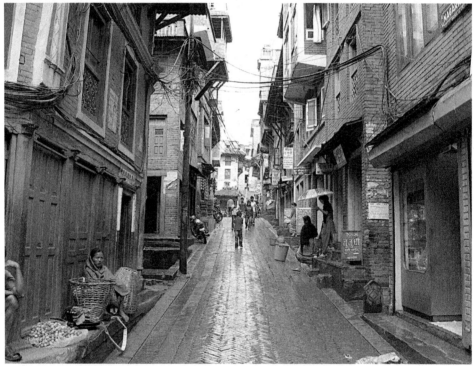

The red brick streets outside the shops of the Old City, wet from a sudden downpour.

On this shopping excursion, he took Jaime to a small shop he'd found where the owner made musical instruments. With the considerable help of David's bargaining skills, Jaime (a music major in college) would leave Bakhtapur with a beautiful little, hand-carved four-string Nepali sarangi.

A traditional Nepali sarangi looks a bit like a fiddle or lyre but more boxy. They are usually carved from a very light wood, locally known as khiro, and have a neck and hollowed-out body. The body is carved into a frame with two openings, the lower one covered with dried sheep-skin. The sarangi has four strings and is played using a bow. Horse-tail hair, which is still used by violin players, was originally used for the bow string, but these days nylon strings are common. Jaime thought her sarangi was worth ten times back home what she paid for it in Bakhtapur, but on the plane ride back, it was damaged, and she has yet to find someone to repair it.

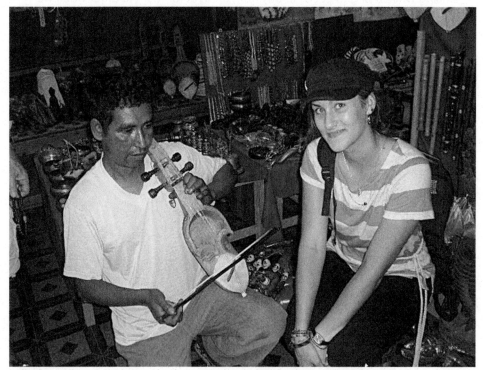

A shopkeeper shows Jaime how to play the sarangi that she bought. Photo courtesy of Jaime Furda.

The rain which continued to fall during our shopping did not diminish our desire to bargain hunt, or our appreciation for the old town's amazing architecture. It also had little effect on the other main "attraction" of Bakhtapur — street hawkers. Street urchins might be a better description once they were through with us. They followed us everywhere, hawking everything from singing prayer bowls, to handcrafted change purses, mala beads, and every other knick knack under the sun. Most of it looked like tourist junk, to be honest, but since this was our first excursion into the real Nepal, most of us bore the barrage of little salesmen with as much patience as we could muster. The oldest of them couldn't be more than twelve or thirteen, the youngest five or six. Their constant, relentless requests to buy, buy, buy however soon became as excruciating to listen to as fingernails on a chalkboard.

Once we got within the walls of the [old] city, it began to rain. I'm not sure if that was it, or just the medieval vibe of the architecture and dark narrow alleyways, but there seemed to be an ominous feel to that place. The merchants were so intense they would follow us for long periods of time; and many of the children we saw would follow us (trained as young merchants), and go from sweet and smiling while trying to get us to buy from them or for them to bitter when we were unable. This was difficult to see in their faces because we were in Nepal on this journey mostly because we are caring people, and I wanted to help them all, but how can you possibly buy from all of them?

Deanna Lee

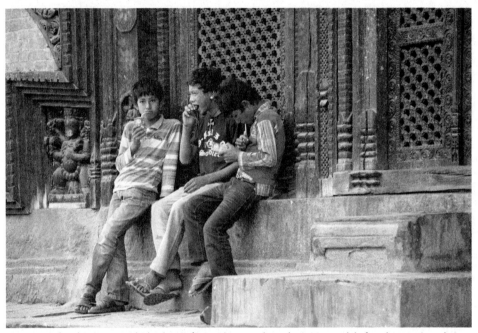

Young street hawkers rest outside the doors of an ancient temple, gathering strength before they continue their relentless pursuit of tourist dollars. Photo by Candace Koslen.

Two boys in particular stuck out amongst the hawkers following us around. One was taller than the others, with a sweet sad face, and a bandage around one hand. He spoke softly, but earnestly. "You buy something, please? I know good place, sir. I get you good deal." He was doing the soft sell and doing it pretty well. The other was probably the shortest amongst this little group of eight or ten boys. He was also the most aggressive. "I get you best deal. You follow me. This way." To both of them we kept repeating, "No thank you, not interested. Sorry."

At first we were all excited, but then we became overwhelmed. After we saw the beautiful temples in the square, we were overcome by the streets. The streets reminded me of Fez in Morocco – full of vendors peddling trinkets, and narrow streets.

I understand that people need to make a livelihood and respect the people selling us things, but after an hour of walking and turning down the trinkets, I was exhausted and wanted to go to bed.

_____ *Minling Chuang*

The first boy shrugged off our negative answers almost like he didn't hear them. He just kept repeating his same pitch. "You buy something, please? I know good place, sir. I get you good deal." The second boy however didn't take all the "no thank you's" too kindly. After a while he started becoming more aggressive, almost belligerent. "You have money. I know you have money. You American. You rich. Why you not spend money?" If you opted to give him a little friendly attitude back, or to educate him to the fact that not all Americans are rich, it only made him more aggressive. He would curse you in Nepali, and you got the point despite not understanding the language. There is a universal lingua franca we all understand when someone says "Fuck you, asshole", no matter what dialect they happen to speak. I had to give the kid his props though. For a little guy he had balls.

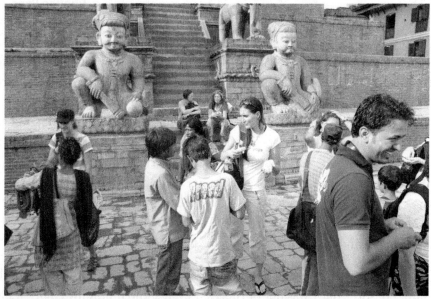

The street hawkers hard at work. The YFF crew out of money. Photo by Minling Chuang.

These two boys jostled subtly for position, one taking the lead, then the other. It seemed at first that they were competing for our business. The truth, I'd guess, is that they were working together, for someone else. Some Fagin-like character from a Dickens novel was running them. When they realized they weren't making any progress hawking souvenirs to us, most of the boys wandered off to look for other customers. These two boys took another tack. They asked us to buy them Nepali-English translation dictionaries. They said they needed them for school.

Now if you think it was easy telling all these poor kids "no" over and over and over for hours on end, even the little guy with the big attitude, I can assure you it wasn't. We had only just arrived in Nepal and none of us wanted to come across as 'Ugly American Tourists'.

June 22, 2010 _____

Is there a polite way of declining? Is there a respectful way to say no? I accept that it is just a fact of life here that the people have to resort to this in order to survive and maybe that means they are very pushy. If you were hungry and your kids were too – wouldn't you be? So why be sarcastic just to be mean to these people? They don't understand the subtleties of the English language, but they can tell your harsh tone of voice. They did nothing wrong to be where they are in life. So why must we treat them nicely only when we need something from them?

_____ **_Tingting Peng_**

Even though Basu and Jesse had told us to do our best to ignore these little street hawkers, that we would find better quality items to buy later on in the trip, most of us ended up buying something from the street merchants, as well as from the more legitimate shop owners we encountered. I ended up spending all the money I'd exchanged from dollars that day on various trinkets and souvenirs. And, I finally gave in and offered to buy the tall soft-sell artist a dictionary. He took me to a bookstore, and in seconds had a 400 rupee dictionary in hand. I could see the manager eyeing us as we made the cash for book swap. I wondered if he was the Fagin I had been seeking. I wondered if the kid would return the book to the seller, split the money, and then move on to the next customer.

When the short kid saw me make this purchase, he asked for the same deal. I told him, no, sorry but I was out of rupees. I even showed him my empty wallet.

He cursed me in Nepali, and went off in search of new business opportunities. I smiled and waved to him as he left. Strangely enough, I think I respected his honest reactions more than the false sweetness of the taller boy. Part of me was annoyed with myself for being so cynical and jaded. But I also did my best to remain polite to both kids. They were after all just trying to make a living, and under much tougher circumstances, I imagined, than anything I'd ever had to do. Ultimately, I guess I was just more of a sucker for the soft sell than the hard sell, and if the short boy had been a good student of human nature, or a better, more experienced businessman, he would have figured that out, and come away with some rupees too.

The whole experience left us very conflicted. Every young hawker, with their pleading eyes and persistent voices, was an assault on our psyches, a twinge of Western guilt which quickly became a full-blown assault as the day progressed. Our brains told us they were all putting on an act, but our hearts angrily refused to listen to that kind of cynical logic. These little merchants were experts at playing on that internal war. One minute they would be softly pleading with us to buy something, and then, when we refused, even politely, they would get angry, even insult us, for being too cheap with our money. The result was an internal war of logic and emotion that ultimately left us exhausted. By the time we got back to Norling, we were all so exhausted that we actually asked to skip yoga practice for the evening...

June 21, 2010_____

It's funny, not even two days in Nepal and we already wanted to skip practice because we were tired. How easily we break. ☺

_____ *Minling Chuang*

Tingting, Jesse, and Subash talked us out of that. As much as anything else we didn't want to disappoint Tingting, who was supposed to be teaching the group that evening, so we sucked it up, and did what we had come to do. Practice yoga. It turned out to be just the thing we needed to soothe our tired bodies and battered spirits.

June 21, 2010 _____

Luckily, we had practice and Tingting led us in a rejuvenating power yoga class. We practiced on the rooftop that overlooked [the] lush golf course that was full of wild monkeys. I seriously think the monkeys were wondering what we were all doing as some sat on the golf course and watched us.

It was the perfect way to end the evening.

_____ *Minling Chuang*

After the sensory overload that was Bakhtapur, and after our rejuvenating sunset yoga practice on the rooftop, we gathered in the dining room of the hotel for dinner. Then we went straight to bed. Our first full day in Nepal had left us all in need of a good night's sleep.

June 22, 2010

Day 3 of the trip

Boudhanath

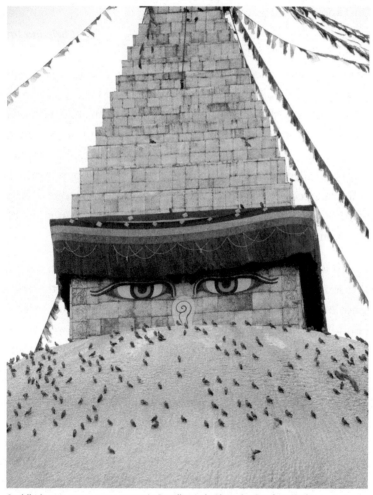

Buddha's eyes, open, atop a stupa in Boudhanath. Photo by Candace Koslen.

The next morning, refreshed and rested, we slipped into what would become a routine for us on our two week journey: morning yoga, breakfast, sightseeing, lunch, more sightseeing, evening yoga, dinner, and finally sleep.

June 22, 2010

We are awakened at 5:30 a.m. with a knock at our door to get ready for 6:00 a.m. yoga practice. Our guru Subash, for a 25-year old man, seems to have an old soul.

He took us through a 1 ½ hour practice that was very complete in waking up every part of my body. There were some really hard poses that I have never done before like duck walking. I don't know if that's the proper name of the pose. I just know I felt as graceful as a duck doing it!

Christina Jankus

The morning yoga practice that day put me in a very open and positive place after the emotionally difficult afternoon we spent in Bakhtapur. I went to the hut where the massage therapist and his family lived, and had an amazing Thai massage. Afterwards, I felt better than I had since I left Cleveland four days earlier. I showered and then went to grab some lunch. Once there, Jesse told us about our next excursion: a place called Boudhanath. We finished eating, hopped on our always ready bus and navigated our way through the hectic, chaotic streets of Kathmandu. Soon we found ourselves in another world from Bakhtapur — not just physically, but emotionally and spiritually.

Boudhanath is one of the holiest Buddhist sites in Kathmandu. Located about 11 km northeast of the city center, the area is dominated by one of the largest spherical stupas, not only in Nepal, but in the world. A stupa is a dome-like structure containing Buddhist relics, and used by Buddhists as a place of worship. The stupa at Boudhanath was white on the bottom and topped by a tall brown and gold spire. Hundreds of colorful prayer flags hung from the top, gently waving in the breeze.

The use of prayer flags actually pre-dates Buddhism, going back thousands of years. Tibetan Buddhists like the ones at Boudhanath began using them around 800 AD to promote peace, compassion, strength and wisdom. The practice then spread throughout the region. The flags do not carry prayers to the gods, a rather common misconception; instead the Tibetans believe that by hanging the flags in high places the prayers (mantras) written on them will be blown by the wind to spread peace and goodwill to all. As the wind passes over the flags, the air is purified and sancti-

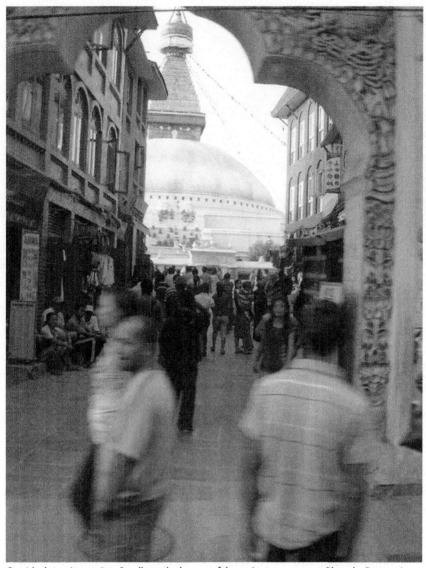

Outside the main gate into Boudhanath, the eyes of the main stupa peer out. Photo by Deanna Lee.

fied by the mantras, and in this way the prayers become a permanent part of the universe. Tibetans renew their hopes for the world by continually mounting new flags alongside the old. This act symbolizes a welcoming of life's changes and an acknowledgment that all beings are part of a greater ongoing cycle.[5]

At the base of the great spire atop the stupa at Boudhanath, on all four sides, giant eyes looked upon the people in the square below. The open eyes symbolize the

[5] Source: http://en.wikipedia.org/wiki/Prayer_flag

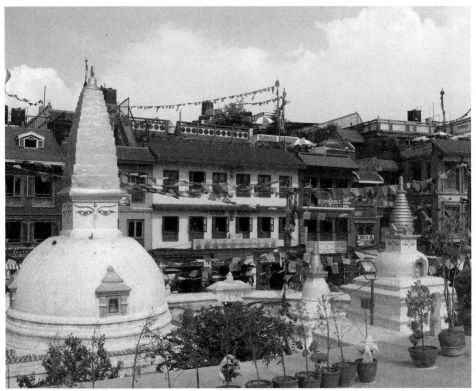

The main square of Boudhanath—clean, orderly, peaceful—in sharp contrast to Bakhtapur.

awakening of the Buddha, and are the unique feature of many Buddhist holy sites in Nepal. It was in Nepal, legend has it, that the Buddha's mind was first "awakened", his eyes first "opened", to the pain and suffering of the world.

For centuries, traveling Tibetan merchants rested and offered prayers at the stupas in Boudhanath, and when refugees entered Nepal from Tibet after the Chinese occupation in the 1950's, many decided to take up residence in the area. Their influence could be felt, as much as seen in Boudhanath. Despite its close geographic proximity to Bakhtapur, the vibe in Boudhanath was peaceful, more joyful, and more happily alive than Bakhtapur. Here in Boudhanath, there was still poverty, still the odd character following us around, hoping to make a few rupees, but life seemed more natural, more relaxed. I kept thinking I had a better chance of running into the Dalai Lama than a character like Fagin in a place like this. Commerce was still important here, but it was balanced; and everyone, travelers and locals, seemed happier.

What strikes me is, this is a very sacred place with an amazing energy. Yet they built a shopping center around it! Ha-ha!

… What also struck me as interesting is the only expectation I had of the Nepali people is I thought they would be sad. They are far from sad! They have only the clothes on their back, ramshackle homes and if their belly is full, they are very happy and happy we came to visit them. They are as curious of us as we are of them.

Christina Jankus

The temple and the Buddhist monks who lived and worshipped in the area probably had a lot to do with that feeling. While Bakhtapur is a very ancient historical place, its residents seemed devoid of spirituality. The struggle against poverty, the fight for commerce by the street peddlers, the negative, dark energy of Bakhtapur, seemed to have buried or snuffed out the spiritual side of that place, instilling in it instead a fevered need for commerce. But not in Boudhanath.

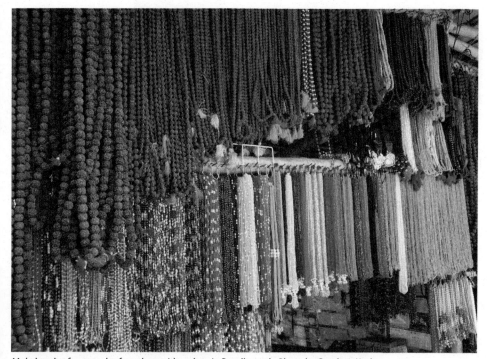

Mala beads of every color for sale outside a shop in Boudhanath. Photo by Candace Koslen.

In sharp contrast to Durbar Square and the crazy hawkers at Bakhtapur, Boudhanath was a very real taste of the olden days unspoilt by over-eager tourist hunters. The whole pace of the place was slower and I found myself getting lost in the movement of visitors, people in prayer and elderly monks giving blessings.

Tingting Peng

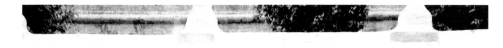

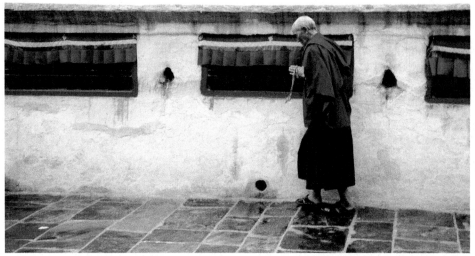

A Buddhist monk turns the prayer wheels outside the main stupa in Boudhanath. Photo by Candace Koslen.

A mere two days into our trip, and we were already starting to move out of the hectic pace of Western life, into the slower, more natural rhythms of Nepal…

June 22, 2010

I'm totally a day or two behind on journaling and that's because I've transferred over to Nepal time, where there is no time…

…at some point, I stopped trying and just sat in my own meditation. As I floated away into my sacred space, I kept coming back to the thought of this whole trip and how the group has bonded so quickly and even though I'm the only one not from Cleveland, I felt so much warmth from everyone on this trip. It's really nice too, that we yogis have something in common.

Tingting Peng

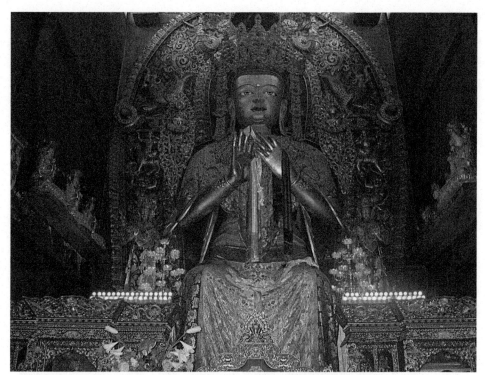

The giant golden Buddha, bathed in candle light, inside the temple at Boudhanath.

We explored the shops and temples that had been built around the main stupa, and inside found some of the most beautiful Buddhist art any of us had ever seen.

June 22, 2010_____

The temple across from the shrine has doors similar to our hotel. We admired them but realized we wouldn't be entering. Guess again...our guide flings open the doors. We see a huge gold Buddha filling the space behind the altar. The radiance, energy coming from it was staggering. No suffering Christ, but a big, gold glowing welcoming Buddha. The small temple was overshadowed by this huge piece — the scale of it was so wrong for the room from a design perspective as we know it, but so perfect from the aspect of an energetic design. The prayer mats surrounding the main area asked you to pause and reflect and take a minute to be with your prayers.

_____ *Kathy Hayes*

Everyone seemed very genuine and friendly here, especially the omnipresent monks. One moment that typified this thought was when the Tibetan Llama of the main Buddhist temple at Boudhanath saw Jesse. The tall, confident, serene man with his head shaved, and wearing the gold and red robes of a monk, walked right up to Jesse and started talking and joking with him. Even though the Llama spoke almost no Nepali, and Jesse almost no Tibetan, they somehow managed to under-

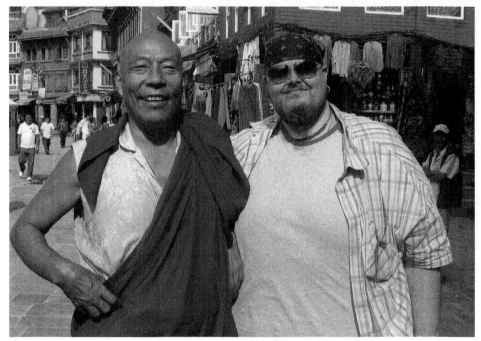

The Tibetan Llama, leader of the Boudhanath temple, and Jesse, who the Llama affectionately called Jambala.

stand each other just fine, joking with each other; Jesse teasing the Llama about his Nepali, and the Llama teasing Jesse about his size. The Llama kept calling Jesse "Jambala" and laughing playfully.

Jambala, I later learned, is the Hindu god of wealth. His form is stout, fat and strong, which probably comes from a time when it was widely believed that a substantial girth was synonymous with wealth and luxury. The Llama must have assumed that someone as big as Jesse must indeed be very rich. Jesse took it all in stride, having experienced this reaction often in his travels in Nepal. But I think it was also Jesse's happy joyful energy that resonated with the Llama — kindred spirits the two of them. They embraced and stood for pictures together before we all regrouped and headed to the bus for the drive back to the hotel.

On our way back, Jesse told us we were going to be making an unscheduled stop. Everyone's interest was piqued. What sort of unscheduled stop, we all wondered. A very special one, it turned out:

I couldn't have imagined what a special day today would turn out to be. It was the perfect way to end our stay in Kathmandu.

It started all the same – yoga practice in the morning, breakfast and a trip to Boudhanath to see the great Stupa…

When Kathy, Tingting, Marc and I went up and visited one of the temples overlooking the Stupa, a monk came and invited us into their prayer session. He was adorable. I had my big professional camera and all he wanted to do was take pictures with it of us, and of all the ornate decorations. If he weren't a monk, I think he could have been a photographer…

After the prayer session, we all went outside to observe the beautiful views and to talk with the monk. In our conversation, I found out he studied in California at the Hsi Lai Si Temple, which is the same temple my parents go to, and where I have been many times to pray. This is such a small world.

Being here in Nepal and meeting this monk has made me want to know more about my heritage. My grandparents and my dad are Buddhist, but I know very little. Besides knowing what to do when you pray, I don't know much else, which is sad. Guess I've always felt more spiritual than religious, but maybe this trip will change all that.

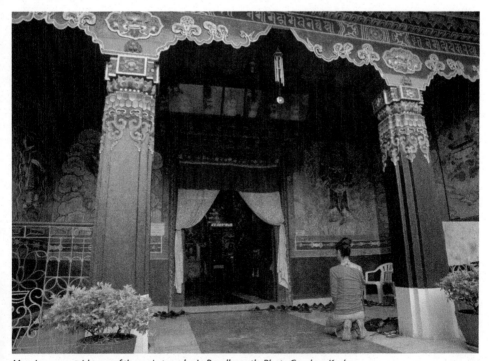

Marni prays outside one of the main temples in Boudhanath. Photo Candace Koslen.

But I digress… I thought going to Boudhanath would be the highlight of the day, but Jesse had a surprise for us. He told us he was going to take us to a magical place where miracles occur. I was curious to see what kind of surprise he had in store for us, especially with such an introduction. But boy did it live up to what he said.

_____ **Minling Chuang**

As the bus left the main road back to the hotel and began winding its way up to what looked like a more residential neighborhood of Kathmandu, we all began to wonder aloud where we were going. Jesse refused to answer, remaining silent, almost stoic. Why all of a sudden had Jesse become so serious, I wondered?

June 22, 2010

Day 3 of the trip, cont'd

NOH

Not long afterward, the bus pulled to a stop at the bottom of a narrow street, and Jesse stood up.

"Okay, we're here," he said. A very slight smile seemed to cross his lips. "Follow me."

We followed him off the bus, trailing behind as if he were our very own pied piper. After a short walk, we came to a gate that read "Imagine House". And then it hit us; we all understood. Jesse had wanted to surprise us, and he had succeeded. Suddenly everyone realized exactly where we were going:

June 22, 2010_____

As we wound our way through the streets of Kathmandu, we stopped in the middle of the road and met Carola, one of the board members of NOH and Michael Hess's sister-in-law.

Suddenly, it hit all of us...we're going to see the children of NOH!!!

We arrived at the gates of the Imagine House and got out of the bus. This overwhelming sense of emotion came flying at me and I could hardly contain myself. "Don't cry" I kept on saying to myself.

We entered through the gates to an open area where we waited with Vinod and Anita. Then, the kids came out of the houses and started walking down the stairs to come greet us.

It was at that moment I completely lost my composure and cried uncontrollably. These kids had smiles on their faces and greeted each one of us by saying "Sister, what is your name?" or "Brother, what is your name?"

With each handshake, more tears rolled down my eyes and snot rolled down my nose. I probably looked ridiculous because some of the kids asked me why I was crying. All I could say is, "I'm just so happy to finally meet all of you."

All I could think about is these children and what they must have gone through to be here. I've been anticipating this trip for 6 months and meeting these children, but even though I knew they were real children, they were only images in pictures and videos until this point. Now, they stand before us, next to us, all around us. I cannot describe the mixture of emotions that I felt.

_____ *Minling Chuang*

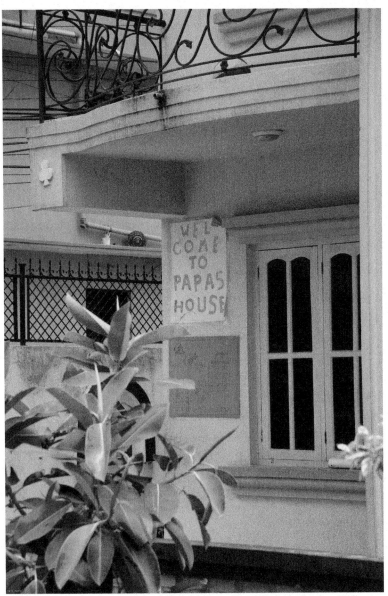

The handwritten welcome sign outside Nepal Orphans Home. Photo by Candace Koslen.

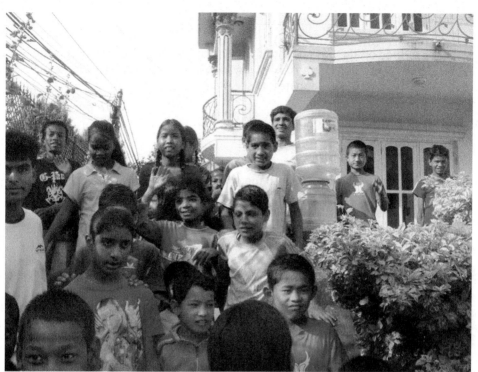

The children of Papa's House rush out to meet us for the first time. Photo by Tingting Peng.

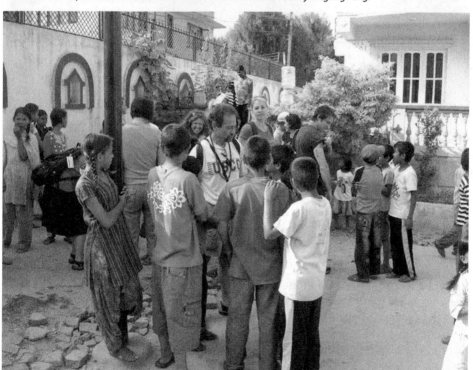

Robb Blain, center, surrounded by the sweetest kids I've ever met. Photo by Deanna Lee.

June 22, 2010

We all hurried off the bus and into the courtyard. As the boys and girls came out... my tears couldn't be held back any longer. The kids were smiling at me and here I was crying in happiness to see them.

Tingting Peng

June 22, 2010

We all hurried off the bus and into the courtyard. As the boys and girls came out... my tears couldn't be held back any longer. The kids were smiling at me and here I was crying in happiness to see them.

Tingting Peng

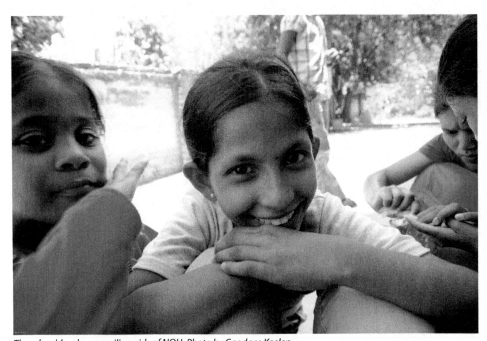

The adorable, always smiling girls of NOH. Photo by Candace Koslen.

June 22, 2010

When the bus pulled up at the orphanage for the first time, and I realized we were finally there, I was overcome with emotion. After more than two years of working to raise money, and looking at the beautiful faces, and hearing stories from Jesse, I was finally going to meet them. I would actually be able to hug them and breathe them in.

It was a little crazy at first with the kids coming out. Some were running to greet us, while some were very shy, and holding back a little. My eye caught [a] little [girl], and I scooped her up into my arms. What a cute sweetheart she is. It was so amazing to see how welcoming they were to us.

Terri Bahr

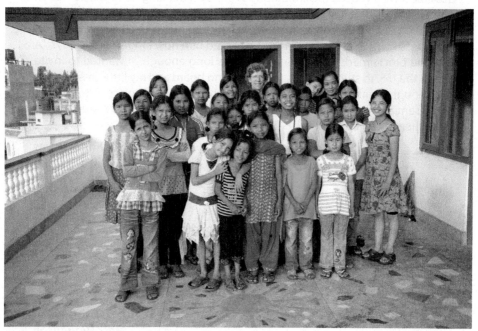

Carola Drosdeck, Michael Hess's sister-in-law and our volunteer den mother, with her beautiful baby chicks at NOH. Photo by Candace Koslen.

June 22, 2010

Sweetness when meeting the kids. It was sheer sweetness -- their faces anticipating -- their desire to connect, sometimes through language, other times through the touch of their hand in yours, and sometimes just by looking into their eyes and meeting them as another soul on its journey. One girl in particular stood by me after meeting, unusually close by our standards of personal space. Then I felt her hand slowly take mine, softly as if to say hello without words. Our shared words had run out -- me having no ability in Nepalese due to my lack of effort. And her running out of English after our conversation. Without words she said "don't go", stand here with me in this moment and share my presence. So we did and slowly more words came and more moments of connecting through glances and smiles. An understanding we had about where we were right now, how powerful both our presences were to one another.

An older boy came and sat by me at the wall, carrying the conversation for the other shy children who watched with big eyes wondering about us all. He asked about my family, who was my family. I didn't need to ask who his was as they were all standing around us and had already exchanged our hellos. He told me he was going to college next year and that I should return again. I laughed and said "ah shall it be at the time of your graduation?" He smiled, saying, "Yes, next April and bring your mother and your brother." Funny thought, not likely but I appreciated his wild possibility and realized that it was entirely possible if we removed the limitations of our own thinking. After all, he was an orphan who had no family and actually didn't know his real age. No birthday parties, no middle school graduation, no new bike...but here he was anticipating a possibility that was powerful. So I asked him how long shall we stay? "A year," he proclaimed, "a year -- no one stays long enough." I wanted to invite him to the U.S. to study in Ohio, free room and board and my little casa. But, as that thought floated through my brain another came in its place. He's here to be present to the other kids, to show them the possibility of a different life, to show them it can be.

Kathy Hayes

June 22, 2010 _____

I have done everything, learned everything, and experienced everything, just for this moment. I am so fortunate to be physically and financially okay to have done this. I went through all my stuff in order to share my pain, if only for a second, to share with the kids. We shared in a touch. We shared in a glance. We shared in a knowing. So I felt one with them. Thank you God: for this path, pain, knowledge, and understanding. What a gift...

Marc Nathanson

June 22, 2010 _____

This is why we are here -- for the children! The beautiful smiling faces of the children!

Christina Jankus

Nepal Orphans Home is really four houses, Imagine, Possibilities, Sanctuary and Papa's (aka Michael's) House, all located within walking distance of each other in a residential neighborhood in Kathmandu. There are about 100 girls and 20 boys living in these houses. All the children are either orphans or had parents who could no longer care for them. Many of the children were Kamlaris and had been rescued from child slavery, by NOH and its sister organization in Nepal, SWAN. We had been told that the Kamlari system was still a sad fact of life in Nepal. We'd heard how it is especially prevalent in the poverty-stricken rural areas that border India. We knew from reading Sold that some Kamlari girls tragically end up taken to India and sold into prostitution, imprisoned in brothels. Knowing all this, we feared the worst, but these kids completely surprised us.

June 20, 2010[6] _____

Words cannot begin to explain the way I felt when walking down the street with Jesse and Jaime. The girls were exiting the school, enthusiastically introducing themselves to us, shaking our hands, calling me "sister", as they walked by in a single-file line with braided hair tied with yellow ribbons...and faces full of smiles and wisdom...and beauty...

...Papa's house – five stories of playfulness, fun, learning, freedom. A yard with kids EVERYWHERE. Kids laughing, jumping rope, playing basketball, soccer, doing arts/crafts inside, and dancing. It was a "playground" that you could only find there or in heaven... We went into room after room; kids flowing in and out, all wanting you to join them... AWESOME...

Those kids are some of the most remarkable, encouraging, inspiring people of any age that I've ever met. They welcome you, open their hearts up to you, connect with you...without even knowing you. I am certain I will learn more from these children than I could ever teach them. Some of them are barely at my waist in height and their eyes hold more experience, wisdom, history than mine at age 31. Many had been beaten, tattered...or SOLD ...and yet are so full of life...

_____ _Rachel Vincent_

Before we knew it, Marc, Robb, David, and I were taken by the hand and led into the boys' quarters, a small annex next to the main house, where they proudly showed off their room to us. About eight or ten of the younger boys shared a 10 x 10 room with bunk beds for each of them crammed into every space possible.

School supplies and a few personal items were stored in small boxes under each bed. Each boy had decorated around his sleeping area with pictures they had drawn or taken from old magazines. Some were of cars, some of rockets and planes, some of sports figures. One boy proudly announced that he wanted to be an astronaut. They queried us intensely, asking where we were from, how old we were, what jobs we did, if we were married, if we had kids. They all loved sports, soccer and basketball being their favorites. They knew who Michael Jordan and Kobe Bryant were, and the Lakers seemed to be their favorite team. They reminded me of myself when I was their age — eager, energetic, excited, inquisitive. And most surprisingly, they appeared to be truly and genuinely very happy.

---

[6] _Rachel, Jaime, and Jesse arrived 2 days before everyone else and got to see the children the morning of June 20th before the rest of us had arrived._

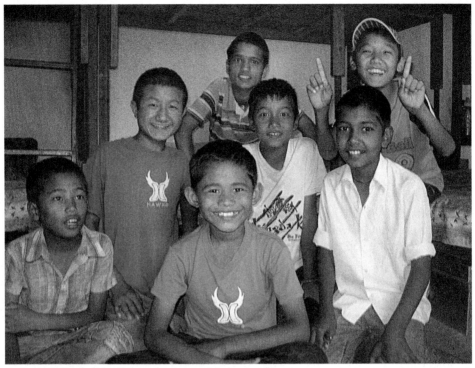

The boys of NOH showing off their room to us, and their sense of humor.

The women in our group were having their own adventure with the girls of NOH, who of course wanted to show off their part of Papa's House to their American visitors.

June 22, 2010_____

...I remember being taken upstairs to the girls' bedrooms. One room had seven beds, hardly any room to walk. But it seemed like one constant slumber party. I noticed the respect they showed one another. If a girl who did not sleep in that room wanted to come in, she would knock on the open door and ask, "May I come in, sister?"

_____ ***Terri Bahr***

June 22, 2010_____

A few of us went inside the house. This beautiful little girl led me to her room, which she shared with four others. She then took me to the study room and we sat down to work on her math assignment, subtractions. She calculated 24 minus 18 in her hand by borrowing 1 from the 2 and subtracting 14 and 8 on her hand. She wrote down 6 and proudly showed me her answer. We would celebrate after she calculated the right answer for each problem. We ended up celebrating a lot because she is a smart little girl, and very good at math as she got all the answers right. Apparently math is her favorite subject and I can see why. When I asked her what she wanted to do when she grows up, she said, "I want to be a teacher."

It was so amazing to me that all these kids are so ambitious at such a young age. They loved studying. Maybe it's because they know life without school, and how hard their life would be without an education. These kids seemed to appreciate the chance they have been given to study, something that I think kids in America take for granted.

For the rest of my life, I'll never forget today and these kids. They will forever be in my heart. I can't wait to see them again.

_____ **Minling Chuang**

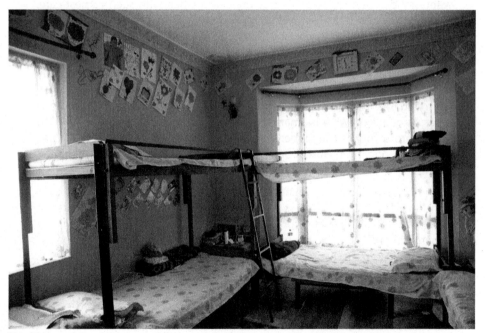

The girls' room at Papa's House colorfully decorated with their own hand painted pictures. Photo by Candace Koslen.

June 22, 2010_____

One of the girls took my hand, and led me into the girls house (Imagine House) and I got a peek inside how these girls live. On the ground floor was one bedroom with three girls sharing; she jumped on the bed and proudly posed for my camera. The walls of the room were covered in drawings; it was probably a very happy place for those girls.

The back of the first floor was the kitchen where some of the older girls were preparing dinner. There was also a study room where the desks were covered in books and pencils. These kids study hard!

[Another girl] came up to me and took my hand. Her big hazel eyes looked up at me and smiled. She led me outside to the back of the house and showed me their garden. Even though the garden was full of crops and corn, it still made me a little bit sad to see the trash littered around the edges of the garden. Every few seconds, [she] would look over at me as we leaned over the ledge of the garden, her eyes full of curiosity and hope. "How old are you?" I asked her. "Twelve," she replied. What was I doing when I was twelve?

I told her that I really like her hair, a chestnut color braided down both sides of her small face. She pointed to my single braid and smiled. Suddenly I got an idea! I pointed to my hair and made the gesture for two braids, then grabbed her hand and led us back to the courtyard. There I sat in between two of the sweetest kids I've ever met and they braided my hair with such earnest care, looking over at each other's work to make sure that the braids were perfectly equal in length. When they finished, we took a picture.

... I haven't felt this much joy or seen this many smiles, so genuine and so heart-felt. I think back to the street kids of Bakhtapur, who were asking me to buy them a dictionary but would then return the books for cash. Those kids were also trying to survive. They would run up to me and announce the world cup scores, "America drew!" It is amazing how a sport can unite the world, even to this remote corner of the globe. And the kids, from back home in the States or in Hong Kong, from Durbar Square, and from Papa's House, they are all still just kids.

Born into very difficult circumstances, it is clear to see what kind of lives each of those kids will have. Unless there is intervention, unless there is outside help, by people like Nepal Orphan's Home, those street children will end up perpetuating the vicious cycle of living on the streets, peddling for themselves or others – just to survive.

Tingting Peng

I never imagined in my wildest dreams that these orphan children, some of whom had been sold into child slavery before coming to NOH, could be so happy, so unjaded. There didn't seem to be any sullenness, or anger, or wounded psyches in this group. They teased each other, and wrestled around, like boys will do, but not mean-spiritedly. You could literally feel the love they had for each other right there in that little room. It wasn't just the boys, though. The sensation of joy, the look of wonder on all their faces at these Westerners who came here from some faraway land just to see them was overwhelming.

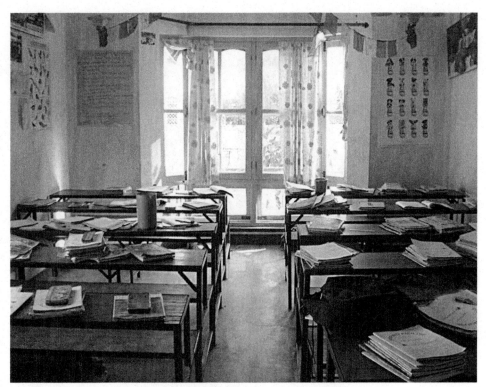

The classroom at Papa's House at recess. The kids study 6 days a week. Photo by Tingting Peng.

We went back outside to rejoin the bigger group, and soon more fun ensued. We showed the kids our digital cameras, and snapped photos of them. Immediately they asked if they could take pictures, too. Soon photos were being snapped everywhere. The kids got a huge kick out of checking out the results on the digital displays of all these newfangled cameras. Laughter echoed throughout the little courtyard between the girls' home and the boys' annex as they took pictures of us, of themselves, of the ground and their feet.

June 24, 2010_____

… One of my favorite moments was when Marc decided to do a pull-up contest against a 14-year-old boy who is very strong. When the boy was about to beat Marc's score, Marc playfully pulled him off the pull-up bar and said "Ok, that's enough." Everyone got a good laugh at this.

_____ ***Minling Chuang***

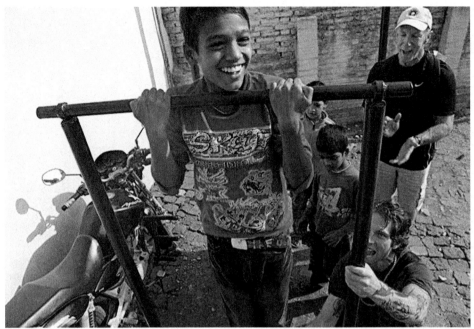

The pull-up contest between Marc and the NOH boys. Photo by Minling Chuang.

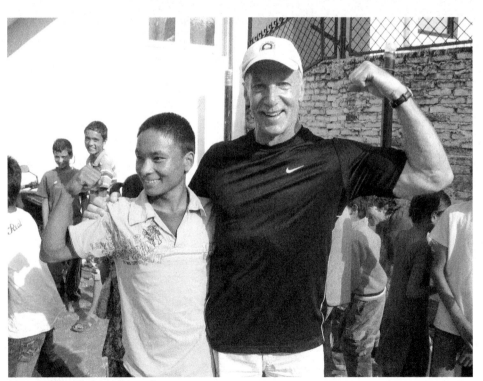

Marc with the real winner of the pull-up contest.

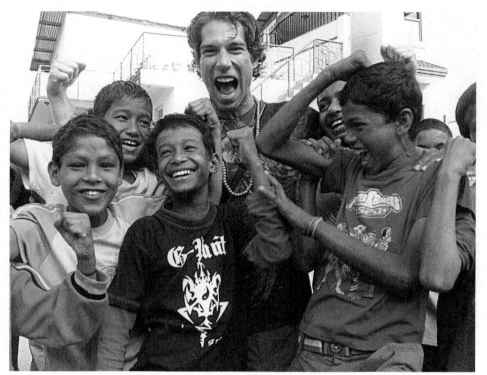
David and his new best buddies showing off their muscles. Photo by Terri Bahr.

As we were all hanging out in the courtyard taking pictures and shooting hoops, Carola offered to show some of our group where the volunteers were staying. So a few of us, Minling, Tingting, myself and couple of the others, walked up the street to check out the Volunteer House. The place was newer than the Imagine and Possibilities houses we'd just visited. There was even a sit down toilet, which the ladies were happy to see and utilize. We took off our shoes, and climbed three flights of stairs to the rooftop. On the way up, Carola showed us a sheet of paper taped to a door. It was the electric power schedule for the city of Kathmandu, explaining when power was supposed to be on, and when it was scheduled to be off. From what I could tell, they barely had power for half of any given 24-hour period. That had to be a challenge, I thought.

Once we were on the roof, we had a full view of the surrounding area. You could see several small houses under construction nearby, and some really fancy-looking ones not too far away. The whole area was surrounded by rich farmland. Clearly this was one of the better neighborhoods in Kathmandu. We then left the Volunteer House and took another quick walk up the hill to Michael's House....

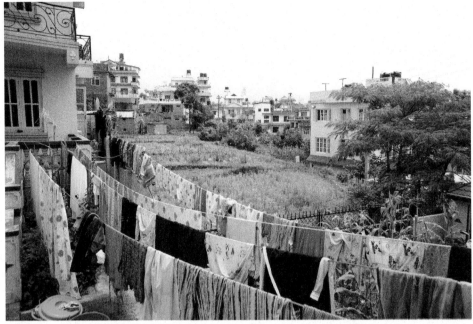

Laundry hanging out to dry behind Papa's House. No Maytag™ washers and dryers here. Photo by Candace Koslen.

June 22, 2010

There, another 33 kids were busy studying after their classes had finished for the day. Inside the study room, I was greeted by another round of enormous smiles. The kids were studying social studies, math and English. Here, in my heart, I knew that I wanted to continue fighting for their cause, their welfare and their future. I want to give them the life that I had when I was growing up – my childhood was simple but sweet. My parents didn't make a lot of money being new immigrants to America, but they focused on my education and tried to provide for me whatever I needed.

I never had a Christmas tree, but I did always get presents, my parents had generous friends. I slept on a steel table for a bed for 4 years until my parents could afford to move and buy me a proper bed. This was nothing compared to what these kids I've just met have gone through; at least I had parents who loved me and didn't abandon me…. This makes me even more committed to these kids and how I can provide for them, even the littlest things. Everyone needs to hear their story.

Tingting Peng

I don't have kids of my own, but if I did, I'd want them to be just like these kids at NOH. I think that's the highest compliment I could pay them. In the short period of time, no more than an hour or two, that we got to hang out and talk with them, my whole perspective on Nepal changed. Like Minling, and Tingting and all the others who were there that day, I thought about those kids for weeks and months after our visit. Reflecting on them made me reflect on myself, and I made a vow that no matter how tough things ever got for me, I'd remember these kids and their amazing attitude toward life, and be grateful for everything I had.

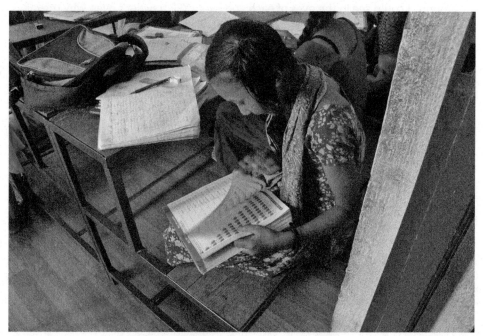

Working on her math homework... her favorite subject. Photo by Minling Chuang.

June 24, 2010 _____

Life in Nepal is so different from America. The kids at NOH appreciate what they have and each other. There were no TVs and video games for them to play. They had each other and it seemed to be enough for them. I also didn't see any of the kids fight, which is amazing considering there are over 150 kids at the orphanage. They loved each other and it clearly showed.

_____ ***Minling Chuang***

There was a darker side to this joyful, intense, emotional encounter with the kids, though. The fact that we only got to spend a very short time with them hit some of us pretty hard. The trip itinerary clearly stated that we wouldn't be spending more than a day or so total with them, but the overwhelming emotion of that first visit drove many of us to want more interaction with these kids:

June 22, 2010_____

When it was time to say goodbye, it was sad. And even though we told them we would be back, I felt disappointed that we weren't going to be spending more time with them. But as we were all interacting on the playground, I looked around. I could see in the eyes of each and every YFF traveler's eyes, why they were on this trip. I could see and feel the passion in everyone's heart….

They live with so much order, respect, and love for each other. I just wish we could have time to really get to know some of them better. I wanted to know what their life was like with their family, and [how] they entered the [Kamlari] system. How long were they in it, and how was their rescue arranged? It leaves me feeling like there are missing pieces to understanding the whole situation.

_____ ***Terri Bahr***

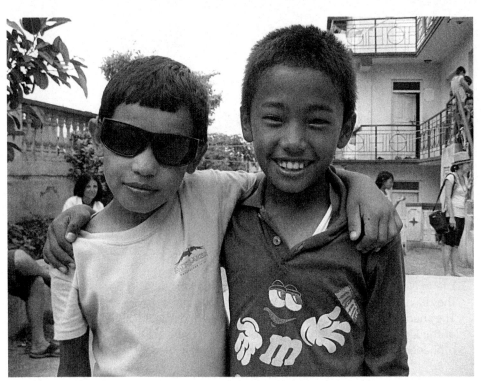

Best buddies. The boy on the left is looking James Dean cool wearing my sunglasses.

June 22, 2010_____

So it was disappointing to hear that of two weeks we will be with the kids such a short time -- a day. Really??

It's about the kids, connecting to their hearts. I guess we'll need to be wide open for our connections to be made so quickly.

_____ **_Kathy Hayes_**

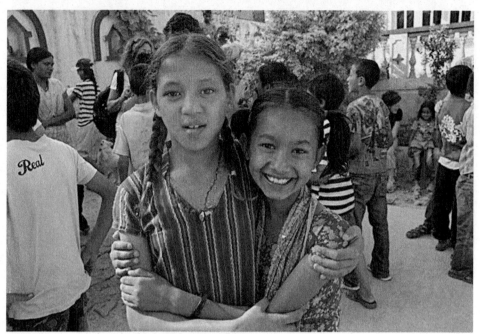

Best friends. The NOH kids love and take care of each other like the closest of brothers and sisters. Photo by Minling Chuang.

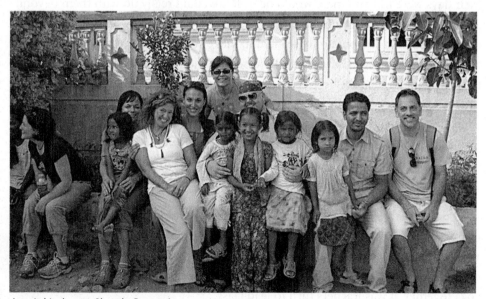

Jesse in his element. Photo by Deanna Lee.

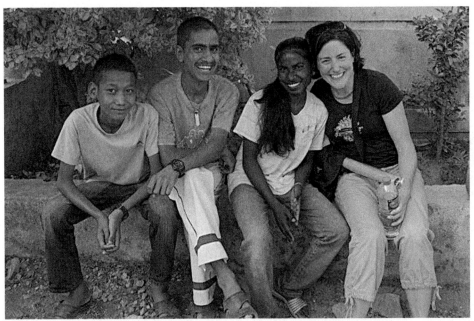

A few of the older kids at NOH with Kathy. The children can stay until they are 18 years old and finished with school. Some have come back to work for NOH after they've "graduated" to adulthood. Photo by Minling Chuang.

On the bus ride back to Norling, Jesse was bombarded with requests to change the itinerary so that the group could spend more time with the children. He patiently tried to explain to us that the kids were in school six days a week, and that their days were full and there would be little we could really do with them beyond a short visit. We were leaving Kathmandu in the morning and wouldn't be back for over a week. That response only seemed to make some in the group more adamant about changing things. Carola came to Jesse's aid and reiterated what he'd said about the kids being in school. She even stressed that Michael Hess, who ran NOH, would never allow a day off for the kids because he felt so strongly about the importance of educating them. Jesse and Carola said they would try to arrange another visit when we returned to Kathmandu, but nothing seemed to soothe the shock of realizing we wouldn't have nearly as much time with these amazing little people as some of us now desired.

I didn't realize it at the time, but this first little fissure in our group solidarity (our journey from 'me to we') was a split that, as the journey became more difficult, would grow to become a chasm. But that fracturing would come another day. This evening, we all gathered in a large building behind the main hotel and practiced yoga together. It was Rachel's turn to lead class...

I taught yoga to a group, for the first time since almost 1 year ago! It was wonderful; fulfilling. I missed it and it felt great. Jesse gave me one of the best compliments saying it was one of the best classes he's ever taken because I teach from the heart...Wow. I know I need to do this again. Yoga is a part of me. "Hello part of me, nice to see you again."

Rachel Vincent

After yoga practice, Jesse and Basu arranged for a local tailor to stop by to take measurements for those of us who wanted to buy traditional Nepali clothing. The men received simple red long sleeve yoga shirts and loose fitting yoga pants, like those worn by Subash, which the tailor had brought with him. All we had to do was find the right size for each of us. The women chose from various colored fabrics and styles, as the tailor took their measurements. Not surprisingly, they seemed to revel in their many choices. The garments would be ready when we returned to Kathmandu in ten days. Once the tailor was finished, our group assembled for dinner and stayed up late into the night eating and talking, despite another early scheduled wakeup call. It was our last night at Norling, and the conversation buzzed around the events, sights and sounds of the last two days. By the time I went to sleep, my head barely touched the pillow before I was out like a light.

June 23, 2010

Day 4 of the trip

Everest Flight

Wednesday morning, we woke before dawn and packed our bags. We had to skip yoga, not because we wanted to, but because the weather had cleared and Jesse had altered the itinerary slightly. We were about to undertake our next big adventure: a flight to Mt. Everest. There was some grumbling about the change in plans, but an hour later we boarded the bus, excited and ready to go, and Buddha drove us to the airport. Candy, Jennette and Marni met us there, and we all boarded a good-sized twin turbo-prop plane and strapped ourselves in.

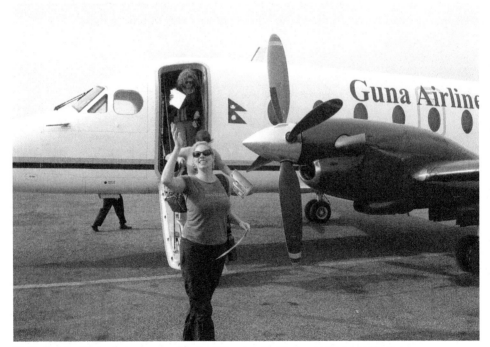

Eve Ennis doing the movie star wave as she gets off the plane that took us to Everest and back.

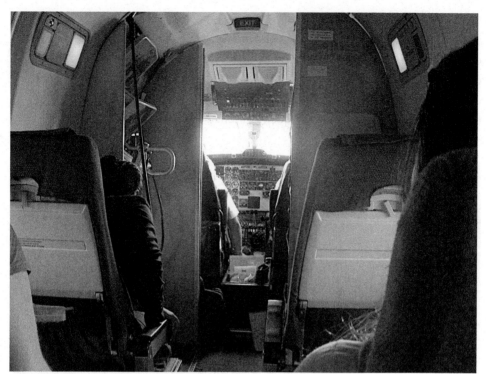

The cockpit of the Guna Airlines turbo-prop plane. Up close and personal.

Just as the last of us were seated, one member of the group had what can only be described as a sudden panic attack. Kathy, as it turned out, suffered from claustrophobia. As she entered the small cabin of the plane, and walked down the narrow aisle between the two rows of seats, I saw the expression on her face begin to change. In a few short moments, she went from smiling and happy to almost hyperventilating. "I can't do this," she said out loud. No one was sure what was happening as she stepped off the plane and walked around outside, taking deep breaths. Eve and Jesse went to check on her. A moment later, she came back onboard, but the small tight quarters inside the plane triggered her anxiety in seconds, and once again she was hyperventilating.

Everyone was onboard by now, and the pilot was ready to taxi onto the runway for takeoff. I felt bad, we all did, but Kathy wouldn't be able to take this flight with us. Ever the trooper, she assured us she would be fine, just as long as she got off the plane immediately. Jesse escorted her back to the terminal so she could wait in the airport lounge, where we'd pick her up upon our return.

We took off, minus Kathy, for a chance to see what it looked like at the top of the world. In a few moments, we were soaring high above the clouds. About twenty minutes later, we were approaching the Himalayas. The flight attendant pointed out our flight path on a small map that she passed around. As we approached the highest mountain range in the world, I stared out the window, transfixed with genuine, child-like excitement. Seeing Everest had been at the top of my list of reasons for taking this trip. The others were equally psyched for this moment:

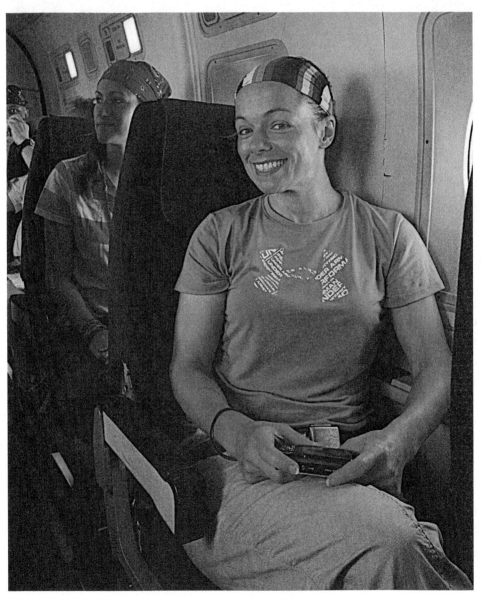

Joyce is all smiles as she buckles up for the Everest flight. Photo by Minling Chuang.

June 23, 2010_____

For 20 years, I have read about, seen pictures of, and wondered about Mt. Everest. It was surreal to be actually looking at it… When it came time to view Everest – or Sagarmatha, as the Nepali call it – we were each called up into the cockpit to see it through the front window. It was unbelievable.

_____ *Gabrielle Stickley*

June 23, 2010_____

My fear of heights went out the window, replaced with an emotional kind of excitement. At the first sign of Everest, the flight attendant ushered me to the open cockpit. "Go look," she said with a smile. And there it was, looming high above the clouds at over 29,000 feet. It was magnificent. I was soaring above the clouds within reach of Everest. The first officer was explaining to me the other peaks, Lotse for example, the one right next to Everest. I wanted to open my arms like wings and yell out at the top of my lungs. It was one of the most exhilarating moments of my life. Ahhhh =)

_____ *Tingting Peng*

Try as we might, words can't really describe the view of the Himalayas we had that crisp, clear morning. Pictures won't really do it justice, either. It's something you have to experience, there, in the moment — a long, long line of snow-covered peaks stretching across the entire horizon, reaching up from the earth to the heavens. Awe-inspiring, majestic, natural beauty as far as the eye could see. Like getting a glimpse of Valhalla or Olympus. For me, looking out the cockpit window when my turn arrived, it was truly a dream fulfilled.

June 24, 2010_____

…in my prayers, I always thank God for the roof over my head. Well, the roof over my head has now changed, as it has been put in a whole new perspective by the flight. God's roof just grew. Now when I say thank you for my roof, it will now be the bigger roof, and the bigger picture. It will still include the bricks, but will now also include the creations and the heavens.

_____*Marc Nathanson*

When we landed, it felt like a letdown, returning to this mortal coil, to borrow a phrase from Shakespeare; back in the real world, on terra firma, with all its strife and suffering, after just a brief glimpse of what immortality must look like. Yoga and Buddhism both talk about detachment, about letting go, not holding on to worldly things, experiences or emotions. Between the short visit to NOH the day before, and now this short flight to Everest and back, we were all getting a hard lesson in that concept.

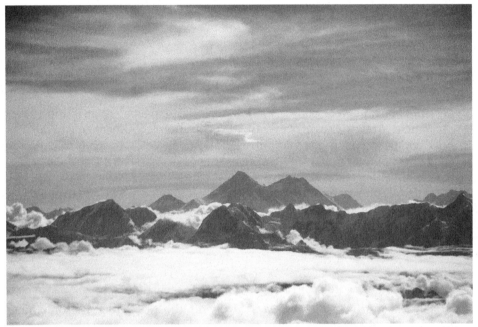

The stunning view of Mt. Everest amidst the Himalayas from the cockpit of our plane. Photo by Candace Koslen.

There was a quick bathroom stop at the terminal, and then we were back on the bus for the drive from the airport to the hotel, dropping off Candy, Marni and Jennette near NOH. We wouldn't be seeing them for more than a week. Much was to happen in that time, not only to those of us who would continue traveling through Nepal, but also to these three ladies, who were about to embark on their own difficult emotional journey as volunteers. After a quick breakfast at Norling, we moved to the next stop on our Nepal adventure: Lumbini, birthplace of the Buddha.

June 23, 2010

Day 4 of the trip, cont'd

The Road to Lumbini

Jesse told us it would be a long ride to Lumbini from Kathmandu, and man was he right. Though it was only about 220 km as the crow flies, on the winding roads of Nepal it was a 10 ½ hour long trip by bus. We began our journey driving through the chaotic frenzy of Kathmandu once again — sounds of horns, engines, cars, motorcycles, and a crazy tractor-like contraption that had to be seen to be believed filling the air. Noise, noise, noise. Inescapable noise. But it didn't bother us. We were excited as we drove away from Norling, talking our heads off about all kinds of things — Nepal, home, work, music, books, food.

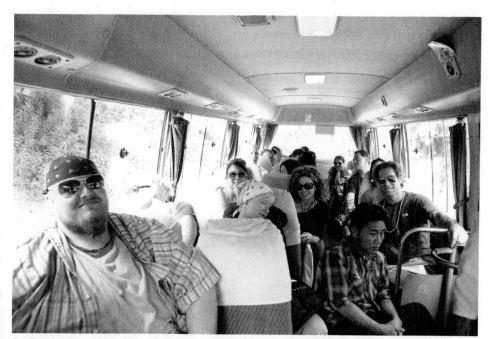

Sun Tze, our trustee porter, front right, relaxes on the long bus ride to Lumbini. Photo by Candace Koslen.

We left the city and all the noise, and moved out of the Kathmandu valley into the countryside. The roads were good as we wound our way down from the foothills of the Himalayas into the Central Valley. The twisting, turning two lane highway was packed with trucks and buses, the main modes of transportation in Nepal. Travel was slow, but for the most part we moved at a steady pace of 30 or 40 km/hour. Soon enough, the roads opened out into breathtaking views of the valley below.

Low mountains and the beginnings of the Trishuli River (named after the trident, or trishuli, of the Hindu god Shiva) dominated the landscape. The river was popular with white water rafters, and from a few vantage points on the drive, we could see big rubber 8- and 12-man rafts floating downstream. I had done some rafting in my day, and from what I heard, this river had class 1 to 3 rapids. Nothing too dangerous, but loads of fun no doubt, especially during the hot days before the monsoons.

We played some music as we drove on, plugging various iPods into the bus's sound system. David's and Deanna's playlists seemed to be the most popular. People started singing along to the tunes. The vibe was joyful. The AC hummed softly, keeping us cool. The lush green scenery seemed to give us life and energy. We laughed and joked and sang as we watched villages small and large go by. A few members of the group who were suffering from the Nepali version of Montezuma's revenge were quietly curled up in their seats, next to the windows, fast asleep. As the bus rolled on, we could see from the windows the people who lived here, and the poverty.

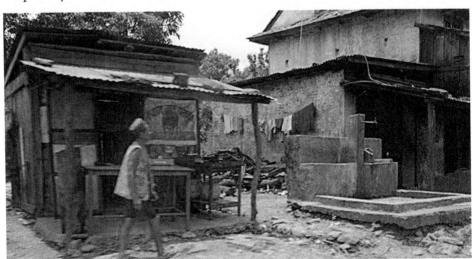

The "miniscule, wood, tin and concrete boxes" described by Gabby. Photo by Minling Chuang.

We went over the mountains and through beautiful valleys, gorges coupled with unimaginable poverty… watched hut after hut after hut pass by, perched on the side of the road – people's homes. Hard to take in, that they actually live in these miniscule wood, tin and concrete boxes. You could close your eyes at one point, and 20 minutes later, open them up, and see the exact same poverty….

Gabrielle Stickley

Some of these dwellings had little shops in front of them that sold all kinds of Nepali goods and other staples, such as water, Coke, Sprite, bananas, potato chips. They looked like the 7-Eleven's of Nepal. Colorful buildings dotted the highway, many with signs for Tuborg and San Miguel beer and Playboy Whisky painted on the sides. There were open air farmers' markets along the way too, with all types of vegetables for sale. We stopped the bus at one of these little markets and Basu bought a big bunch of bananas, which a few of us happily ate. They were small, sweet and delicious.

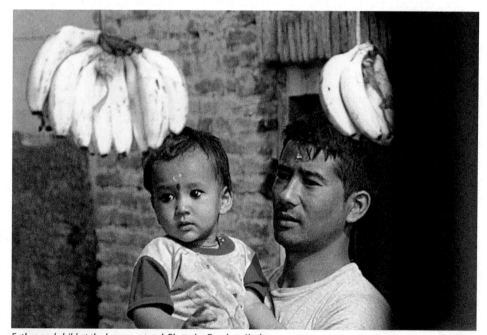

Father and child at the banana stand. Photo by Candace Koslen.

The bus trip, though it certainly started out fun, had some unexpected challenges in store for us:

The ride started out great, everyone was talking and laughing. We were starting to bond. At one point we even had a singing contest where Basu, Subash and Jesse showed off their skills. Basu sang a hilarious song about Monkeys and Donkeys..."You are a donkey, I am a monkey..." Subash did a chant, and Jesse showed his rapping skills.

The ride was fun, but the bathroom breaks were a different story. I must admit I didn't even think about or question where we would take restroom breaks. I just assumed that there would be rest stops where we could use the facility. I've been to many developing countries and the tour groups usually had places for us to go.

We were on a winding road on one of the many mountains we'd have to pass to get to Lumbini when someone said they had to go to the bathroom. Buddha, our bus driver, pulled to the side of the road and stopped. I did not see a bathroom anywhere near us. All I heard was Jesse saying girls on one side, boys on another. I looked at all the ladies and they were running to the side in the bushes. I could not believe what was going on here. Do they expect us to go on the side of the road? Seriously? I've never been camping before and definitely never went to the bathroom on the side of the road before. The whole idea disgusts me. Guessing I had no other option, I just went for it. To make matters worse, there were all these cars, buses and trucks zipping by. I'm just hoping I don't flash any passing driver and don't pee on myself. This is going to be a long day...only 9 hours to go.

_____ **Minling Chuang**

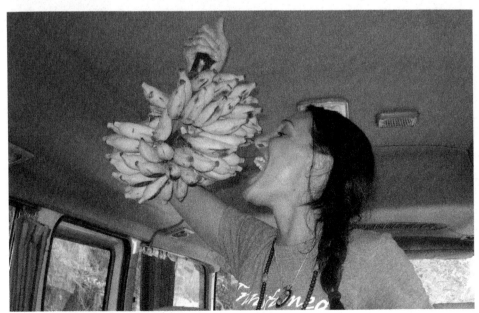

Deanna is one hungry monkey. The bananas were sweet and delicious.

At first, the conversations were very lively as everyone was excited after our morning flight along the Himalayas. I was stuck in the back of the bus on a wheel well. I was never so jostled around so much. I enjoyed getting to know David, Kathy and Joyce better as we were together for such a long bus ride. We took many bathroom stops. I can't remember the last time I went to the bathroom in nature. I'll have to do a better job as I think I went on my hiking sandals. Thank goodness someone invented antibacterial wipes!

*Christina Jankus*

Some time after noon, we stopped for lunch at the Blue Heaven Restaurant overlooking the now much wider, muddy brown, fast flowing Trishuli River. Food was served hot and delicious, this time including French fries. We happily chowed down on the local grub while gazing out at gorgeous views of the river below, as it wended its way down from the hills above and past the restaurant's outdoor patio.

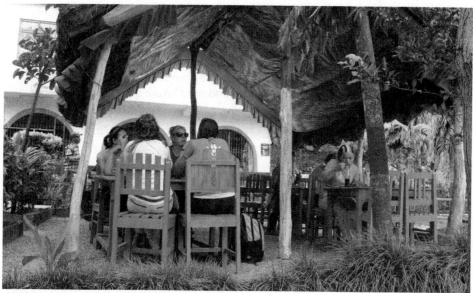

The Blue Heaven Restaurant, our lunchtime stop on the road to Lumbini.

I noticed that the Nepalis here, away from Kathmandu, though poor, working class people, appeared quite happy. Happier than the people we had encountered in Bakhtapur, that's for sure. Maybe the natural beauty of where they lived, surrounded by lush green mountainsides, terraced hillside farms, rice paddies, and the large flowing river, provided a soothing balm. In a way, it seemed to have a similar effect on them as the Temple and the monks had on the residents of Boudhanath. Grace comes in many forms, I suppose. Our bellies, at least the healthy ones, now full, we were soon back on the bus again, back to the long, slow, bumpy ride to Lumbini, interrupted only now and then by the odd bathroom break. The vibe on the bus was quieter now, more contemplative...

June 23, 2010 _____

A few hours later, we were back on the road again, this time heading out of Kathmandu to Lumbini, the birthplace of Buddha and our next destination... It was a 10-hour bus ride, sprinkled along the way were several bathroom stops at some interesting toilet facilities (roadside) and we all got to know each other on a whole new comfort level.

The whole energy level of the group, after 10 or more hours on the road, was completely spent. I probably slept more than halfway through the ride, no idea how, since my head kept banging against the window. When I did wake up for several brief periods, I was greeted with magnificent scenery of the Nepalese countryside.

From the lush green mountains down to the plains, I hadn't seen something so beautiful in terms of landscape since I was a young girl in China. To see the way of living of the locals, stone huts, wooden lean-to's, shared public water faucets, it all felt very real. As real as my childhood in China, it brought me back there, and I felt empathy, an understanding, a compassion for these people. One day, their country will pull out of this and their future generations will see, live something better.

_____ ***Tingting Peng***

As the day wore on, the ride grew exceedingly tedious and difficult. Ten and a half hours in a small bus, even surrounded by great people and great natural beauty, is no walk in the park. It's tough. Very tough. Eventually we got tired, and as the roads got rougher we all took a pounding, getting bounced, rattled, jarred, shaken and jolted by every single bump.

June 23, 2010 _____

...By the end of our bus ride I felt so ill. I usually don't get car sick unless I'm in the back seat with a crazy herky-jerky driver. Our driver is not to blame. The roads are not well paved and are very winding. Nepal reminds me of Pittsburgh with rice paddies.

_____ ***Christina Jankus***

We finally arrived in Lumbini, located in the south central part of Nepal not far from the border with India, at sunset. The winding roads, steep mountainside cliffs, and deep valleys carved by the ever widening river had given way to a gentler terrain. The town that surrounded it was loud and chaotic like Kathmandu, though smaller, and with more bone-rattling bumpy roads. A day that had begun with bright, white, breathtaking beauty was ending in darkness and exhaustion. We arrived too late to eat at the Korean monastery where we'd be staying, so Jesse and Basu arranged for us to stop at Siddhartha House, a small hotel about 15 minutes away, for some food and to stretch our aching bodies. It was around 9:30 or 10 p.m. when we, a bedraggled bunch of road-weary travelers, finally got off the bus to eat.

Dinner was little relief, however. The native bugs seemed to be everywhere, in our hair, in our food, in the very air we were breathing. By then, total exhaustion had set in. We were cranky, aching, and really, truly, completely fatigued. My back was a wreck. Dave tried to crack it for me, but he was too tired. Then Jesse stepped in and answered my prayers with a back-cracking for the ages. I swear the sound of my vertebrae unloosening actually echoed through my skull for a good minute. Subash helped loosen some of our aching shoulders as well. Everyone appreciated the relief. There was one more small pleasure we got to enjoy at the Siddhartha House after the brutally long trip here. At least momentarily, as Christina so nicely described:

June 23, 2010

I was grateful to find a proper toilet... only to find that when I flushed it the water came [up] from the floor. Well I guess that takes care of my sanitized hiking sandals.

Christina Jankus

I was so tired I couldn't bring myself to eat much. After a bit of food and two cups of tea, I dragged myself back on the bus for the short drive to the Korean monastery where we would spend the next two nights. We were all at the end of our physical endurance, and no one seemed in a good mood.

We arrive at the Korean Monastery in Lumbini which looks very eerie in the dark. I room with Tingting and Joyce. The room was very minimalist and clean. The "beds" were on one long platform with linoleum. We were provided rollout mattress and a pillow, and we were encased in colorful mosquito nets. Joyce was so tired she fell asleep on the linoleum.

Christina Jankus

We were done; all of us utterly spent. Unfazed by the austere accommodations, Dave and I happily crashed for the night under our mosquito nets and whirring fans, a gecko guarding the door from any insects who might try to sneak in.

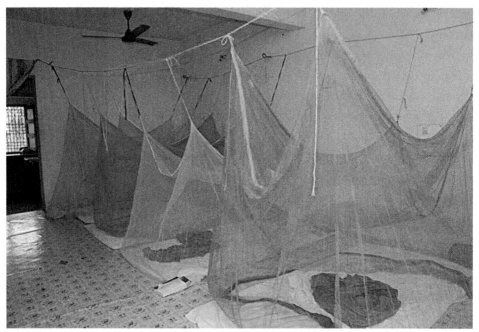

Mosquito netting over our "beds" at the Korean Monastery in Lumbini. In a country where malaria once killed many thousands, these nettings were not decorations, they were a necessity. Photo by Minling Chuang.

Like Jesse with his back-cracking skills, like the natural beauty on the drive here, like the Buddhist temple and monks of Boudhanath the day before, our gecko friend served us well. We didn't see a single bug anywhere in our room. For that little bit of good fortune, I said a quick thank you before succumbing to my own complete exhaustion and falling fast asleep.

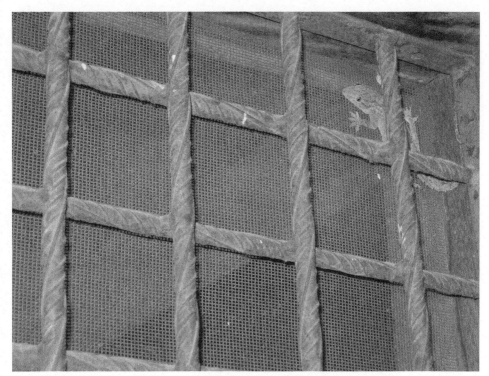

Our bug-eating friend, the gecko. His suction cup feet allow him to walk on walls — and ceilings.

June 24, 2010

Day 5 of the trip

Lumbini

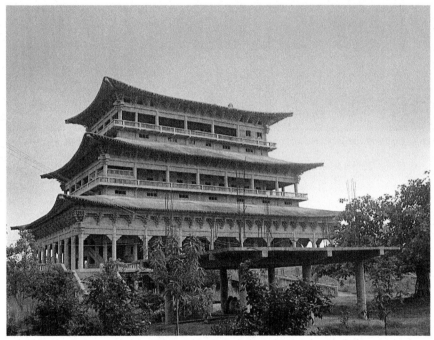

The unfinished main temple at the Korean Monastery in Lumbini. Monasteries like this are very expensive to build, even in Nepal. Though this one was in its 10th year of construction, it still retained a sense of real austerity. The monks here, however, were gracious enough to let us stay with them at very reasonable rates, for which we were very grateful.

June 24, 2010 _____

Today woke up at 5:30 a.m. to sound of bells and the soft humming of the monks.

_____ ***Tingting Peng***

Morning began for me at the Korean monastery with a soft, persistent clacking together of sticks. Clack… clack… clack… There was a gentle, steady rhythm to the sound that stirred me from my deep slumber in a much more respectful way than any alarm clock ever did. Soon the clacking of the sticks was joined by the sound of bells and the chanting of monks, calling their brethren to morning prayers.

I rousted myself out of bed and went to the simple sink in the back of our room and washed my face. I looked around the room we were staying in, and was struck again by its simplicity: unpainted wooden shelves for storing clothes and personal items, a large bucket for washing clothes, a thick string stretched across the back of the room for hanging the clothes to dry, several smaller plastic buckets for bathing. There was no shower, just a spigot to fill up the buckets in a small area behind the sink.

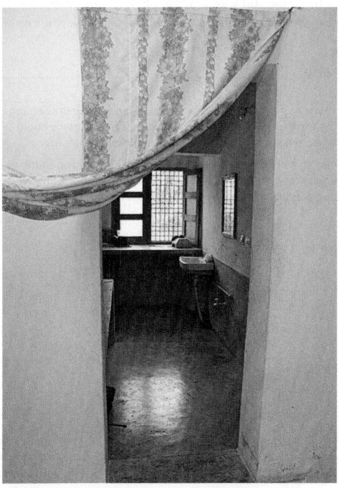

A typical bathroom at the Korean Monastery. Photo by Minling Chuang.

I put on a pair of shorts and a t-shirt, and stepped outside into the cool, pre-dawn air. It looked like it might have rained a bit the night before, but I hadn't heard a sound. I am usually a long sleeper, 8 or 9 hours a night, but I found myself in Nepal not needing more than 6 or 7 hours at the most, before feeling awake and refreshed. There's something about sleeping in a place where time is kept by the rising and setting of the sun, rather than clocks and watches, that is truly more restful than spending the night on the best mattress covered with the highest thread-count sheets.

Sleep also improved everyone's impressions of our surroundings. In daylight, we could see that the temple itself was huge, made of poured concrete, and still under construction. The monks and local builders had begun work on the giant multi-story structure over ten years earlier. Only now was the basic outer structure nearly complete, and there was still a lot of finishing work to be done. The construction workers we saw labored on the building from dawn to dusk while we were there.

June 24, 2010

I slept well last night. I think I am getting the hang of the time change. In the daylight the monastery is beautiful. It is not yet finished as we could see workers walking up the stairs with trays of cement [for] the roof.

I like it here. It is very peaceful... That's most likely because there are a lot of rules. A sign tells us that drug taking, card playing, drinking, smoking, singing and dancing are prohibited at the monastery... there is [also] a dress code.

Christina Jankus

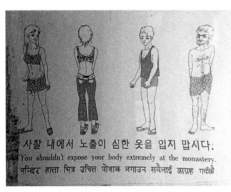

Monasteries have their rules. Photo by Christina Jankus.

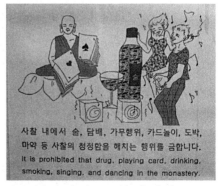

Most of these rules, however, are for the foreigners who come to visit.

Jesse had brought a satellite phone on the trip, and this morning he offered everyone the opportunity to call home. A satellite telephone, for those who don't know, is a kind of mobile phone that connects to a satellite orbiting the earth, instead of a ground-based cell tower like the ones dotting the U.S. They are a lot like regular cell phones, but more useful to those who travel a lot in underdeveloped countries where cell service is sporadic at best, and often non-existent. Jesse's satellite phone reminded me of a walkie-talkie, or an early 80's model cell phone. What it lacked in aesthetics, however, it made up for in functionality.

It had been almost a week since we'd left for our trip, so we all took advantage of the 'sat' phone that morning to call home. When it was my turn, I punched in the code that Jesse had given us and then my parents' phone number. I waited for a moment, and then heard the line ringing on the other end. When my mother answered, she sounded both very near, and at the same time strangely far, far away. Her voice was remarkably clear, given that it was traveling halfway around the world, but faint. She was surprised and thrilled to hear my voice, and happy to know I was safe and sound, even though I'd checked in with my sister via email the first day in Nepal to let my family know I had arrived. We didn't talk long. With the time difference it was early evening in Ohio, just after dinner. She and my dad had just watched the U.S. win a game in the World Cup, she told me excitedly. I gave her a quick rundown of where we were and where we were going. I would have talked longer, but there was a line of others waiting to use the phone, so I told my mom I loved her and to say hi to my dad. I would check in with them again, via the satellite phone, if and when I could.

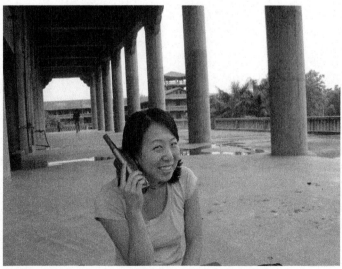

Minling calling home on the satellite phone. Photo by Kathy Hayes.

After I hung up, I became very emotional. I don't know if it was being so far away from my family here in Nepal, but in that moment I felt an overwhelming love for my mom and dad. Hearing her voice that morning nearly brought me to tears. Sometimes we don't realize how much we truly care about the people in our lives until we find ourselves on the other side of the planet from them.

June 24, 2010

Jesse has a satellite phone. We each took turns using it. I was so grateful to hear my parents' voices....

Christina Jankus

After we had made all our sat phone calls, we gathered on a raised patio area at the back of the large temple in the center of the monastery grounds to practice morning yoga with Subash. Monasteries tend to draw pilgrims, and this place was no exception, especially given its location in Lumbini. Thousands of Buddhist devotees made the pilgrimage to Lumbini each year, and many of them stay at affordable places like this monastery. As we practiced yoga that morning, we drew a small crowd of these pilgrims, taking pictures and talking and laughing amongst themselves as they watched us, strange westerners doing up dog and down dog poses outside their place of worship.

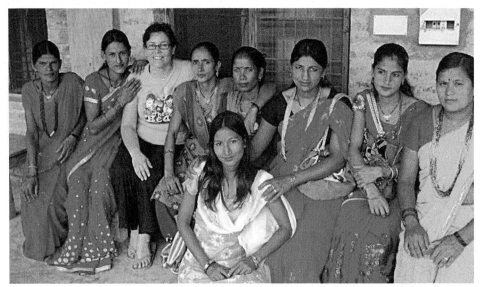

Indian Pilgrims at the Korean Monastery. We weren't the only foreigners in town. Photo courtesy of Christina Jankus.

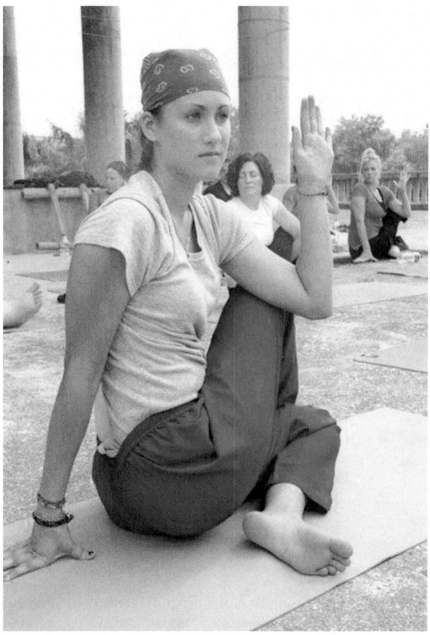

Jaime Furda in Ardha Matsyendrasana (Half Lord of the Fishes or Half Spinal Twist) pose. We practiced yoga twice a day, every day. By the end of the two weeks we were in amazing shape. Photo by Minling Chuang.

You would think that monasteries like this one would also draw a lot of monks, but our little YFF group, along with all the gawking pilgrims, seemed to greatly outnumber the actual monks who lived there.

I ... imagined the [Korean] temple to be full of monks. I only saw 4 monks living there and one monk was German. He was always very pleasant and smiled as he passed by. I don't think I've ever seen a non-Asian monk before. Guess I've been ignorant to think that all monks were Asian. It's funny how we have so many images and pictures of "how things should be" ingrained into our minds. We have so many judgments about everything, even when we don't even mean to judge. This is probably human nature, but I do wonder why we judge so much. Do animals judge?

Minling Chuang

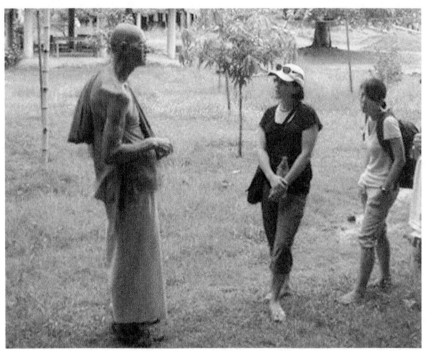

A German monk at the Korean monastery in Lumbini. Photo by Jaime Furda.

By the time our 1 ½ hour practice was over, I was pretty sweaty. Although it was still fairly early in the day, it was already very hot. I asked about showers, but Jesse told us there were no shower facilities at the monastery, and that the monks here took bucket baths. It actually sounded fun to me, so I went back to the room and checked out the bathing facilities. In a room behind the sink area were some plastic buckets, one large and one small. The large one you filled with water, and the small one you used to scoop the water out and dump it over you. I took my soap and filled the big bucket from a spigot coming out of the wall. Then I stripped down and scooped up some water and dumped it over my head. Whoa! What a shock! The water may have been lukewarm to the touch, but when I dumped it over me, it felt downright freezing cold. I shivered vigorously. Undeterred, I dumped more water over my arms and legs, to get used to the temperature. Then I quickly soaped up and washed my hair, all the while scooping and dumping water as necessary.

As I was bathing, I noticed in the back of the bathing area, on a slightly raised platform, there was a squat toilet, consisting of a small, flat porcelain area with a hole in the middle and two ridged spots, one on each side of the hole, to plant your feet and keep you from slipping on the concrete floor. while doing your business. Behind the toilet was a small water pipe with a faucet handle, that you opened to send water rushing into the toilet to clear things out and wash the waste away. Very interesting, I thought to myself. Wonder if I'll be able to use it. Soap was running into my eyes, so I dumped more water on myself. By the time I was done with my bucket bath, I felt invigorated, not to mention a whole lot cleaner. I happily dried off, and felt so good, I decided to shave as well. Afterwards, I put on a clean change of clothes and went to eat.

Breakfast was a Spartan, almost military-like affair. We stood in line with a couple of the monks and a few of the pilgrims, and spooned out food from a few hot steamers filled with potatoes, oatmeal, sliced mango, and a large pot of tea, all served in tin cups and plates. Afterwards, we rinsed our plates and cups at a long low sink in the back of the dining area.

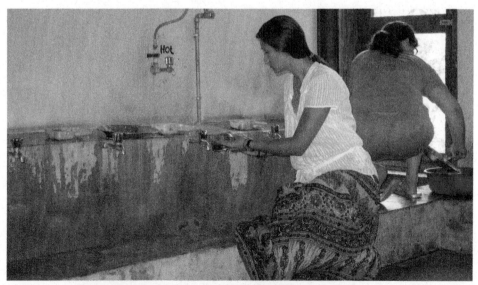

Like everyone else, we had to do our own dishes here. Thankfully the signage helped.

As we ate, we all talked about our adventures taking bucket baths — and also about the squat toilets. Jesse had warned us even before we left Cleveland that we'd encounter these primitive by Western standard conditions, and it had caused more than a few eyebrows to raise. But I'd been to China before, and had some experience with squat toilets, unlike most of the people in our group.

Using a squat toilet can be quite a challenge to those unaccustomed to them. First of all, there's the squatting. You're much lower to the ground than you're used to when sitting on the porcelain thrones back home. You can easily lose your balance and need strong quad muscles to keep yourself steady while making the effort to evacuate your bowels. Luckily for all of us, we'd been doing yoga for years, so we had the quads and the core muscle strength to be able to successfully squat and poop, should we need to—or want to.

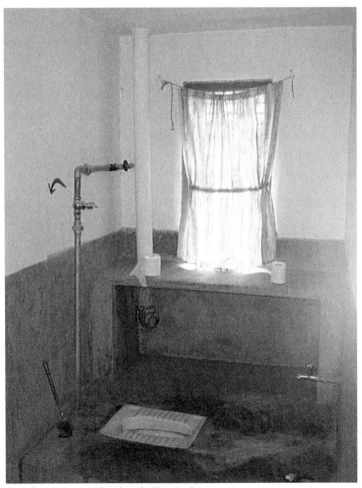

The infamous squat toilet. Photo by Tingting Peng.

The bigger challenge for some of us, though, was psychological more than physical. If you haven't squatted before, it can be a challenge to convince yourself that you can successfully pull it off. So many people just put it off, "holding it", to use a common bathroom phrase, until better accommodations come along. We were going to be at the monastery in Lumbini for a couple of days, and then we would be traveling even further out into the back country of Nepal, so putting it off wasn't going to be an easy option. Nature has its own timetable, and we were eating fresh, healthy meals made up mostly of vegetables and lentils, all high in fiber, which made "holding it" impossible, at least for me.

The other, more urgent factor coming into play was that Jesse had told us early on, that on a trip like this most people were going to get sick, by which he meant, intestinally challenged. He said that this was because our bodies would be detoxing from all the red meat, preservatives, sugar and alcohol we consume in the west. Most of us, however, were pretty healthy eaters, and a few among us were vegetarians. My feeling is that this stomach illness had more to do with our biological clocks being turned upside down by the 12-hour time difference, than any detoxing that was happening. Either way, virtually everyone on the trip came down with varying degrees of a stomach ailment during our first few days in Nepal.

Regardless of how sick you got, even the mildest upset stomach can keep any of us from "holding it" for any extended period of time, whether we want to or not, and whether we like our toilet facilities or not. When you gotta go, you gotta go. And this first morning in Lumbini, right after a pleasant breakfast of potatoes, rice, mangoes and bread, and bathroom talk, I had to go. I gave Dave a heads up as I headed back to our room, as there were no real doors in the bathrooms in each room. And then I went to the squat toilet in our room and squatted.

At first I didn't have a good sense of balance, and worried I might miss the target area completely, or worse still fall over backwards mid-turd. Then I saw that there was a water pipe running down the wall in front of me, close enough to hold onto, so I grabbed hold and steadied myself. And just like that, I went. Excretion, like exhalation and perspiration, is a very normal, natural thing for a human being to do. And naturally, you feel good when you do it. This morning, not only did I feel good, I felt proud. Proud that I had accomplished what others had feared to even try. I reported my success to Dave, and he clapped me on the back.

"You're my hero, dude!" he said overjoyed at my accomplishment.

"It was nothing," I said. "You should try it."

"No thanks," he said, the joy leaving his face. "I can hold it."

I laughed. From that point on, I was a good little squatter and David's personal hero just for doing what came naturally.

The rest of the day we spent exploring the area around Lumbini, one of the most sacred places in Buddhism, and designated a World Heritage site by UNESCO. There are dozens and dozens of Buddhist temples, shrines and statues in the area. Many of the temples have been built by and represent various countries where Buddhism is practiced around the world. Japanese, Chinese, Taiwanese, Malaysian, and I think even one sponsored by Americans, each temple was uniquely beautiful.

June 24, 2010 _____

Buddha here, Buddha there, Buddha everywhere watching with open eyes.

_____ *Christina Jankus*

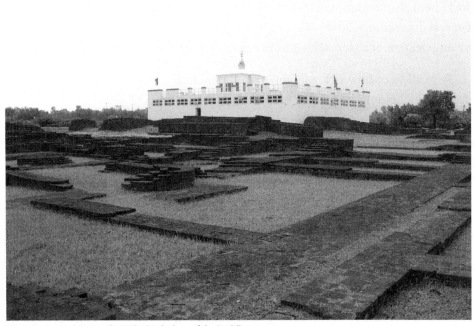

Maya Devi temple in Lumbini. The birthplace of the Buddha.

The Mayadevi temple is located on the actual spot where Maya Devi, the Mother of Buddha, gave birth to the child that would grow up to found one of the world's great religions while holding onto a low hanging branch of a tree. There are depictions of the scene all around Lumbini. It's the Buddhist version of Christ born in a manger, and there are many similarities to the two stories, including an "immaculate" conception. When I first heard the story of Maya Devi, I imagined that this poor woman must have sought shelter from the heat, and there, under that tree, had given birth. A rustic image not unlike Bethlehem came to mind. But when I read up on the story I discovered that Maya Devi was a Queen, nine months pregnant and traveling from her palace to her hometown to give birth, as was the custom. When she stopped her procession in a beautiful park in Lumbini, she was so taken by the spot that she decided to give birth to her child there.

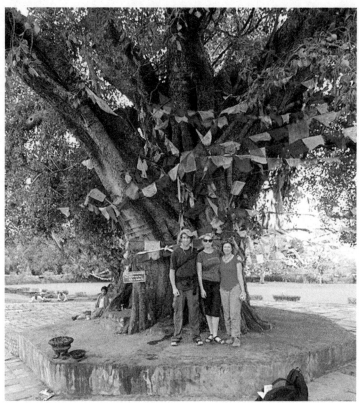

David, Eve and Terri, under a giant Boddhi tree much like the one under which Maya Devi, the Mother of Buddha, gave birth to the founder of one of the world's great spiritual philosophies. Photo by Eve Ennis.

We joined a long line of pilgrims outside Maya Devi waiting to enter the simple, beautiful temple that is now constructed on the site of the Buddha's birth. The surrounding area was covered by sculpture gardens and huge trees strung with prayer flags that provided some shade from the hot noonday sun. Once inside, we found ourselves in a much cooler space. The line of pilgrims moved quietly along a walking bridge path made of wooden planks that led finally to a ledge from which you could look down and see the stone that marks the exact spot where the Buddha was born. Taking that slow walk, with all those devotees, moving quietly and speaking in hushed tones, was a very moving experience.

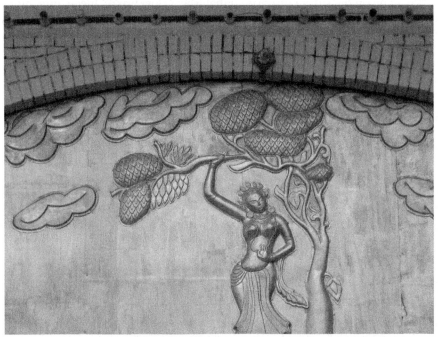

A gold bas-relief adorning a temple in Lumbini depicting the moments before the Buddha's birth.

Afterwards, we toured several more temples, each one incredible in its own way. It was a great way to spend an afternoon, despite the unrelenting heat. I'm sure people have similar experiences when they travel to other holy places like Bethlehem or Mecca, or the Ganges River in India. These places somehow put you in touch with your spiritual side, with that fundamental quality that makes us all better people when we allow ourselves to tune into it. My personal favorites were the exquisitely striking Thai temple, completely white, inside and out, and the Maya Devi Temple, which we visited after lunch.

June 24, 2010_____

... What this trip has done for me so far is to further open my eyes to what's already inside of me. I feel more connected to the people around me, to the world as a whole, without a controlling need to fully understand everyone or everything. I can accept things as they are. This trip has tested my footing, taking me deeper into the unknown and I am loving every minute of it; I know there is nothing to fear. Whatever happens, happens; I am happy to be continuously exploring and discovering on my journey into the unknown and it is beautiful.

_____ ***Tingting Peng***

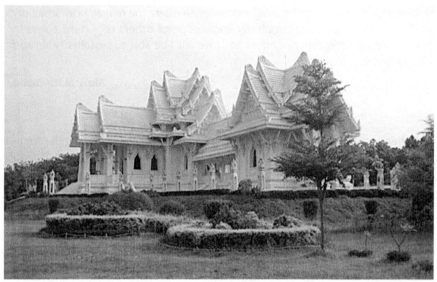

The beautiful alabaster Thai Temple at Lumbini. Many Buddhist nations around the world have built temples here. Photo by Kathy Hayes.

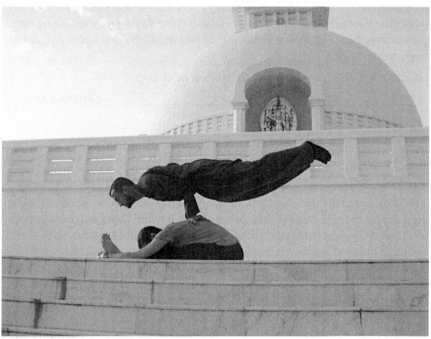

Subash in Mayurasana (Peacock) pose, balanced on Deanna, who's in Paschimottanasana (Seated Forward Bend). Photo by Jaime Furda.

June 24, 2010 _____

We left Kathmandu for the ten-hour bus ride to [Lumbini]. And along the way we saw mountains, rivers, valleys, and many villagers. It was like a ten-hour movie filled with so many sights, wonderments, and questions. There were so many questions. But the whole experience made me realize how small my world has been, and how small my knowledge of others is. I have come to realize that only through openness and love will I be able to sustain my life and relationships.

_____*Marc Nathanson*

But there was, once again, darkness here along with the light. Maybe that's just Nepal. Or maybe that's just how it should be. Always a yin to the yang — joy and happiness walk hand in hand with pain and suffering. That is the way of the world, is it not?

June 24, 2010 _____

There was an elderly woman, tiny and frail with pleading eyes and hands clasped together that followed us from temple to temple to beg. We were discouraged from giving beggars money. This woman has been haunting my thoughts. I understand the rationale behind discouraging us from giving beggars money but, I don't see how 100 rupees would do any harm and could really help her out.

I don't know. This is as confusing as it is overwhelming.

_____*Christina Jankus*

June 24, 2010 _____

... Outside one of the temples, an old lady and her son (or maybe grandson) were begging for money. Both of them were skinny beyond belief and her leathery weathered face was contorted with an expression of sadness and despair. We'd been discouraged from giving beggars money, probably because then it'll create a frenzy, but I still can't help but wonder if we can help one, even just one person, why don't we? Recognizing our limitations to play Mother Teresa, yet at the same time, not limiting ourselves to the people whom we can help; even if we just have $1 for each person...

_____*Tingting Peng*

Buddhism isn't the only religion practiced in Nepal. Hinduism is also prevalent, especially in the south of the country, which is where we were. And Hindus, as most people know, have a certain reverence for cows. Although they follow no single set of rules, Hindus' reverence for these creatures can be found throughout all the religion's major texts. Some writings trace the cow's sacred status back to Lord Krishna, one of the faith's most important figures. He is said to have appeared 5,000 years ago as a cowherd, and is often described as bala-gopala, "the child who protects the cows". Another of Krishna's holy names, Govinda, means "one who brings satisfaction to the cows". Other scriptures identify the cow as the "mother" of all civilization, its milk nurturing the population. Just as in Kathmandu, cows traveled wherever they wanted to here in Lumbini. No one ever disturbed them, even if the animals wandered into the middle of an otherwise very busy boulevard.

But cows aren't the only cattle that are important in Nepal. Oxen and water buffalo are equally important, but for much more practical, earthy reasons. Oxen and water buffalo are used throughout the country to pull carts and plows, turning over fields for farming, moving goods, people and produce to market, and for their milk. And in Lumbini, water buffalo were everywhere. As we walked to and from Maya Devi, we could see herds of them off the side of the road.

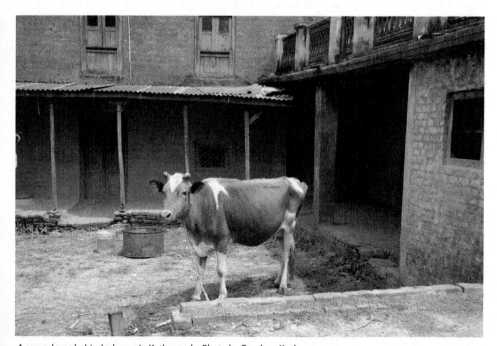

A cow relaxes behind a home in Kathmandu. Photo by Candace Koslen.

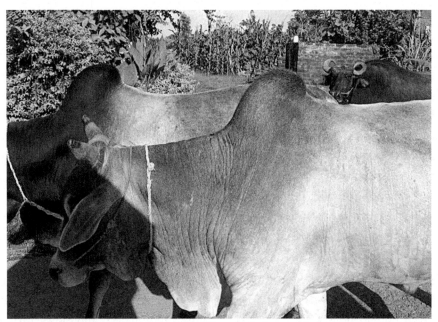

Oxen do much of the heavy lifting in rural Nepal. These are Brahman cattle, recognizable by their large shoulder humps. Photo by Terri Bahr.

Seen from a distance, water buffalo are quite impressive animals. Up close they look downright mean. Jesse and Basu warned us to give them a wide berth. These beasts have giant curved horns made of very hard, very sharp bone shaped like handlebar mustaches that sit on the tops of their heads. Their bodies are huge, sleek, black like gunmetal, and powerfully muscled. Their heads are big, with long flat snouts, and their faces have a perpetual scowl that makes them look constantly annoyed, if not downright pissed off. Yet the funny thing about water buffalo in Nepal is that these fierce creatures, unlike cows, get no respect. They are the Rodney Dangerfield of cattle (with all due respect to Rodney).

To illustrate, as we were heading back to the monastery from Maya Devi, we saw a small woman herding a group of large water buffalo. She carried a walking stick, and if the buffalo strayed too far from the herd, she would swat the biggest of these beasts right across their backsides. It was the funniest thing I think I saw on the whole trip. This tiny woman would whack a water buffalo for getting out of line, and the huge beast would turn its head only slightly toward her, scowl, and then move along back to the herd. Given their sheer size and orneriness, I definitely wouldn't mess with a water buffalo, walking stick or not. But given a choice, I wouldn't want to mess with that little woman with the big walking stick either. She might give me a swift crack on the butt if I did.

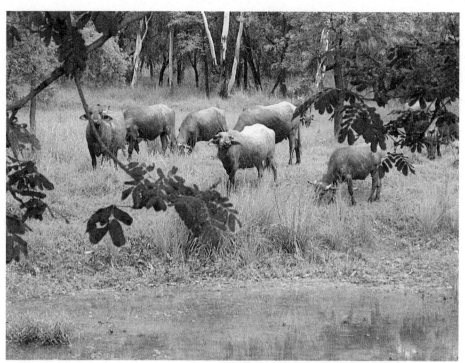

A herd of water buffalo gazes menacingly at the photographer. Thankfully there was a river between us and them.

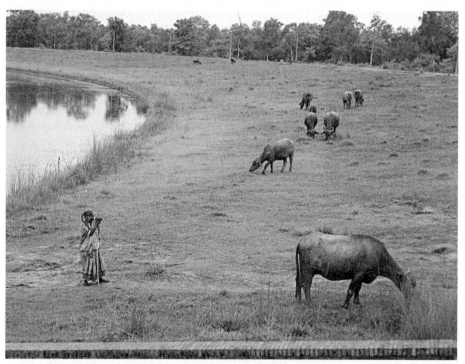

A tiny but fearless older woman herding water buffalo like they were sheep. Photo by Terri Bahr.

One week into the trip, things had gone swimmingly thus far. We'd had some amazing experiences already, and on this day we were really enjoying taking in the sights in Lumbini. This place, like everything we had seen so far in Nepal, was having a positive effect on the group as a whole. We really seemed to be bonding, much like an extended family:

June 24, 2010_____

In the last two days I have seen a group of people who barely knew each other become a family. A family who doesn't even comprehend the power they possess, the changes they can bring about…

I hope everyone understands why they are here. Yoga for Freedom isn't just about the freedom of children but the participant's freedom as well. Many of us are locked inside a cage of our own making, too afraid to leave. Afraid of the very things that allow us to truly live.

_____ ***Jesse Bach***

June 24, 2010_____

What I have truly seen is a bonding. A bonding with harmony. Being blessed by an 85 year old Buddhist nun and asked to walk with a Buddhist monk. I saw a majestic mountain in harmony with other mountains (including a virgin mountain that is forbidden to be climbed). I saw a busload of people who came into harmony on a long journey. I saw a gate opening to harmoniously welcome a busload of foreigners into a Korean monastery. I saw a yoga practice lead by a Nepali to a group of foreigners, while a Korean prayer service was going on and a group of Indians were looking on with smiles on their faces. Wow. I saw harmony but better yet I felt harmony. No better yet, I became one. I felt the God in me mesh with my group, with the Nepali people, with the smiling faces of the Kamlari children, with Mt. Everest, with the bus, with the incredible yoga practice.

_____ ***Robb Blain***

After just four days together, we had settled into a happy rhythm, a harmonious contentment with the adventure at hand. You could see it reflected in the journals:

June 24, 2010_____

Over lunch break, I had a really nice conversation with Marc and David about how the last two days have been for each of us.

For me, experiencing everything has humbled me beyond words. Somehow, the magnificence of the stupa and Mount Everest, as well as the smiles of the children and the bus ride through the villages, have really given me a new appreciation for my life and all the people and things in it.

To be here (Yoga for Freedom) for the kids means much more than to just see them, spend time with them or give them things they don't have. Over the last two days, all of the sights and sounds as we travelled to Lumbini have made me realize that everything I see here on this trip is a part of the kids' lives – the living traditions and culture are an ingrained part of their circumstances. To really get to know them, to really understand them and to then do whatever I can to support them, means that I have to fully comprehend the factors that have shaped their lives, and that has been shown to me every moment I'm in Nepal.

How can anyone say that one person can't change the world? If each of us on this trip comes out of it more empowered, more inspired, and more connected to all of humankind, then every one of us has the potential to change the world. And that is what we're here to do. Be agents of change, be selfless in service, be the eyes of the world, and the voice of its people.

What I've seen here so far is already affecting the way I see the world and the people in it. How can I ever get angry at someone, really, for doing something that may be intrinsic to their survival? How can I ever judge another through the colors of my own lens? We are all the same at the end of the day and when I stopped trying to simply survive, I finally began to live. At the level of true humanity, there is so much fear, but also hope, and I have seen that in the kids at NOH and the kind people of Nepal. When you strip down to the bare necessities of life and still find contentment there, then there can be growth, possibilities and creation. To build a life from nothing (or rebuild) can be one of the greatest gifts in the world, and we are doing that here for the kids and we are (or at least I am) taking this away with me when I get home – every day is as precious as the previous and the next, so make every day count.

_____ *Tingting Peng*

June 24, 2010 (I think... :-)) _____

The past 48 hours... Every time I try to actively realize I'm here, it doesn't resonate. I think it won't become real until after the fact. It's a blur, a vision...it'll settle at home...

Home feels so far away. It seems like an out of body experience. In the temple in Lumbini now. Everyone else has left. I swear I hear footsteps on the marble floor. It would not surprise me to be surrounded by all that's been here. I look up- no one. Again and again this happens. Echoing Om's...but no one chanting. Yesterday I was sick. Really sick...

Then the 10 hour bus ride to Lumbini, which almost didn't happen. After getting off the bus, post-mountain flight, I almost collapsed, a few times. Tears flowed uncontrollably from my eyes. [Marni?][7] cooled me down with a rag, Jesse drew a cold bath and carried me to it, Jaime was there EVERY step of the way. We've become like sisters; taking care of each other, sharing secrets. She's wonderful. 19. Hard to believe. Everyone was so caring yesterday and I'm so grateful.

_____ *Rachel Vincent*

We finished the day with another great yoga practice, a nice simple meal in the temple commissary with the monks, and then we drifted back to our rooms for a

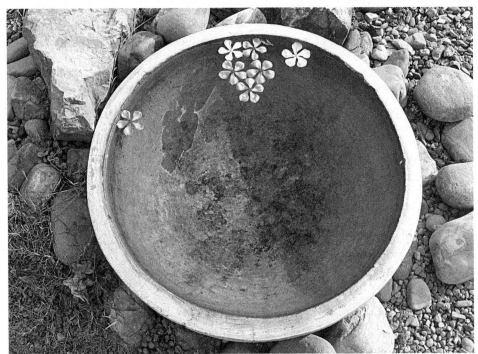

Flowers floating in bowl of water — a traditional Zen Buddhist style of art which creates an idealized miniature landscape meant to express the harmony that should exist between man and nature. Zen is derived from the Sanskrit word dhyāna, which can be approximately translated as "absorption" or "meditative state." [8]

bit of journaling and a good night's sleep. People were happy. Jesse and Michael's vision of what this Yoga for Freedom trip should be was taking shape nicely. We were absorbing a lot on the trip so far, and the experiences of the last few days, coupled with this day in Lumbini, inspired the poet in one of us again. This time it was Jaime:

---

[7] *It wasn't Marni. It couldn't have been, because Marni wasn't on this part of the trip with us. Rachel was so sick however that it's no surprise she couldn't remember exactly who it was who did apply the cold compress.*

[8] *Source: http://en.wikipedia.org/wiki/Zen and http://en.wikipedia.org/wiki/Chinese_garden*

What I've Seen

Women carrying babies
And young children
With black smudges around
Their eyes—
What's left of the eyeliner
That decorated their
Young, innocent faces.
Kind of symbolic,
Those smudges—
You know?
What some of these
Kids
Have seen...
Their idea of how
Life should be
Is probably
Smudged,
Too.

= = =

Rachel was sick
(she's like a
sister
to me), so
I told her she should at least
try a banana.
I walked back to the van
and grabbed a couple.
On my way back
toward the river,
I saw a little boy.
I didn't know where he'd come from,
but I decided that
he should have a banana, too.
Flying above and around
the Himalayas
was cool, but
the impact of
that boy's smile
made Mount Everest seem like
an anthill.
-j

June 25, 2010

Day 6 of the trip

Narti

The moon shines brightly outside the Korean Monastery late at night. Photo by Deanna Lee.

June 25, 2010_____

Last night we lay on our backs looking at the evening sky with the temple looming above us, weighty and heavy, like it could come down and bury us under a mountain of cement.

_____ *Kathy Hayes*

I woke up to the sound of clacking sticks once again calling the monks to prayers. It was very early, just past 5 a.m. I threw some water on my face and, dressed in shorts and a Cleveland Browns t-shirt, I went outside. It was still cool and the pre-dawn sky was a reddish pink as I quietly closed the door to the room so as not to wake David. As soon as I stepped out, I ran into Gabby and Kathy coming out of their room. They were going to the big temple for the morning service, and I quickly decided to join them. It was a short walk from the dormitory, across the small courtyard, up the concrete steps and into the temple. We entered through the main doors, and quietly walked into the prayer area, which we found softly illuminated by a few dozen small hanging lanterns that glowed red, orange, yellow, and green, casting a warm light into the otherwise dark space. A large bell and gong hung near the entrance, across from which was the main altar to Buddha. The monks who had arrived before us were all dressed in their traditional red and yellow colors, their robes reflecting the light from the lanterns.

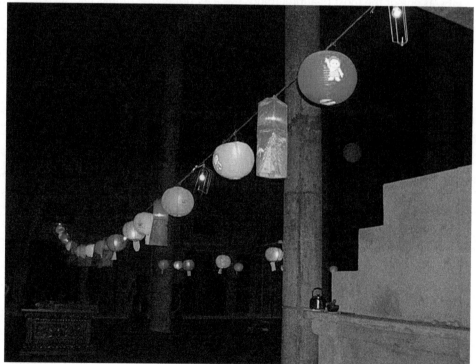

Inside the unfinished main temple at the Korean Monastery; lanterns light the space where morning prayer services are held. Photo by Deanna Lee.

We stood on one side, and watched as the rest of the monks appeared. There were no more than a couple dozen people living at this monastery, and maybe only ten of them in the temple this morning. As they filed in, they took mats and pillows from one corner of the room, and laid them out before the altar. They knelt facing the large statue of Buddha, and an older monk began to lead them in prayer -- softly, rhythmically chanting the words in a low humming voice. Gabby, Kathy and I grabbed some mats and joined them. We tried to follow the chants as best we could despite our lack of facility with the language. I actually recognized some of the words of their prayers; they were words I had heard many times in yoga classes. As the chanting continued, the monks would all turn in one direction, then another, continuing to pray as they moved. The effect of the gently glowing lanterns combined with the monks' deep chanting and throat-singing of verses was hypnotic, peaceful, relaxing.

June 25, 2010

It was one of the most beautiful things I've ever done. The monks had such a lovely harmony. It was intoxicating.

Gabrielle Stickley

The whole service lasted less than an hour, and the three of us left feeling exhilarated and ready to attack the day. We joined the rest of the group for yoga behind the temple, followed by another breakfast in the commons. Then we packed up the bus, checked that we hadn't left anything behind, and headed off to the next stop on our trip, Narti.

Narti is a small, poor, rural village located about 120 km northwest of Lumbini, on the edge of Nepal's western plains at the base of the foothills of the Himalayas. We were going there to visit an orphanage called Lawajuni. Lawajuni means "New Beginnings" or "New Life" in Nepali. It was a sister orphanage to NOH, and the man who ran it was familiar to both Jesse and Michael Hess. Jesse told us that all the girls at Lawajuni had been Kamlaris, all rescued from child slavery, some as recently as just a few weeks before our arrival. The Kamlari girls who had no parents, or whose families could not care for them, were given a place to live at Lawajuni. A few of the girls at NOH had come from this orphanage, and had gone to NOH because it had more educational opportunities and better healthcare than the remotely located Lawajuni was able to offer at that time.

Narti was in many ways the real reason we had come to Nepal. It's located in the epicenter of the Kamlari system, and we were going there to see for ourselves the consequences of that system, and its effect on the innocent children of the country. We would spend two days there, living and interacting with the kids in order to immerse ourselves in the experience. That was the plan anyway.

Jesse warned us that in Narti we'd really be roughing it. Now, some people in the group thought the austere accommodations at the Korean monastery had been less than ideal, but this was going to be more challenging still. The idea that the conditions could get rough on this trip had been discussed several times during our preparations and during the first week in Nepal, but I didn't feel any real concern. None of us did. We felt like we were ready for anything. I had gone camping many times before, slept outdoors in tents, even in sleeping bags under the stars, and fearlessly done my "business" in the woods. I was not afraid of roughing it. Not in the least. At the time, we all seemed up for the challenge...

June 25, 2010

We are heading to Narti today to visit recently rescued Kamlari girls. I have heard the housing situation will be tents and sleeping bags, but as far as this whole trip has been, going with the flow is really the best part. Staying open, stepping into the unknown and just trusting all will be good.

Tingting Peng

The bus ride west to Lawajuni was a short one, at least compared to the monster trek that got us from Kathmandu to the Korean monastery. A mostly uneventful 3 or 4 hours. The group was quiet that morning. Deanna was suffering from a migraine and tried to get some sleep on the bus, while others read, or listened to their iPods. Everyone seemed to be in a contemplative mood.

June 25, 2010

The monastery [had been] intense, the "beds" we slept on were thin mattresses over a stone floor and the electricity would be out most of the time, so the rooms we were in were very hot and quite uncomfortable; all these things and the full moon keeping me up at night led to a very bad migraine. Once in a while I will get one, and when I do they are devastating, so the bus ride to our next destination was painful.

Deanna Lee

There was little discussion about what we could expect in Narti, or what we'd encounter at Lawajuni. I stared out the window, taking in the landscape -- steep hillsides, some terraced with rice paddies, others completely covered with jungle forest. Finally, as we turned off the main highway onto a smaller paved road, Jesse, who had been especially quiet up to this point, stood up, asking for our attention. We were very close to Lawajuni, he said. When we got there, he went on, we'd be meeting a group of 150 or so girls, many of whom had been child slaves, some until quite recently. He told us these girls did not speak English, they had never been to a big city, and their view of westerners, especially men, was fearful at best. They had been traumatized by their experiences as Kamlaris, he said, and we should expect them to be very shy, very reserved when they met us. He reiterated the fact that Lawajuni was not Kathmandu, not even Lumbini. It would be very rural.

It wasn't so much what Jesse said, as how he said it that affected us at the time. Even though our expectations about orphans in Nepal had been completely up-ended by our visit with the kids at NOH, after hearing Jesse talk about Narti, we began to imagine the worst. I had visions of Dickensian misery in my head, maybe spurred on by the experience I had in Bakhtapur, maybe from reading the harrowing account of Lakshmi in the book, Sold. However, as we drove through the gentle, rolling hills and rice paddies that dotted the countryside, my concerns began to ease. It really didn't look that bad. Sure it was rural, but the road was paved, there were convenience stores and small farmers' markets on the way, and a few small homes along the roadside. The area looked quite beautiful, really; gentle rolling hills and verdant farmland mingling with acres of tall, thick trees. I'd seen worse places in my travels.

Just before noon, we arrived in the village of Narti. As we turned off the main paved street onto a dirt road, our bus suddenly bottomed out crossing a fairly deep drainage ditch. It was quickly apparent that we were stuck. Our driver, Buddha, appeared only mildly perturbed; he had obviously handled worse crises. He assessed the situation with Basu in soft, measured Nepali, and Basu then explained to us in English that if we all got off the bus, lightening the load, Buddha would be able free the bus. We clambered to the passenger door, but it wouldn't open. It was wedged shut from the outside. A little drama ensued as we recalibrated our choice of exits.

The bus got stuck and we had to jump out to release the weight. Because the passenger door was stuck, we had to climb out of the driver's door... some jumped out of the windows. Nothing seems to surprise me anymore on this trip.

**Minling Chuang**

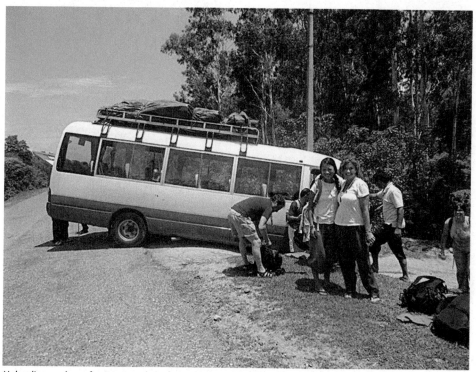

Unloading our bus, after it got stuck on the way to Lawajuni. Photo by Eve Ennis.

Everyone managed to scramble off the vehicle, either through the driver's side door or out a window, with little difficulty. Outside, the sun was shining directly upon us, high in the bright, blue cloudless sky. Because we were shaded by some very tall trees, we didn't feel the heat right away. The group was in good spirits, laughing at our momentary little predicament in the ditch, as we followed Jesse and Basu down the dirt road and through the jungle forest. I wasn't exactly sure where we were going, none of us were, but I was happy just to be off that damn bus. I'd had enough of being bounced around for a while.

After four to five hours on the bus, we arrive in Narti. Jesse seemed to like the element of surprise very much. The bus gets stopped by a steep drop, and we find ourselves walking into what we think is the village of Narti.

_____ *Gabrielle Stickley*

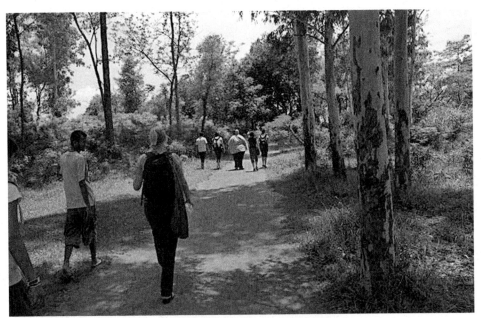

Following Jesse up the dirt road through the jungle to…? Photo by Minling Chuang.

The road through the woods led out into a large open field… but this wasn't the village of Narti we were entering; we had actually just walked to Lawajuni itself. I took a quick look around the place to get my bearings. On the left, there were two dormitory style buildings of simple concrete construction, with white-washed walls and wood framed windows with no glass, just steel bars. A few light blue wooden shutters were all that kept these buildings from looking utterly bleak. There was, however, a relatively new Yamaha motorcycle out front, which struck me as a little curious. Straight ahead was a small brick barn filled with hay, a large milking cow taking shade inside. Next to the barn and down a small dirt hill was a large water pump, which apparently drew water from a nearby creek. Behind the dorm buildings and the barn, a big backhoe sat idly in the sun, with many recently felled trees lying around it.

On the opposite side of the field was a very large, two-story, unfinished white-washed concrete building that I later found out was part schoolhouse and part dormitory. Between the building and the water pump were piles of dirt and gravel, and behind that, one single large outhouse, about the size of a small chicken coop. The conditions were primitive, without question, and a little jarring…

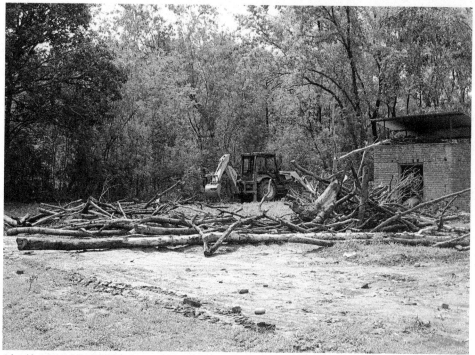

A backhoe sits idle behind felled trees at Lawajuni. I wondered how such a piece of heavy equipment ended up there, in the middle of nowhere.

June 25, 2010

Once I had a chance to look at the campus, it seemed like a prison to me. The buildings were cement as most buildings in Nepal are except the windows were barred. There was no glass or screens in the windows, just bars. I guess to keep out wild animals. There was some construction going on with bricks lying everywhere and trenches dug for the cement supports.

Christina Jankus

As we looked around, trying to take in the place we'd be calling home for the next two days, a small group of girls came out to greet us. Several of the older girls who had come out of the dormitory building presented our group with flowers and bindi. A bindi is a traditional forehead decoration worn throughout South Asia, a dot of red color applied in the center of the forehead close to the eyebrows. It can also consist of a sign or piece of jewelry worn on this spot.

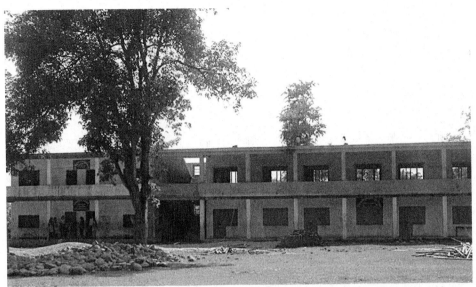

The unfinished two-story school building at Lawajuni. I slept our first night there in the room partially visible on the top right. Photo by Tingting Peng.

June 25, 2010

We ... saw at least 50 girls. A few walked up to us and started putting this red dot on our foreheads and gave us these beautiful and fragrant flowers. Other girls shyly watched us and stood to the side.

Minling Chuang

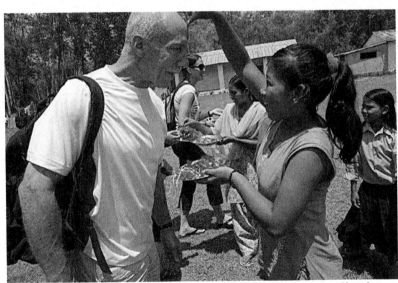

Marc receives traditional blessings, called bindi, from one of the girls of Lawajuni. Photo by Minling Chuang.

Nowadays bindis are worn by women, men, girls and boys, and no longer signify age, marital status, religious background or ethnic affiliation the way they did in earlier times. The bindis in this case were made of powder from crushed red flowers, and the girls were using them as a way to formally greet us and give us blessings. In the mid-day heat, as we began to sweat, the bindis quickly began to run red, down our noses, creating a rather comical effect.

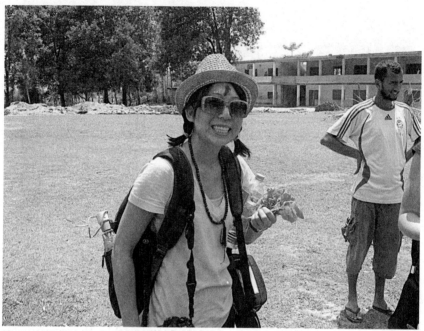

The sweltering heat is already melting Minling's bindi.

While we were being greeted with bindi, Basu, Buddha, Sun Tze and Subash had managed to get the bus out of the ditch, driving it up the dirt road to where we were all gathered. They parked it under the shade of a lone, small tree in the center of the large grass-covered field, a courtyard and playground for the home, where they unloaded our packs. We helped them as best we could without getting in their way. All the while, the noon day sun continued to beat down, baking the courtyard to a crispy, dry brown. Soon even the Nepalis were sweating.

While this unpacking was happening, Jesse asked us all to sit next to the bus so the rest of the girls could meet us. Again, we were all a bit unsure what exactly to expect. A couple of the older girls greeted Jesse with a hug, smiling and laughing as he spoke Nepali with them. In a moment, about 30 or 40 more girls ranging in age from about 5 to 15 were led out to meet us. Unlike the Nepal Orphans Home, there were no boys in this group. The girls appeared to be in good health, well-groomed, dressed mostly in traditional Nepali saris. A sari, for those who don't know, is a strip of unstitched, dyed cloth, about four to nine meters long usually worn with one end wrapped around the waist and the other draped over a shoulder. The sari is very popular in this region of the world.

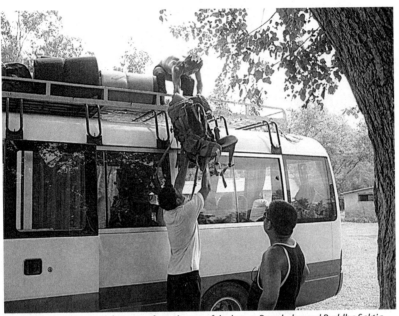

Sun Tze unloads the rest of our gear from the top of the bus as Basu helps and Buddha Saktia watches.

The girls were quiet, so quiet it was almost uncomfortable. They were obviously very shy, even around Jesse, except for the few older girls who must have known him from his previous visit. We all sat down around the bus, quietly staring at each other, not really sure what to do next…

June 25, 2010 _____

We were greeted with flowers and Bindi. Then there was a stare-down between us and the girls. It was odd as neither we nor the girls knew how to react.

_____ ***Christina Jankus***

June 25, 2010 _____

While traveling for four to five hours [to get here], there was ample time to make a speech to the group. But not one word was said, prior to arriving in Narti. We were driven into an area where girls ran out to welcome us. Nothing was said by Jesse, and we eventually just sat down across from each other on the ground, staring like Indians and pilgrims, dumbfounded by each other.

Finally, we distributed the toys and presents we came with, and the girls started to relax. There was no way to communicate, except by smiles. After a while, all turned into awkwardness. Jesse said nothing.

_____ *Gabrielle Stickley*

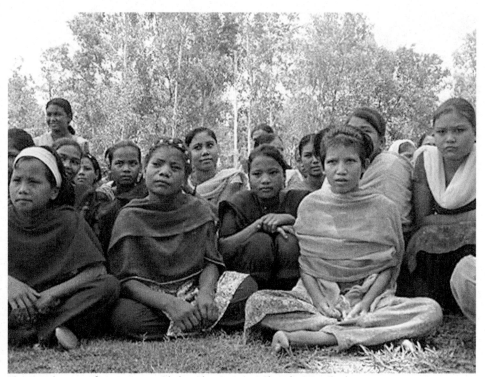

The stare-down, our first encounter with the girls at Lawajuni. Photo by Jaime Furda.

We had brought a large number of small gifts to hand out, and a couple of the women in our group, along with Jesse, took the initiative and began giving out presents. As we handed out the little earrings, fun rubber-band bracelets, beanie babies, beach balls, Frisbees and other items we'd brought for them, the girls would shyly say, "Thank you." We took the opportunity during this brief exchange to introduce ourselves and quickly learned that very few of them spoke much, if any, English, one or two of the oldest girls being the exception. The rest could say 'hello', 'how are you', and tell you their name and ask yours, but that was about the extent of the communication.

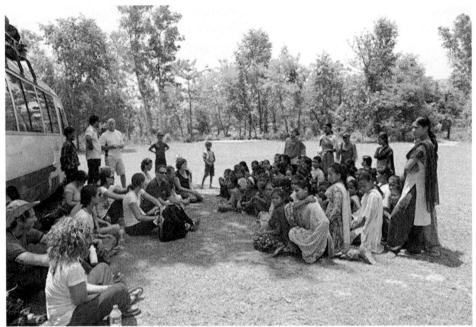

Introducing ourselves to the girls of Lawajuni. Unlike NOH, there were no boys at this orphanage. They were all rescued Kamlari girls. Photo by Minling Chuang.

June 25, 2010 _____

Each of them would say "Thank you Auntie" or "Thank you Uncle"... I wondered why they didn't call us sister or brother [the way they did at NOH]. Are they showing more respect?

_____ ***Minling Chuang***

Aside from Jesse, our Nepali was even more rudimentary than their English. I had hardly bothered to read the Nepali primer more than once or twice since Jesse emailed them out before the trip, and I was basically stuck with saying, "Namaste". This made for some awkward initial moments as we tried to find ways to communicate with each other. What made it more difficult for me was that many of the younger girls were extremely wary around the men in our group. It was understandable, since what we'd heard and read is that some Kamlari girls had been horribly mistreated by men. But these kids, like the children at NOH, seemed to be remarkably resilient and resourceful. Children understand the one language that's common to everyone, the language of laughter and fun. The braver girls along with the women in our group took the lead, and soon we all began to open up and become friends...

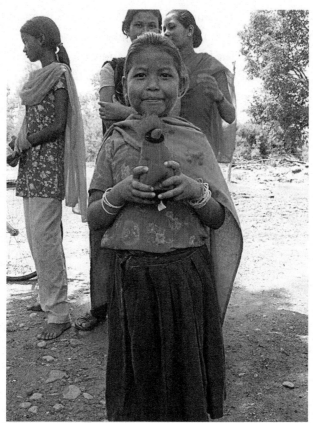

Little girl smiling with beanie babe. Photo by Deanna Lee.

June 25, 2010 _____

We had no idea what we were supposed to do. It was an interesting contrast to our time at NOH. The girls here were really shy and didn't speak to us. We all felt uncomfortable because we didn't know what to expect. Jesse told us to sit down as they unloaded the bus. The girls sat on one side and we all sat on the other side. It was a bit awkward and some people tried to sing songs… I think "Rudolph the Red Nose Reindeer" was one of them. Kathy and Rachel started to do some handstands off to the side and the girls clapped. David took out his mini fan that squirted water and went up to the girls. They were so curious [about] the fan because they didn't know what to expect when he came up to them and all of a sudden they felt the water squirt and the fan's breeze. They giggled as he went from girl to girl.

_____ *Minling Chuang*

After the exchange of bindi and gifts, we were escorted to an upstairs room in the partially completed school building where Jesse said we could relax and just let the girls hang out with us. The room was nice and cool compared to the sweltering heat outside. From the time he had stood up on the bus and first addressed us about Narti, Jesse seemed very apprehensive, especially about how these girls would react to us. He tried to articulate his worries, but without any real clarity, so we all sat around confused as to how best to interact with these kids. Jesse's advice was to "just let them be with us" for a while, just hang out without any agenda, so that the girls could get used to our presence. Some of the braver girls came right into the classroom and joined us. We sat around tossing the Frisbee with them for a while, and then they disappeared, to where we had no idea. We all marveled at how quickly the girls' shyness was disappearing. They really seemed to like the fact that we were here, at least the ones we had met so far.

A few minutes later a different group of girls returned with lunch — white rice, peppers and potatoes, paneer and vegetable curry — which the girls had prepared themselves. The food was excellent. Despite the harsh conditions, and the major language barrier, perhaps Narti would turn out be just as great an experience as our short time at NOH had been.

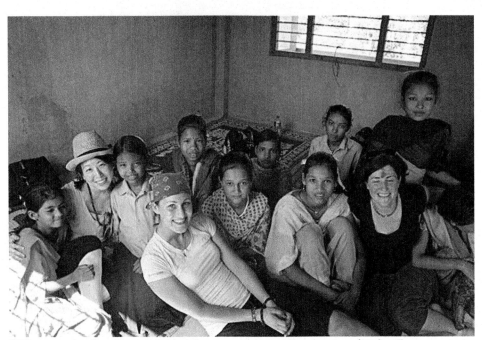

Chilling out and cooling off in an unfinished classroom at Lawajuni. Photo courtesy of Minling Chuang.

Through all of this the girls seemed happy, very happy. If you're happy then I'm happy.

_____ *Christina Jankus*

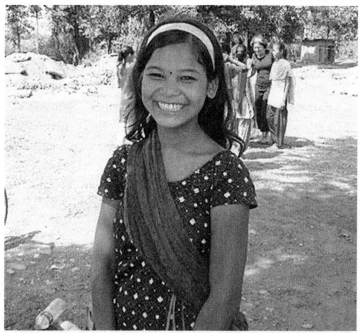

It didn't take long for these girls to start smiling. And when they did, it was remarkable. Photo by Jaime Furda.

The girls might have been happy, but I was having a small crisis right about then. I had been taking some pictures of us eating lunch when suddenly my camera began blinking a warning — the memory card was full. When I realized I hadn't brought another card with me, I panicked for a second. I had tried to buy one at the airport in Newark but they didn't have the right size card for my camera. I had brushed it off then, thinking it wasn't very likely that I'd take more than 500 pictures on this trip. Of course now I had, and we were barely halfway through the trip. I can't take anymore pictures, I thought. That totally sucks.

My mind raced for a solution. I dug through my backpack, found my little camera bag, and inside discovered that luckily I had brought along the camera's data transfer cable and a flash drive. I remembered too that Tingting had a small netbook computer with her. Two plus two equals four, and I quickly asked her if I could borrow it. She was nice enough to let me use it, so while the others finished eating, I went to one of the empty classrooms down the hall and dumped the hundreds of photos I had taken onto Tingting's laptop, then transferred the pictures onto my thumb drive. The whole process took maybe half an hour, and worked like a charm. "Happy happy joy joy," as I often say, quoting Ren & Stimpy on those occasions when things actually work out. Happy and relieved.

After lunch, we were left on our own to do as we liked. Memory card now empty, and belly full from lunch, I wandered the grounds, camera in hand looking for something to photograph, or someone to talk to. I like kids, but having none of my own, navigating among sixty young girls who spoke little English was a bit intimidating. I didn't know what to say to them other than "Namaste." They always returned the greeting, some with a laugh or a smile, others shyly. Watching them play, such sweet, beautiful children, it was difficult for me to comprehend the exploitation many of them had suffered.

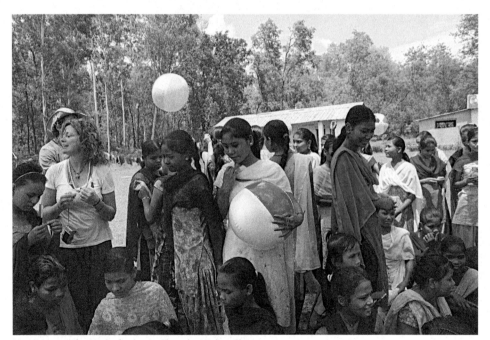

Handing out gifts. Let the fun begin. Photo by Minling Chuang.

June 25, 2010

After a delicious lunch, which included the best fresh goat cheese paneer I've ever had, Kathy and I took the ribbons we brought and started tying them in the girls' hair. We had an assortment of ribbons that we bought and let each girl choose the one she liked. We enlisted the help of Chris and by mid-afternoon we gave each girl her own ribbon for her hair. I think we became known as the ribbon ladies because the girls who had ribbons would bring their friends over to us so we could tie ribbons in their hair. It was so nice to see the girls smile and open up to us…

Minling Chuang

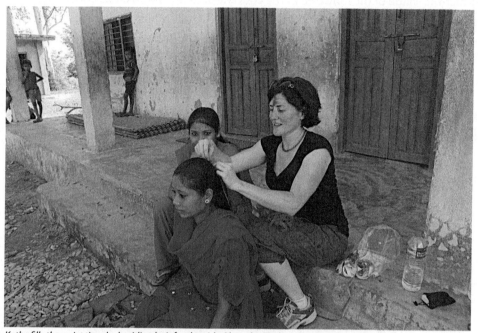

Kathy fills the quiet time by braiding hair for the girls. Photo by Minling Chuang.

June 25, 2010

…One thing I wish I had done before the trip was to brush up on my schoolyard games. There was a language barrier between the girls and us. We had to rack our brains to think of games that we could teach them and play together. At one point Gabrielle and I showed the girls patty cake and it took a while for us to remember that game and the words (still not sure if we had the words right).

Kathy showed the kids Duck Duck Goose. I played "volleyball" with the girls and the beach ball. We also did wheelbarrow races and sang songs – we would take turns and the girls would sing a Nepalese song and we would sing an American song. However, I was convinced that their songs had more traditional value, as the only songs I could remember were current pop culture songs or easy songs like "Take me out to the ball game." Tingting and I even sang a grade school song in Mandarin. At one point, we broke out into dance. The girls showed us some traditional Nepalese dance and we just danced crazy inside the circle.

The whole experience made me realize how young our country is and that it doesn't have the same deep-rooted traditions as other countries. I wish we did and that we could show the girls our traditions.

_____ ***Minling Chuang***

The rest of us searched for some shelter from the sun wherever we could find it, under the shade of the lone tree in the courtyard, in the unfinished school building. Deanna hadn't been feeling well since before we left Lumbini, so she took shelter in the bus, hoping to get a little sleep. Basu, Subash, Buddha and Sun Tze had rolled out some sleeping mats and were resting as well.

As I sat watching Tingting and Minling dancing with the girls, a Nepali in his early 30's carrying a small backpack walked into camp. Jesse introduced him as Charlie. Charlie worked for SWAN, the Social Welfare Association of Nepal. One

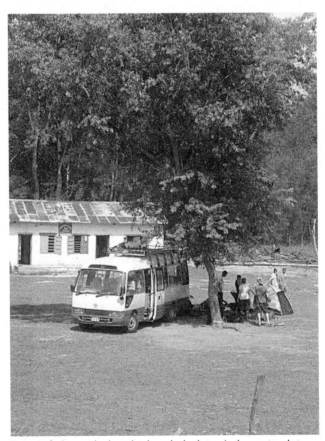

Trying to find some shade under the only shade tree in the courtyard at Lawajuni. Photo by Eve Ennis.

of SWAN's main missions was the eradication of the Kamlari system in the western part of the country. This was the first I had heard that the Nepalis themselves were actually making an organized, concerted effort to change things. I knew that the Kamlari system was against the law in Nepal, but I had naively thought that somehow it was just westerners who were trying to do something about the terrible plight of these kids until I met Charlie. Makes perfect sense now. Who better to change things than the Nepalis themselves? Seems pretty obvious, I know, but when the light bulb went off that afternoon I actually felt relieved. Maybe the situation for these kids wasn't hopeless after all.

We sat down in a circle around Charlie, in the shade provided by the bus and the tree, and listened as he gave a brief talk about the work going on at Lawajuni and at SWAN. We had a lot of questions for him about the Kamlari system, which we were still trying to wrap our heads around, so he did his best to answer. Charlie spoke English quite well, though he was very soft spoken. You had to lean in close at times to catch everything he was saying…

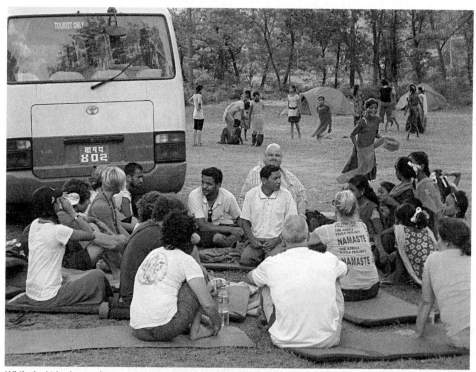

While the kids play, we listen to Charlie tell us about SWAN's work rescuing Kamlaris.

It was midafternoon by now and swelteringly hot as we sat talking with Charlie.
Hotter than anything I'd ever experienced in my life, and I've done Bikram yoga
during heat waves in the summer in Los Angeles. In all this heat, Basu, Subash,
Buddha and Sun Tze began setting up the tents we were going to be sleeping in for
the next two nights. When Charlie finished his talk, a few of us got up to try to help
them work, and that was when the first real stirrings of trouble in the group began.
We had heard before the trip that we were going to be sleeping in "communal" tents
in Narti, which we assumed meant big tents.

These tents however turned out to be quite small, two-man North Face tents.
They were new, and very good quality, perfect for trekking in the Himalayas where
it was cold at night, even in summer. But to me, these little tents looked like they
would make the perfect sauna if we tried to sleep in them in this weather. I asked
Basu if he'd ever slept in these tents in these conditions, and he said, "No problem."
Whenever I hear someone in a foreign country say to me, "No problem", I know
there's going to be a problem. But I liked Basu a lot, and trusted him completely.
He was smart, experienced, and a native. Who would know better how to deal with
these conditions?

Playing it cool, I asked Basu how hot he thought it was here in Narti. He said it
was easily 115 degrees. That sounded about right to me. I guessed that the humidity
was upwards of 50% as well. My t-shirt was stuck to my skin like a wet towel, my
hair was matted down on my head, my face was slick with sweat, and my lips tasted
of salt. Jesse and Basu had provisioned plenty of water for us, but I quickly realized
that drinking water didn't do very much at all to cool you off in this kind of blistering heat. Soon the tents were up, and each of us picked one to sleep in. Dave and I,
being roommates, grabbed one. Robb and Marc did the same. Jesse took one of the
one-man tents, and the women divvied up the others. We stowed our gear inside
and then were left to wander around, a bit to our own devices.

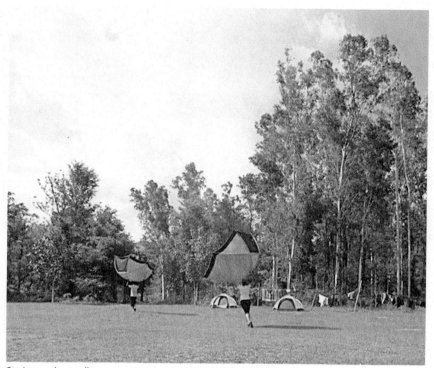

Setting up the small two-man tents we would be sleeping in. Photo by Eve Ennis.

Nothing much else was happening at the moment, and I found myself wandering from shady spot to shady spot, trying to keep my mind off the heat. At one point, I noticed Charlie talking to another man near the water pump behind the small barn with the milk cow in it. I hadn't seen this man before. His name, it turned out, was Krishna Chaudhary, and the red Yamaha motorcycle parked in the courtyard was his. Krishna worked for SWAN as well. He he ran things here at Lawajuni, and had given a little speech at lunch which I'd missed because of my memory card problem. Krishna looked older than Charlie. He was probably in his 40's, and had thick black hair and eyes that appeared to size you up even as he smiled and greeted you warmly.

As I watched him chatting with Charlie, a group of girls carrying plastic jugs walked past me down the small dirt hill toward the two men, and I decided to follow. When the girls arrived at the pump, Krishna began to work the lever, and the young women filled their plastic jugs with water as it gushed out of the nozzle. Jesse had wandered over by now, and he warned me not to drink this water, which he said came from a nearby river, because the bacteria in it could make you sick if your body wasn't acclimated to it. I had a different idea. I walked over to the pump,

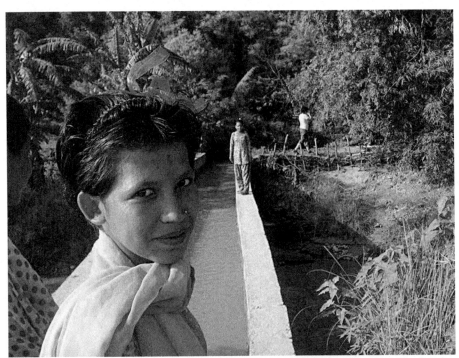

Hiking along the irrigation canal at midday in the rice field behind Lawajuni. Photo by Tingting Peng.

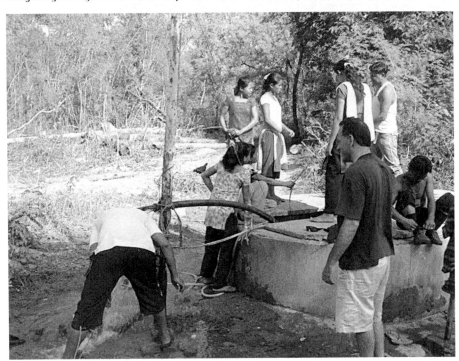

Looking for some temporary relief, Basu and I soak our sweltering heads under the cold flowing water pump at Lawajuni. Photo by Tingting Peng.

smiled at Krishna, and then stuck my whole head under the clear flowing water. The sense of relief I felt was immediate and profound. The water turned out to be nice and cold, and the soaking I gave my head was incredibly refreshing. Krishna laughed and smiled as I walked away shaking my hair like a wet dog, feeling at least momentarily a whole lot better.

At this point in the day, it felt like it was 120 degrees easily. The sun was still high in the sky, still beating down on us, relentless and oppressive. There was no running water, only the well and the pump. Not even squat toilets. A few people ventured to the very rustic outhouse and came back with their eyes watering. The conditions were a far cry from what we were used to in the US. They were even a far cry from the conditions we'd experienced at the Korean Monastery. We thought we had been tested in Lumbini, but between the heat, the raw rural poverty, the primitive outhouse, the dirt and dust, the unfinished work-in-progress nature of Lawajuni, and the realization slowly dawning on some of us that these small tents we had to sleep in were going to be a real problem in these temperatures, Narti began to look like more than just roughing it. It looked like this place would be really tough to handle for two days and nights.

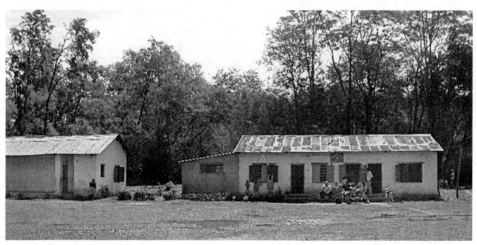

Just trying to find some shade, outside the girls dormitory at Lawajuni. Photo by Jaime Furda.

6-25-10 _____

We then proceeded to wander about aimlessly for several hours, punctuated by small, sweet encounters with the girls. "Hello, Auntie. How are you?" But that was the extent of it. Then we just stood there… befuddled by what to do next.

_____ *Gabrielle Stickley*

June 25, 2010 _____

I noticed some of our members breaking into smaller groups, talking – about what I don't know. Someone from the small group motioned me over and asked what I thought about all of this. I didn't really have any thoughts as I was just going with the flow. It seemed to work for me.

_____ *Christina Jankus*

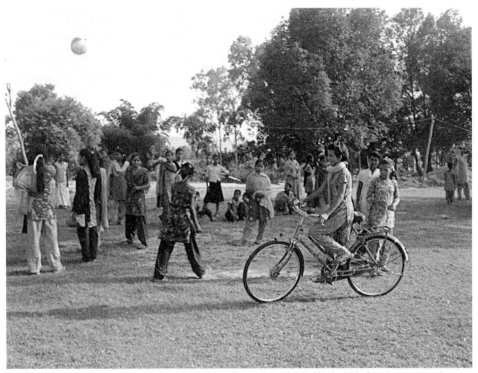

The girls break out the bicycle and keep on having fun. In the center, dressed like a Catholic school girl, her hand resting on her hip, is a very shy young girl who rewarded our interest in her with the most amazing smile I've ever witnessed. Photo by Tingting Peng.

June 25, 2010 _____

…while some of us where playing with the girls, I couldn't help notice that a lot of people on the trip were not… they were sitting off to the side in the shade. I started to feel a sense of sadness that more people weren't engaging with the girls. These are the girls we are here to help and show them our love. Yes it's hot and the conditions are really rough, but we are here for the girls. How could people waste an opportunity to be with these girls who have been through so much? I really don't get it. But I tried not to let the others get to me

188

and tried to focus my attention and energy on the girls. I was just so happy to be there with them.

Minling Chuang

A few of us managed to put aside the tough conditions and make the best of things playing in the courtyard with the girls, bouncing beach balls, throwing Frisbees, meeting and chatting with more of the girls. There was a bicycle propped against the side of the dormitory, and Tingting hopped on and began riding it. The young Nepali girls were soon following her like Mary Poppins as she rode around the large grassy field, the young girls, and one very funny goat, chasing the bike around the courtyard.

These girls were outgoing and friendly, but many of the others remained shy, and apparently others still, at least from what I heard, were too scared or shy to even venture out of their dorms to visit with us. Since there were over 150 children living here, and we could only see about 50 of them around, that meant there were quite a few who hadn't even ventured out yet.

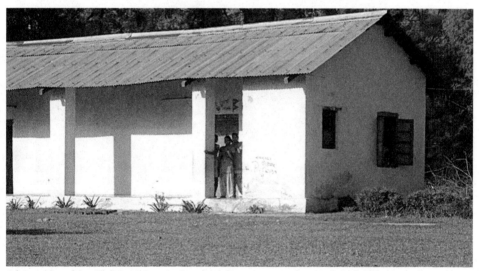

A fair number of the girls living at Lawajuni were too shy to venture out to see what all the fuss was about when we arrived. Photo by Tingting Peng.

June 25, 2010

Over the next couple of hours, as we cooled off from the soaring 100+ degree heat in one of the spare classrooms, curiosity got the better of the girls... several of them, slowly started to make their way up to us. I received a quick tour of their cramped and modest living quarters. Mina,

15 years old and one of the older girls in the group, spoke to me in good English as she showed me her room.

…The rest of the afternoon and evening was spent playing with the girls. I entertained them by riding on a bicycle and chasing them around on it. Then we moved onto playing volleyball with a beach ball, which occasionally turned into a game of football. The girls had so much energy; there was so much life in their eyes. We also had a singing session of American and Nepali songs, which then turned into a dance jam [and] even more singing and dancing and clapping. It was such a joy to see them so happy.

Tingting Peng

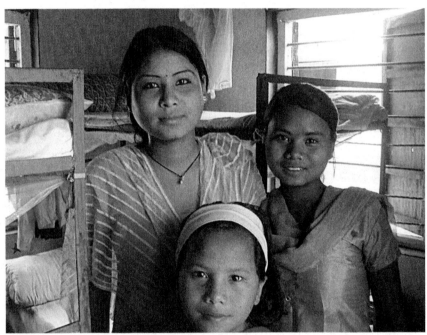

A few of the girls took Tingting back to their room to show her where they slept and studied. Photo by Tingting Peng.

The heat became even more intense as the day drew on, and many in our group could only seek shelter from the sweltering sun in whatever patch of shade they could find, not really able to do much else. The people who lived here, including the girls in the orphanage, were used to this kind of heat. They weren't even sweating. Traditionally, this was not a time to be outside for them anyway. In fact, many of the girls were back in their rooms in the shade of the cooler concrete dormitories. But for us, there was no real escape. The heat was doing a number on us, playing with the psyches of the less experienced campers in the group. We had a wide range of outdoor experience, from none at all to those who had trekked through wilderness far from civilization with just the packs on their backs. There was also a considerable age range in our group, from 19 to 62, and none of us were used to this climate, except perhaps Tingting, who lived in Hong Kong, and Robb, who had served in Vietnam and had experienced these conditions. Gazing at those small one and two-man tents, we all saw the way we were going to be living for the next two days, and it was not going to be 'kumbaya' camping. It was going to be survival camping. A number of folks were getting increasingly uncomfortable, and you could see panic setting in amongst some at the thought of a two night stay in Narti.

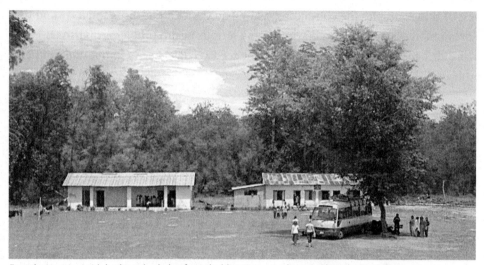

Even the Lawajuni girls had to take shelter from the blistering noonday sun. Photo by Tingting Peng.

Now you might think people were making too big a deal about the heat, that it was all in their heads. I certainly thought so initially. But as the day wore on, I began to sympathize with those suffering. Heat exhaustion and heat stroke are not something that should ever be dismissed as trivial. Often dehydration occurs because a person hasn't replaced the water lost by sweating. We were drinking lots of water, but it wasn't necessarily helping. The body cools itself most efficiently by sweating and then by the sweat evaporating. Should sweating be unable to meet your body's cooling needs, heat-related illnesses can and will occur. And our sweating, profuse as it was, wasn't proving to be nearly enough to keep us cool.

Adverse reactions to heat usually start with minor symptoms like heat rash, but can progress quickly to heat cramps, then heat exhaustion, and finally to heat stroke, which is a life-threatening medical condition. Heat cramps can include heavy sweating, weakness, nausea, vomiting, headaches, and muscle spasms. Heat exhaustion occurs when sweating cannot dissipate the heat generated within the body. Heat stroke, which can quickly follow, is a life-threatening situation where the body's cooling system completely fails. Body temperature spirals out of control, rising over 106F (41C), and sweating stops and mental status changes like confusion, seizure, and even coma occur.[9]

Even doctors can't always make clear diagnoses between the various degrees of heat-induced illnesses. And none of us were doctors here, so we really had no way of knowing how the heat might ultimately affect any one of us. We were a pretty resilient bunch, I thought, perhaps somewhat optimistically, and we'd be able to make the best of things despite the conditions, as we had done in our visits to NOH and the Korean monastery. So far, we'd avoided any serious health problems on this trip, but that didn't mean everything would be fine for two days here. Compounding these problems, there was no real agenda or program we were following at Lawajuni…

June 25, 2010 _____

We spent the rest of the afternoon resting, eating, and wandering the grounds with the girls (who called us "Auntie.") After several hours of this, a few people began to wonder what our purpose here was. Many of us wished we could do something more, like build the girls something, or paint, or pick up trash. And some began to get frustrated.

_____ ***Gabrielle Stickley***

We were all on our own to make up whatever activities we could think of to keep ourselves occupied. This lack of structure, along with the stark accommodations, only added to some people's growing frustrations, unnerving them further. In addition, several of the women in our group were also having issues with the safety of the camp.

June 25, 2010 _____

I'd been asleep off and on all day, the heat was making my migraine even more extreme and it was all I could do. Some of us were sick or getting over being sick, many of us had open wounds and had no access to running water to clean our cuts, and we were sleeping in tents in the beginning of monsoon season in a town where we couldn't be certain we felt safe sleeping so exposed.

_____ ***Deanna Lee***

---

[9] Source: www.medicinenet.com.

Even though Jesse and Basu tried to reassure everyone that it was perfectly safe camping out here, as far as some people were concerned, we were out in the middle of nowhere, and those North Face tents were looking smaller and smaller and more vulnerable by the minute. Safety wasn't a major issue for me with respect to the tents. To me, those tents were starting to look more like little sweat boxes.

The combination of the intense heat, the primitive conditions, the safety concerns and the lack of something else to clearly take our minds off these things was about to prove disastrous to the spiritual journey 'from me to we' that had been the theme of our trip so far. Jesse had told us Narti would be tough, the brochure had said this trip would be a test physically, emotionally, and spiritually, but until we experienced it, we couldn't begin to understand what awaited us. Despite Jesse's warnings, despite what was clearly spelled out in the original flyer and the itinerary for the Yoga For Freedom trip, the reality of Narti was beginning to prove far more challenging than some folks could handle, and under these circumstances, in that moment of intense suffering, things started to unravel...

June 25, 2010

As nighttime fell, some of us walked to the local store, which is little more than a stand with food, drinks and other necessities. This was when everything changed. Marc turned to me and said that a few people were talking about leaving, and asked what I thought and if I'd go along with it. I was completely shocked and immediately said no and that I was here for the girls. I also pointed out that just a few days ago he complained we didn't get to spend enough time with the children at NOH, and now he wanted to go when he has the chance to spend time with the Kamlari girls. I was definitely not happy about hearing this and didn't know that people wanted to leave until now. We were supposed to stay for two days and nights and we haven't even made it through a night and people want to leave?

Minling Chuang

June 25, 2010

...we went to Gunga's to pick up some cold drinks (Gunga is really sweet). This is where it went downhill for me. Some of us were sitting in the back room there talking about what we could do to help the girls. I mentioned that the Philalethean Society at Heidelberg (my sorority at school) would be more than interested in helping in whatever ways we could: writing letters to them, sending care packages... Jesse shot every one of my ideas down. The mail is practically nonexistent. He'd have to take everything himself. We can't give them toys because they break and/or the girls stop playing when we leave (seriously?? ::sigh::). What I got from that is that it's basically impossible to help them. "Well then, why are we here?" "To witness."

I came on this trip to make a difference. To physically do something to change the world, even if it's just a little bit. I'm not going to sit around inside for four hours just because someone thinks it's too hot to move. I'm going to get up on my two left feet and attempt to learn how to dance Nepali style with the girls.

_____ *Jaime Furda*

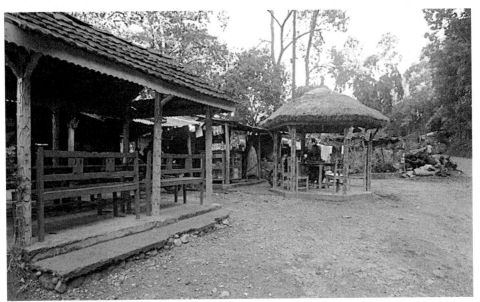

Gunga's local store, just up the road from Lawajuni, where the grumbling first started. Photo by Eve Ennis.

June 25, 2010 _____

Around sunset, a few of the YFF participants decided to walk down the street for some cold soda and snacks. That's when the dispute and complaints started. People were exhausted (ok fine), overcome with heat stress and the poor conditions at the orphanage. The schedule was unclear and people were getting nervous about sleeping in a tent overnight, though I didn't really understand why. It all sounded like a bunch of spoiled brats whining about things that their privileged a$$es are not used to and therefore refused to accept or deal with.

On the way back from the village store, I spoke in a state of disbelief and frustration with Minling and vented [my] feelings.

_____ ***Tingting Peng***

Various people from the group, Marc, Terri, Rachel, Minling, Tingting and several others, came over to talk to me about the frustrations that were bubbling up. I had been at Gunga's for only a few minutes to get a cold soda, but it was cramped and hot in the back room, so I left right away, before the discussion got heated. I hadn't seen anything confrontational happen while I was there, but I could see how upset everyone was as they came back, and it didn't take a rocket scientist to see there was a real problem brewing. We were far out in the back country, miles and miles from the nearest real city, and we were going to be out here for another day and a half. We were all hot, sweaty, and tired. We were in an unfamiliar place surrounded by unfamiliar people, and night was beginning to fall.

Things were becoming progressively more tense, and I thought the only way to get us back on track was to gather together and discuss the situation as a group. Otherwise, these feelings would stay bottled up, boil over and explode, and that couldn't be a good thing. I went to Jesse and explained to him what I was hearing and seeing. He had a concerned look on his face, but agreed that it was better to discuss things now than to let them fester. So we gathered everyone together to talk.

Jesse started things off, asking if there was anything anyone wanted to discuss. Several people said they were feeling very uncomfortable, sick from the heat, and wanted to leave Narti as soon as possible. Some of the women felt unsafe out in the middle of nowhere in small tents. Several others were annoyed at the lack of an agenda here at Lawajuni. They had had enough of Narti and they wanted to go. On the other hand, others were adamant that we should stay. For them, Lawajuni was the whole reason they'd come to Nepal in the first place. They were completely against the idea of leaving early. A few of us, myself included, were either on the fence, or willing to go along with the majority. Jesse felt like it was a bad idea to leave ahead of schedule and said so. There was a lot of sniping and plenty of emotion in everyone's arguments for staying or going, and Jesse seemed at a loss for how to alleviate the tension. He was clearly, firmly in the stay camp. He tried to alleviate the safety concerns by asking Basu to speak, and vouch for the safety here. Basu backed Jesse on this point. Safety was not an issue here, he stated unequivocally, but his assurances did not sway those who felt vulnerable.

June 25, 2010 _____

...we were ushered into a circle to discuss the situation. Jesse started the conversation and said that he would be very disappointed if we left early and that we should work through our own issues and stay. People started talking about how unsafe they felt and how terrible the conditions were. Other people talked about how they wanted to stay and that we should put our own thoughts and feelings [aside] and go with the plan. All I could hear was words passing around. I could barely concentrate on everything people were saying – it was so surreal. Can't we just enjoy being here?

*_____ **Minling Chuang***

June 25, 2010_____

…someone said that we needed to talk things over with Jesse. I thought it was a good idea to get things out into the open. I nodded my head in response to this suggestion…

Many in the small break out group wanted to leave Narti as the conditions were less than stellar. We would be sleeping in very small tents in oppressive 120 degree heat. I said nothing in response to this statement. I just watched and listened to what everyone had to say… It was very confrontational and for me very upsetting as I don't like group discord. I cried and snotted on myself just taking in everything and feeling dread and regret every time the suggestion to leave Narti was made… I cried more thinking of how we would disappoint these lovely people who have shown us nothing but kindness.

I needed a hug from Jesse as I felt like I was falling apart. He and Kathy hugged and encouraged me.

*_____ **Christina Jankus***

June 25, 2010_____

My opinion… was that people needed to just suck it up and make the best of the situation. You know, we signed up for it, knew it was coming (though unaware of the exact conditions)… Why just give up on it and leave?

*_____ **Jaime Furda***

June 25, 2010_____

I didn't chime in and say why I wanted to stay. As the conversation kept going, I knew that people's minds were made up in either direction and there was no convincing anyone to change their minds and the whole exercise was pointless. Can we just stop fighting and spend time with the girls?

*_____ **Minling Chuang***

I knew that leaving early might not be the easiest thing to do logistically, let alone emotionally for those who really wanted to stay. The trip had been carefully planned; hotels and transportation had to be booked well in advance given the relative size of our group. A few of us tried to find some kind of compromise, to work things out, but the two sides were deadlocked, and no one in either faction wanted to budge in the slightest. As the leader of the group, Jesse appeared to be shell-shocked by the intensity of the conflict, stunned by what he must have felt was a complete betrayal of the core mission of this journey. He was clearly, deeply invested emotionally in Lawajuni and in his purpose in bringing us here, and he was clearly at a loss as to how to resolve this sudden wave of tension and animosity that had built up so quickly, like a sudden summer storm. He started to withdraw into himself, and soon the group broke up into various small factions, each debating the merits of the other side's position.

June 25, 2010

Tingting and I started venting about the situation. We really didn't understand why people wanted to leave. We all signed up for the trip and knew it was going to be rough. In my mind, I signed up for whatever was going to come my way – the good and bad. Couldn't other people put their own concerns aside and just be here with the girls and enjoy the moment? Yes, the conditions are difficult, over 100 degrees plus humidity and no running water. But this is reality and how other people live and how these girls live. These girls don't have a choice, but they make the best of the situation and are happy, why can't we? I am going to be very upset if we have to leave because some people can't handle the conditions. This is why we came here!!! It's not fair that some people want to leave and we may have to leave, even if some of us don't want to.

Minling Chuang

June 25, 2010

When we got back from the break at the soda shop in Narti, it was dark already and the group was called together to discuss the issue of some people wanting to leave a day early. I expressed my disappointment and asked for everyone to consider being selfless FOR ONCE TRULY, and to let go of their own insignificant fears because there's really nothing to fear. Those girls needed us to show them that they are the same as us; they are not just a cause for pretentious good little yogis.

As the discussion went on, it became increasingly obvious that the group was bitterly divided. There were those who had signed up for only the fun stuff, the easy stuff, but who were unwilling to acknowledge and fully participate in the difficult aspects of the trip, such as experiencing how these Kamlari girls really live. Those unwilling to be totally open to all aspects of the journey were not going to be persuaded.

_____ ***Tingting Peng***

To try to diffuse the tension, at least a little, we discussed sleeping on the issues and seeing how we all felt in the morning, but we were soon getting nowhere with that idea. As we were arguing the merits of even this modest compromise, a group of ten or twenty villagers suddenly showed up, appearing en masse out of the gloaming. We had no idea in that moment what was going on, or even who they were. A few of these villagers and some of the older girls from Lawajuni began to lead us over toward the dormitory buildings. Not everyone was eager to follow, unsure of who these people were or what they wanted from us. Again, the language barrier didn't help, only adding to the confusion and frustration of the evening. Jesse finally spoke up and told us that these people were from the nearby village, and had come to put on a traditional welcome dance for us.

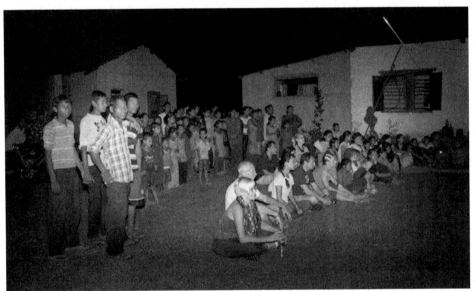

The villagers from Narti arrived just in time to stop our bickering, and to put on a show of native dance and music for us. Photo by Minling Chuang.

How ironic, I thought. Here we were arguing about leaving this place, and a whole bunch of nice folks from town just arrived to throw us a welcome party. The Greeks have a word for this sort of welcome. They call it philoxenia — an

198

ancient Greek concept of hospitality, generosity and courtesy shown to those who are far from home. One of the older girls who lived at the orphanage came over and asked us, in broken English, to please come and watch the performance. A couple of the villagers joined her, prodding us, gently but persistently, to join them. Despite the language barrier, they clearly sensed that something was wrong with our little group, but they didn't let that stop them from their mission. They politely, but firmly herded us to where they wanted us to go. Not wanting to make a bad situation worse than we had already managed to make it, most of us reluctantly followed the villagers over to a spot just in front of the dorms, where they motioned for us to sit down.

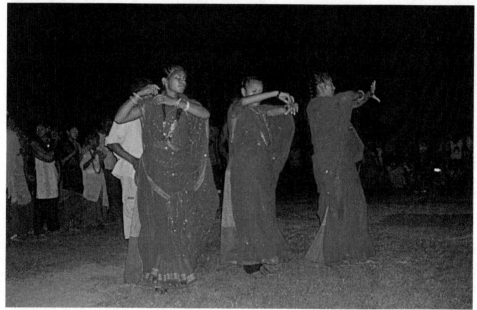

Native dancers in full regalia. Photo by Deanna Lee.

It was dark now, pitch black under a moonless sky. The performers, three men and three women dressed in what looked like traditional village garb, began the show — the men playing hand drums as the women started slowly twirling in their dresses, dancing and singing a traditional Nepali folk song. I looked around from where I was sitting and was surprised in that moment to see at least a hundred villagers, maybe more, who had quietly arrived from the surrounding area to watch the show, and apparently to meet us. All the girls from Lawajuni seemed to have come out as well. There had to be a couple hundred people out in the courtyard. A few lanterns provided the only illumination by which to see the dance, and they cast funky shadows on the dormitory walls, their light dancing and sparkling in the whites of the villagers' eyes and smiles, as if Halloween had been turned into some kind of happy little dance party. It all felt very tribal to me, very much like a Native American powwow I had been to years before, but a little less formal.

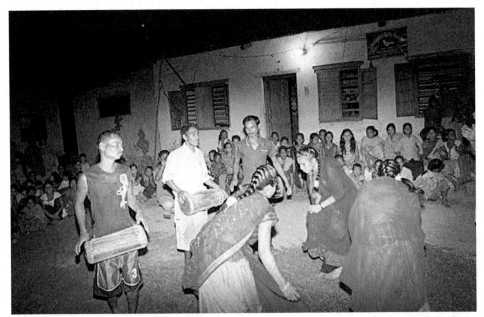

As the men increased the intensity of their drumming, the women intensified their dancing to match them. Photo by Minling Chuang.

The men's drumming grew more energetic and the women's dancing more frenetic as the performers began to increase the tempo. Everyone in the audience was enjoying the show when suddenly one of our group was pulled into the dance circle by one of the villagers. It was a moment of pure spontaneous fun, and before we knew it, a whole bunch of us were being dragged up there to dance along with the performers.

June 25, 2010

Luckily, in the heat of our discussion, the villagers came and started beating their drums and dancing. The whole village came out to welcome us by putting on a special performance. The group dispersed without a resolution and joined the villagers in celebration.

The villagers put on a beautiful performance. The whole town was there to celebrate. As I walked around and took pictures of the performance and the villagers around us, I felt a little sadness because they did so much to prepare for our arrival and welcome us, and we may leave the very next day. Towards the end of the performance, the dancers invited all of us to dance with them in celebration. In that moment, all of my worries went away and I just enjoyed being there with everyone. Everyone was dancing, laughing and having a great time... There was so much laughter and love present. It's actually hard to believe that we were all fighting earlier.

Minling Chuang

June 25, 2010

The townspeople had been arriving during our discussion, and a gathering of sorts ensued; there were drums and dancing and some talking, I say some because there was a language barrier that got in the way. One of the beautiful things about this was just being with another person and not having to feel the need to spend time with much conversation and question asking and storytelling. For a moment, we were all just "being" together.

Deanna Lee

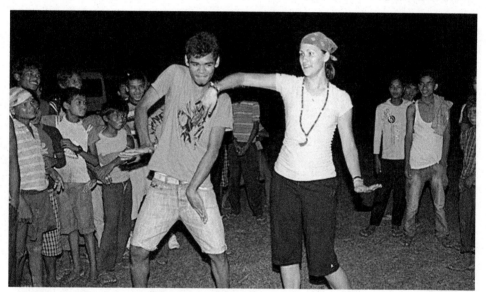

Jaime is one of the first to join in the fun. Photo by Minling Chuang.

June 25, 2010

In the midst of the heated and emotional conversation, there was music being played and some girls had begun to dance for us — it was their showing of appreciation at our visit. A bus had arrived, carrying many of the villagers to the grounds and there was a pretty big crowd surrounding us. The girls dressed in elaborate costumes and danced as some local boys drummed up a beat. The Lawajuni girls sang in unison providing the soundtrack to the dances.

A few of us joined them in the dancing, as some of the younger girls also jumped in. Their faces were lit with bright smiles and laughter, and it was night and day compared to just a few hours earlier when we first met the girls all quiet and shy. We danced and danced and danced... until the singing stopped, until the drumming and the clapping stopped, until our legs and arms were too tired to move, until we were all drenched in soaking sweat.

*_____ **Tingting Peng***

We did our best to follow the villagers' lead, or made up our own dance moves as we went along. The more we danced, the more the audience got wrapped up in the performance, and the more fun we were all having. Soon everyone was clapping and singing and having a good old time. I let myself get pulled into the dance and did my best to spin and whirl and stay on my feet without crashing into anyone else. It wasn't long before I was laughing and clapping and singing words I didn't understand like a crazy person.

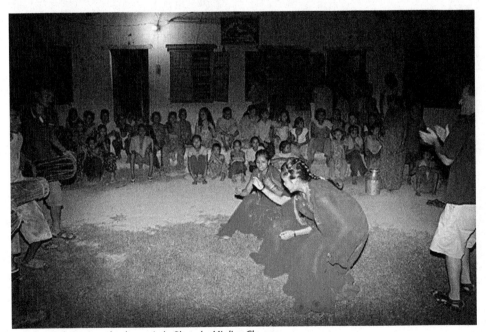

I was being drawn into the dance circle. Photo by Minling Chuang.

We must have danced non-stop for half an hour at least as the drums beat, and the men and women, now joined by the crowd of villagers, clapped to the rhythm and sang along with the songs. It was a sweaty joyous celebration of life. Somehow, right in the middle of the divisive debate we had been having about leaving Narti, we were becoming one with the villagers, part of their community. It was an absolute total blast. By the end of the dance, we were exhaustedly high-fiving people we'd never met in our lives. One teenage village boy even jumped into Robb's arms and gave him a big bear hug, shouting, 'Thank you! Thank You!' I think it was all the English he knew, and all the English he needed. It was a truly beautiful moment at the end of a long, challenging day....

June 25, 2010_____

[The day] turned into fun and joy. A group of teenage boys standing behind me got my attention. A little interaction and the group exploded into total laughter and fun. The evening was something I will never forget. We were all high-fiving when one of the teens just grabbed me and hugged me like a family member I have not seen in many years.

_____ ***Robb Blain***

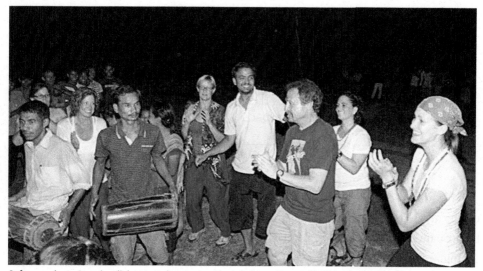

Before you know it, we're all dancing, clapping and loving every minute of it. Photo by Minling Chuang.

As quietly as they showed up, most of the villagers left the orphanage when the performance ended. A few of them stayed, wanting to meet these Americans who had travelled so far to come to their tiny little village. Their English was rudimentary at best, but their excitement and enthusiasm were plainly visible, even on this moonless night. They asked us questions, some of which had to be interpreted by Jesse or Basu. Were we rich? What kind of jobs did we have? How far had we traveled to get here? How long were we staying? That last question hung in the air like

203

a leaf blown from a tree, held aloft, against gravity, by a warm summer breeze. No one had the heart to tell the villager who'd ask that question that we were strongly considering leaving in the morning. One boy declared proudly that he wanted to become a movie director, like Steven Spielberg. He said it with such sincerity and conviction that my heart jumped. I had worked in Hollywood for many years, and I knew what a lofty dream that was. But in that instant, I really hoped that this young man's dream would come true. Finally, when all the questions had been asked, and most of them answered, the last of the villagers left, disappearing into the night as quietly as they had arrived.

By now, we were exhausted, dripping with sweat, and in great spirits. And then the Lawajuni girls called us to dinner. At this point, it was quite late, and I for one was actually growing tired of all the eating we'd been doing. Who wants to stuff themselves in this kind of intense heat this late at night, I grumbled to myself. I just wanted to go to bed. But the girls were so sweet and so eager, it was impossible to refuse.

June 25, 2010

The girls had lovingly prepared us dinner, and even though we were tired, we followed them into the kitchen and dining room and ate the meal they had prepared for us. It was a sign of respect.

Tingting Peng

We followed the girls around the back of the dorm building to the kitchen and dining area. The stove was a make-shift affair, more like a couple of hotplates heated by propane. There were several small long benches and tables, and the floor of the dining area was nothing more than packed dirt. But the food was delicious. I just shook my head as I ate. Is everyone in this country a good cook, I wondered, or are the ingredients they use just so fresh and tasty that anyone can whip up a simple, good meal? I got a little verklempt, to steal a phrase from Mike Myers on Saturday Night Live, just thinking about it. We were here to "feed" them — to serve them somehow — and here they were feeding us again. Amazing.

In the midst of our post dance feel-good buzz, we discussed delaying a decision about leaving early until the morning, to sleep on things. Jesse was clearly still stressed, and expressed it to those in the group who insisted on leaving. He thought it would be poor etiquette, even insulting, to leave early, and he would be very disappointed if we chose to go. This really upset some folks. They felt that Jesse was being self-righteous, and they expressed it. And just like that, our brief moment of harmony ended. It was very late though, and people were so tired that they didn't have the energy to provoke another major conflagration, for the time being anyway.

June 25, 2010

We decided to voice our concerns to Jesse, who became immediately defensive. He reminded us that we should be able to put ourselves in the lives of the Kamlari for two days, and that we can go "home" and they cannot.

He was very disappointed in us. He would not eat with us, or speak to us for the rest of the night. I wanted to try and resolve the differences between us, but Jesse said he needed some alone time. So we all went to bed, with the issue unresolved.

Gabrielle Stickley

Nothing was decided that night, and people were so utterly exhausted that they just drifted to their tents to try to get some sleep. From that point on, my own personal experience began to unravel, too. I changed into an old t-shirt and some running shorts to sleep, and entered the little tent I was to share with Dave. It was sweltering hot inside, just as I feared. When I lay down on the sleeping mat, sweat began to run down my back and puddle beneath me. I took my shirt off, put it back on, and took it off again. I started complaining, and David took out his little fan, the one which had amused the kids earlier in the day, and tried to hang it from the top of the tent to blow down on us. It had absolutely no effect at all. Finally, I just couldn't take it anymore.

Earlier that day, Marc had had an idea about sleeping in the empty classroom where we first had lunch. It was an open space with 10-foot high ceilings, windows on one side and a door on the other. I decided right then and there that I was going to try it. It had to be better than this tent. I picked up my sleeping mat and slipped my sandals on and headed across to the school building and up the stairs to the classroom. Dave came with me, but after a few moments lying on the concrete floor, he personally found it no more comfortable than the tent, so he took his mat and headed back down. I, however, had found respite. I rolled out my sleeping mat on the cool concrete floor, and pulled one of the large wicker mats we'd sat on at lunch over the top of it. This allowed any sweat coming off me to go through the wicker to the mat below thus keeping me relatively dry. The floor might've been hard, but between the sleeping mat and the wicker, I was fine. After a quick shot of bug spray, I rolled over and went happily to sleep.

A couple hours later, I was awakened by lightning flashes and thunder rumbling in the distance. I watched the lightning show through the open window. It was spectacular! Like a Fourth of July display put on by Mother Nature. The bright flashes and rolling thunder went on for about thirty minutes, as the storm drew closer, before it finally began to monsoon. It rained sheets and buckets, harder than anything I'd ever seen in my life, and I was so happy to be up here in my own room, nice and dry. The temperature dropped 20 degrees, too, and a cool breeze picked up as the rain continued. It was blissful. I even had to pull part of the wicker mat over me like a blanket, for warmth. A few minutes after the rain started, I heard the sound of voices coming up the stairs...

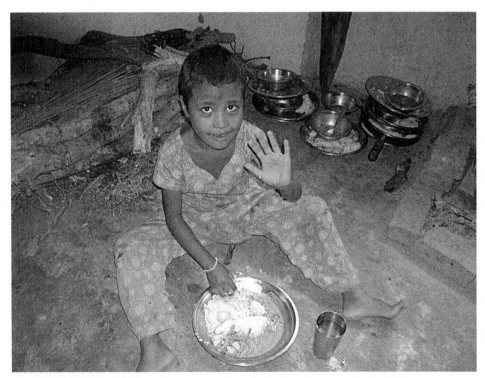

A late night dinner of green peppers, lentils and rice that the girls made for us in the "kitchen" behind the dormitory. Photo by Deanna Lee.

June 26, 2010 _____

... after the village dance party, we retreated to our tents. Kathy and I shared a tent. It was hot and muggy and we both wished there was a fan in the tent to help cool us down. The heat just seemed to be trapped inside and would not escape.

In the middle of the night, I heard thunder and it seemed... it would start to rain soon. Kathy and I made a decision to leave our tent and find shelter at the adjacent school where there was an empty classroom. We weren't sure if the tents would withstand the rain and didn't want to take a chance. So we tightly packed our luggage in the middle of the tent hoping that the middle wouldn't get wet and took our mattress to the classroom where we found John fast asleep. It was actually soothing to listen to the rainstorm as we slept in the classroom... the rain brought some much-needed coolness to the air.

_____ *Minling Chuang*

June 26, 2010

Day 7 of the trip

Leaving Narti

June 26, 2010 _____

We wake in our tents to the sound of rain, and it rains for hours. Each of us makes the mad dash to the outhouse, between the raindrops, retreating back to the tents, lickety split. What will happen today?

_____ ***Gabrielle Stickley***

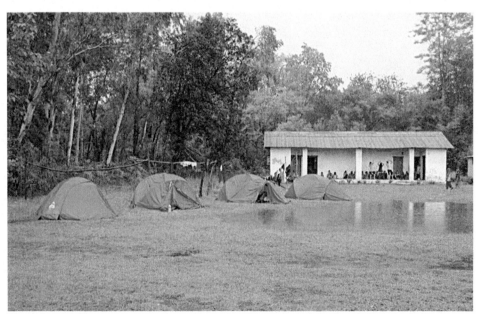

We awake to lake front property after the monsoon rains of the previous night. Photo by Christina Jankus.

June 26, 2010 _____

Somehow some way I fell asleep. I think I may have simply passed out. Even though I slept well I didn't feel right. The dread in me was building. I could already feel the regret over having to break our commitment to stay two nights. I do not like to disappoint people. It causes me a lot of stress.

_____ *Christina Jankus*

June 26, 2010 _____

When we woke up, we saw a huge lake near all the tents and it was only a few feet away from our tent. If Kathy and I [had] stayed, we would have had lakeside property. Kathy and I knew that this rainstorm would seal the deal on our early departure.

The group never came to a resolution the night before, but we knew people would not want to go through another heavy rainstorm in the tents. This thought saddened both of us.

_____ *Minling Chuang*

We awoke around 7 a.m. feeling a little better. We ate (again!) and then had another serious meeting. Those in favor of leaving were still adamant about doing so. I was torn between staying and leaving. I could've toughed out another day and night, I'm sure, but I didn't want any of the others to be completely miserable. There would be no joy in that for me. It was clear now that there was no happy resolution to this problem, so Jesse made an executive decision: he would arrange for us to move on to Chitwan, despite his own, and several others, hurt feelings.

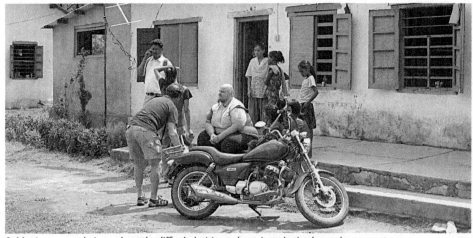

Robb tries to console Jesse about the difficult decision to leave Lawajuni a day early.

209

Jesse and Basu began making the arrangements to leave. The decision to leave seemed to lighten the atmosphere almost immediately. We would have a very light yoga practice and then still have 2 ½ hours of playtime with the girls. Subash led us in some breathing exercises, and then everyone dove into having fun with the girls, and helping out with whatever minor chores we could find. A few of us, led by Robb and Marc, began moving the trees and branches that had been cut down near the backhoe to clear a space for what we found out was going to be a new dorm building.

June 26, 2010 _____

Someone found a scorpion which was a nice temporary distraction. A bright point in my day was the sight of a tiny girl holding the cardinal she received the day before. She brought it with her everywhere. I beamed as I brought the unwanted Beanie Babies from friends and family members and little cutie could not part with it. So precious!

_____ *Christina Jankus*

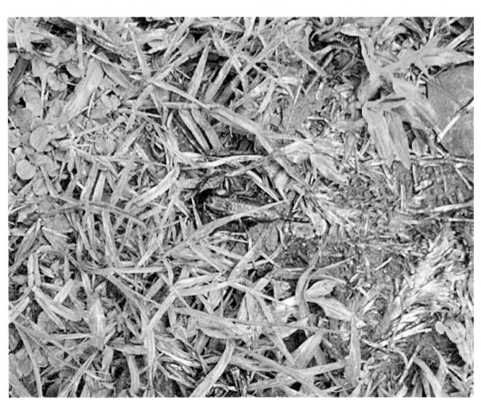

A black scorpion. Apparently not uncommon in these parts. Photo by Christina Jankus.

At one point, as we were clearing the cut-down trees, Gabby got a nasty scratch on the top of her foot. She sat down on the porch outside the girls' dorm to tend to it, when the oldest girl, Dita, came out carrying a bottle of iodine, some gauze and a pair of long-nosed scissors. In no time, she had Gabby's cut disinfected and bandaged. I was impressed at how professional she had been in going about it, and told Dita she would make a fine nurse, or a fine doctor, some day. Her English, it turned out, was quite good, and she beamed with pride, having completely understood me.

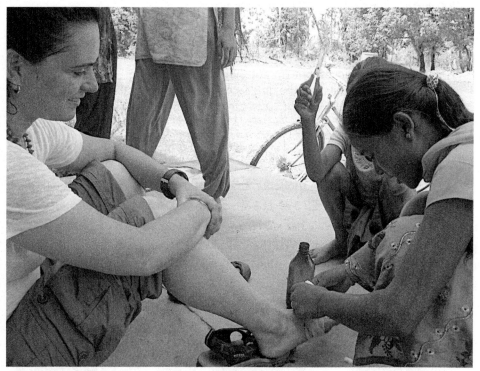

Gabby receives health care, Lawajuni style, from one of the older girls.

June 26, 2010

When we got [here], we didn't know what to do with the girls. Our brains were tapped out of ideas on games we could explain and play with the language barrier. Somehow, we ended up having one of the girls teach us a few Nepalese dances. She was a really good dancer and I was trying my best to follow along. Think the girls liked watching me stumble my way through the complicated steps and sequences. Don't get me wrong, I love to dance, but only freestyle because when it comes to following steps I have 2 left feet. At one point I even tripped on the foot of one of the girls watching and fell over. The girls got a good laugh out of it and we were having a great time! Whenever I got close to one of the girls sitting on the floor watching the performance, she would automatically move back in fear I would trip and fall again.

The time we spent with the girls this morning was precious. Soon after hanging out with the girls on the porch, Jesse decided that we should move on to Chitwan because...the group was falling apart and people were upset at each other because some people wanted to stay and others wanted to go. Logistically it would have been too challenging to separate, as we were 6+ hours away from Chitwan... Kathy had to leave the group for a bit and when she returned she told us that the girls asked her, "Are the Americans leaving?" It broke my heart to hear this and how the girls would be affected. By then it was too late and the decision had been made.

The girls trickled into the room where we practiced yoga and we showed them some more yoga moves – wheel, handstands, acro-yoga and many more poses. They also taught us some more Nepalese dance moves. I wish I could say that I'll remember the moves, but I'm not that good of a dancer. But what I will remember are the smiles on the girls' faces and how happy they were in that moment.

Minling Chuang

As our guides packed up the tents, some of the girls became emotional. One child, an almond-eyed girl of 10 or 11 with a round face and big cheeks, had tears in her eyes, so I tried to make her smile. Somehow I managed to. Her English was pretty good. We laughed and joked. Then she drew a big heart in the dirt and wrote the words "I Love You" inside. I swallowed the big lump in my throat and kissed her hand. She just beamed at me.

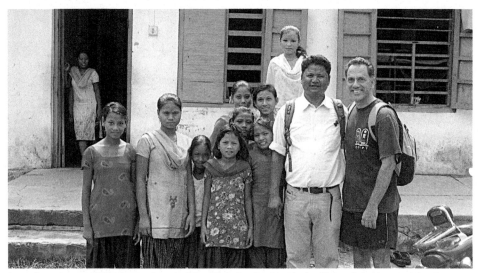

I pose for a picture with Krishna and some of the girls before leaving. He was disappointed by our early exit.

I also made friends with one of the littlest girls there. Her hair was cut very short. She was small, maybe 4 or 5 years old. Her eyes and spirit reminded me of my sister at that age, and I was immediately drawn to her. She was very reserved with me at first, but I drew her out, playing a little game. "My name is John. Very nice to meet you! What is your name?" I said, holding out my hand, and then tickling her hand when she took mine. She smiled wide, and then tickled my hand and started to laugh. Seeing her laugh and smile made me as happy as I'd been the whole time we were in Narti.

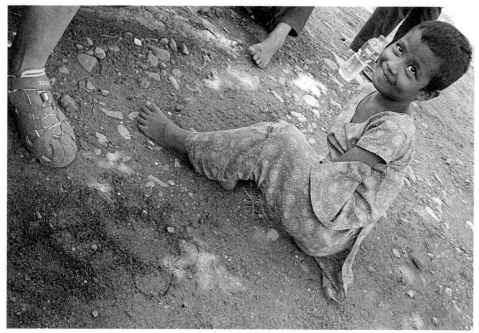

One of our favorite little ones, smiling shyly after drawing a flower in the dirt for us.

Then I noticed another girl standing alone, wearing a worn school uniform — light blue shirt, black dress, knee high stockings — leaning against the wall of the dormitory building. I'd seen her the day before, and she hadn't smiled once. I wondered if she was just shy, or if she'd been traumatized in some way. I was afraid to find out. And afraid if I went right up to her and played the little game I had just played with the other little girl, I might scare her. Then I saw Gabby sitting on the stoop next to the girl. I asked Gabby to ask the little girl what her name was. Gabby looked at the girl, then back at me. I nodded. Then Gabby leaned over and softly asked the young girl her name. At first, she didn't seem to respond, but when Gabby asked again, it was clear she had said something, just very softly. She repeated her answer very softly. Gabby repeated what the little girl had said, trying to confirm the name the girl had whispered.[10] The young girl nodded. Gabby smiled and took her hand. "Hello," she said, then repeated her name. "I'm Gabrielle." Just like that a light went on inside that little girl, and she smiled from ear to ear, a smile as bright as the noontime sun in Narti. The transformation was dazzling, incandescent, unforgettably beautiful.

I walked over to where this little girl and Gabby were, and played the same game with her that I'd played with the other little girl. "My name is John. Very nice to meet you! What is your name?" Then I shook her hand too, and she smiled that most incredible smile again. Her whole demeanor changed, as if someone had turned on a happy switch. I was over the moon with joy seeing her flash that amazing smile. Very pleased with my success, I played this little game with as many kids as I could, and we all got a kick out of it.

Then I got another idea. The day before, I had watched Jesse and Jaime sing songs back and forth with the girls, Jesse and Jaime in English, the girls in Nepali. So I asked the girls to sing a song for me. They did, singing something in Nepali, and then they asked me to sing one for them. The only thing I could think of was "On Top of Old Smokey." So that's what they got. They had no idea what I was singing, but they somehow understood it was a goofy song, and laughed and clapped when I was finished. Then I started to teach them to write words on the ground with a stick. Of course, they quickly grabbed the stick and began to show me all the English words they knew how to spell. They could write their names. I was impressed. Some girls were a little too young to be spelling, so one of them drew a flower in the dirt. It was beautiful.

Just before noon, we were called to lunch. Another feast of hot white rice, potatoes and peppers, and a truly excellent lentil/pea soup, all prepared by the girls. By then the bus had been finally packed up and it was ready to roll. A few people began to say goodbye, and the girls, especially the almond-eyed 10 year old, became emotional again. Sometimes when goodbyes get emotional, I have this flash to an old British World War II song by Vera Lynn that my mom would sometimes sing. "We'll Meet Again…" I asked Basu how to say, "Until we meet again," in Nepali. Peri betola, he told me. So I started saying it to everyone. It became a game. Instead of saying goodbye, we said peri betola. Until we meet again…

---

[10] *We were asked by NOH not to use any of the children's real names, either at NOH or Lawajuni.*

One of the most touching things I witnessed on the trip was here. The kids at this orphanage had been the most newly rescued from slavery and at first they were so shy and timid. It was hard to communicate with them at first but we started playing games to bridge the communication gap. We learned a Nepalese dance and taught them American songs, taught them some yoga and played games. To see these girls open up to us and connect with us after the things that some of them had just been through was touching, and by the time we left we seemed to have gotten so close. The goodbyes were filled with hugs and "I love you sisters…"

Deanna Lee

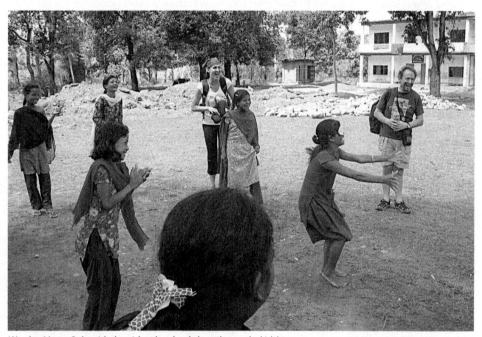

We play Marco Polo with the girls, who clearly love the wacky kids' game.

Meanwhile, the others were playing some fun games like Marco Polo with the girls. It seemed everyone was having a fantastic time.

June 26, 2010

As the bus got loaded with our gear, we said our goodbyes. The girls took some of our cameras and started taking pictures of all of us and themselves. They would motion us to gather around and take our pictures. We continued to play games up until we left. The most popular game was Marco Polo. We gave the girls blindfolds and they had a blast at trying to find an unsuspecting person to become the next Marco Polo player and teasing the current player.

When it was time to leave, I became very emotional. We walked from the orphanage to the road to get on the bus. As we walked, the girls clung onto us. At one point, I think I had about four girls holding onto some part of me during the walk. The look in their eyes turned from excitement and joy to sorrow. It was heartbreaking to say goodbye. They'd ask, "Auntie, are you coming back?" I didn't know what to tell them. I want to come back to Nepal, but not sure if I'd be back to Narti. I didn't want to tell them yes or no and just smiled and hugged them. Why did we have to leave? I kept on thinking. These girls just wanted our love. I hugged them goodbye and one girl pulled me over and gave me a kiss on the cheek. Then she started sobbing. I cried as I left them and when I turned around to give one final wave, they waved goodbye [back] and soon we were gone.

_____ **Minling Chuang**

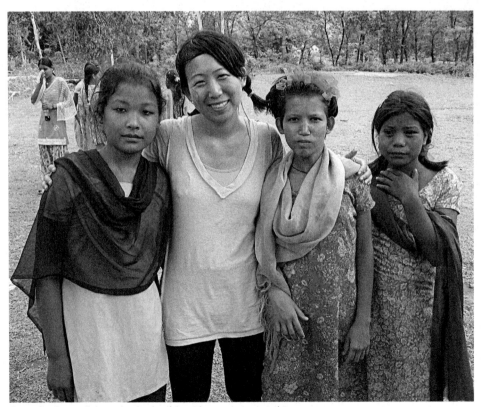

Tears of sadness roll down the cheeks of the girls as we prepare to leave.

The girls took our hands and walked us to the road where we boarded our bus. I hugged each of them, not wanting to let go and leave. One of them pulled me to her and gave me a big kiss on the cheek. It was an incredible sight to see them all waving to us as our bus pulled away. I did not want to leave!!

_____ ***Tingting Peng***

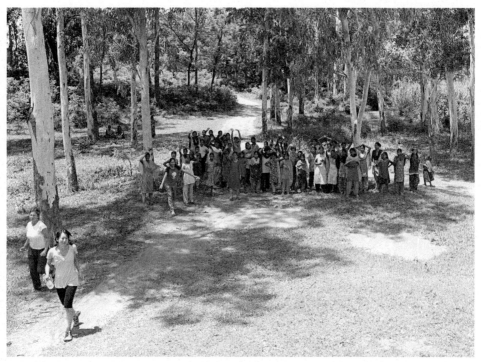

Minling and Terri race to catch the bus as the girls of Lawajuni wave goodbye and shout Peri Betola — Until We Meet Again.

When the bus cleared the ditch in the dirt road from the orphanage and was back on the main road out of Narti, we dragged our stinking, sweaty, tired but content bodies onto it, revived by the air-conditioning. And as the girls waved goodbye to us, we shouted back, "Peri betola!"

We'll Meet Again[11]

We'll meet again, don't know where, don't know when

But I'm sure we'll meet again some sunny day

---
[11] *Music and lyrics by Ross Parker and Hughie Charles.*

Keep smiling through, just the way you used to do
Till the blue skies chase the dark clouds far away

Now, won't you please say "Hello" to the folks that I know
Tell 'em it won't be long
'cause they'd be happy to know that when you saw me go
I was singing this song

We'll meet again, don't know where, don't know when
But I'm sure we'll meet again some sunny day...

June 26, 2010

Day 7 of the trip, cont'd

Chitwan National Park

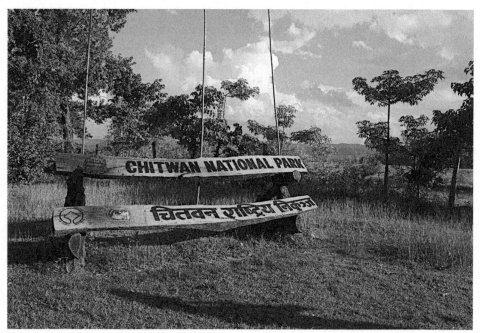

The entrance to Chitwan National Park in the lowland jungles of south central Nepal. Photo by Minling Chuang.

On the way out of Narti, Jesse had scheduled a stop for us at the headquarters of SWAN to hear a talk on what their organization was doing. Krishna, who worked with SWAN, was expected to give the lecture. When we arrived there, we were ushered into a small, air-conditioned room, and the twenty of us sat cross-legged on the floor. Charlie and another SWAN associate arrived, and together they conducted the PowerPoint presentation instead, which turned out to be very informative.

June 26, 2010 _____

The presentation about SWAN and the Kamlari system was interesting. SWAN focuses on not only rescuing the girls, but also [on educating] the locals about the Kamlari system and works with the locals to develop sustainable sources of income. Most of the girls sold are from poor families. Charlie, a board member of SWAN and the local principal, was a Kamlari himself and presented the information with so much passion and love for the cause. I'm so glad that there are so many locals who are taking up this cause and creating a better future for their country.

_____ *Minling Chuang*

It was quite hot outside when we boarded the bus around 1 p.m. and headed east for the next stop in our itinerary. Some people read, some slept, others had their iPods and headphones. One thing that did lighten the mood was Kathy and her bottomless bag of goodies. Every time someone needed something, Kathy invariably produced it from this oversized purse of a bag she was carrying with her. Hand sanitizer, Kleenex, toilet paper, gum, candy, cookies, bandages; she had all of it in there, and amazingly she never seemed to run out of anything. Pretty soon we all learned to just ask Kathy for whatever we needed.

June 26, 2010 _____

The bus ride was much more subdued than our first ride, no singing contest for sure. I couldn't tell if people were tired, upset, or just wanted a break. All I know is I was tired and ready to get to our next destination.

_____ *Minling Chuang*

Our next destination was the Hotel Parkland, a small hotel & resort just on the outskirts of Chitwan National Park. Chitwan is one of the finest national parks in all of Asia. It lies in the lowlands of south-central Nepal, covering an area of about 900 square kilometers and has been listed a World Heritage site since the early 1980's. It's renowned for its wildlife, and is home to such endangered species as the Royal Bengal Tiger, the one-horned Rhinoceros, and the Sloth Bear, as well as monkeys, elephants, Asian deer, crocodiles, many varieties of insects and butterflies, over 500 species of colorful birds, and a wide variety of plant-life.[12]

---
[12] source: wikipedia.com

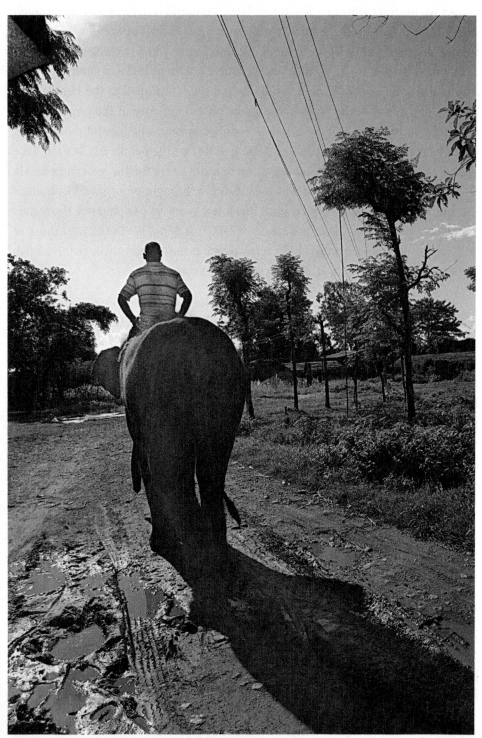

Typical transportation in Chitwan. Photo by Minling Chuang.

As we neared Chitwan a few hours later, we found ourselves driving through a sub-tropical forest. The people we saw from the windows of the bus looked different from the folks in Narti. Before I came to Nepal, I hadn't realized how many different ethnicities make up the country. There are literally dozens and dozens of different peoples, from the Sherpa who live in the Himalayas, to the Humla who live in the northwest, the Newar who make up the majority of the population in the Kathmandu valley, and the Tharu, 1.5 million strong, who inhabit the lowland, jungle-covered south of the country. Jesse told us that the people in Chitwan were Tharu, and that they ran the park and surrounding area for the government. He also reminded us that Chitwan was the reason we brought bug spray. Mosquitoes and malaria were a real problem until just a few years ago, wiping out thousands of people a year before the introduction of DDT spraying. We in the west think of DDT as the toxic destroyer of bald eagles, which it most certainly is, but in Nepal, and especially in Chitwan, DDT is literally a life saver.

We traveled through a small town to get to the hotel, where Jesse said we could shop during the day, and eat and drink at night. He said it was frequented by tourists from all over the world who came to camp and hike in Chitwan. On the road in, we saw a man riding an elephant, and another riding a camel. And all around farmers were planting rice in water-filled paddies. When we finally arrived at the Parkland, we exited the bus with our belongings and were led to a series of little two-story bungalows where the guests of this lodge were housed. The bungalows surrounded a central courtyard with several gazebos in it, one of which housed a small bar.

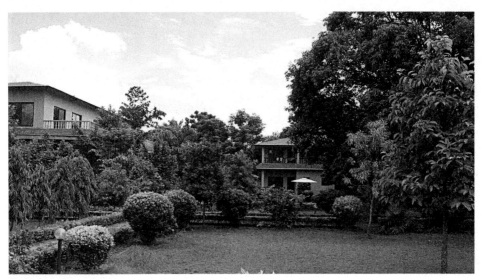

The Hotel Parkland in Chitwan.

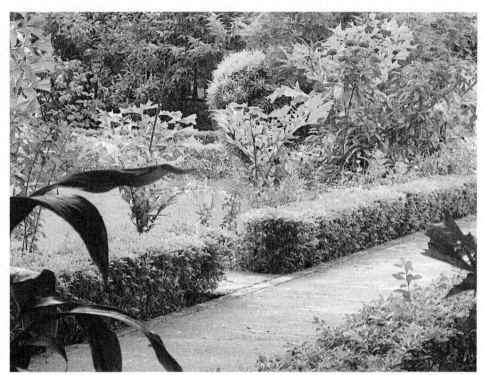
Like the Grand Norling, the Parkland excelled in simple, yet elegant landscaping.

As we checked out the accommodations, it was easy to see that everyone was really pleased. Not surprising, since the Parkland was luxurious compared to where we'd stay in Lumbini and Narti. The landscaping around the resort was gorgeous.

The rooms were small but pleasant, with beds, fans, AC, a TV, a dresser and large wardrobe, and very nice bathrooms with showers, which we all took immediate advantage of…

June 26, 2010_____

It's funny, even though I wanted to stay in Narti longer, I was not terribly upset that we were headed to a resort. After 2 days of not showering (and the rainfall didn't count as a shower), I probably smelled awful! At least everyone else was in the same boat and we all smelled together. After our first shower in Chitwan, Robb said it was the best shower he ever had and it's one that he'd always remember! LOL! The simplest things make us happy!

_____ ***Minling Chuang***

After showering we gathered in the dining hall and had a fantastic meal on the veranda in front of the hall. The weather was warm and humid, but not unpleasantly hot, and there was a soft breeze blowing outside. The food was once again fresh, hot and delicious. The conversation as we ate was subdued, but much of the tension of the previous day had disappeared, at least on the surface.

June 26, 2010

It is Saturday, halfway through our journey and we've just arrived at Chitwan National Park. What a difference 24 hours can make. I think some of us were so excited to see elephants that they've sort of forgotten that we had just been camping on the grounds of an orphanage only 12 hours earlier. This begs the question, why am I here? Why are the others here? Why are we each individually here? For some, their reasons were not compelling enough to overcome spending one more night of "roughing it". For me, I am feeling a tremendous sense of sadness at leaving the Lawajuni girls a day sooner than planned. I am here for an experience, whatever that may be, and honestly, I feel robbed of the full experience right now.

_____ *Tingting Peng*

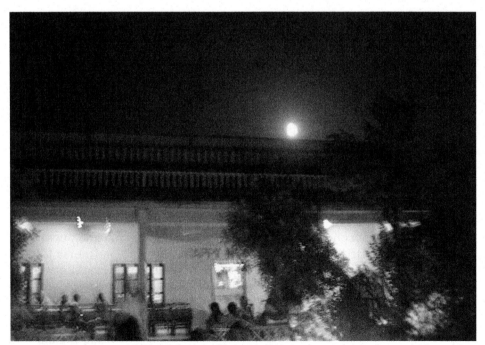

Dining on the patio under a full moon at the Hotel Parkland in Chitwan. Photo by Deanna Lee.

We were all exhausted by the time dinner was finished, and some of the group called it an early night. The rest of us gathered under the gazebo and made small talk for a while, then drifted away to our rooms for a much needed good night's sleep. David and I, who were both big soccer fans, tried to find the World Cup on TV, but just as we figured out which channel, the power went out. It seemed a sign from the Nepali gods that it was time for us to crash for the night, too. As I lay in bed, the fan running on genie power, quietly whirring above my head, I wondered what adventures, and what drama, tomorrow might bring.

June 26, 2010

We hold onto fear, because no matter how bad or scary that fear is, we know it, [we're] familiar with it…. I had many fears about this trip. Many were informed by others, yet none of them have materialized.

Terri Bahr

June 27, 2010

Day 8 of the trip

Chitwan

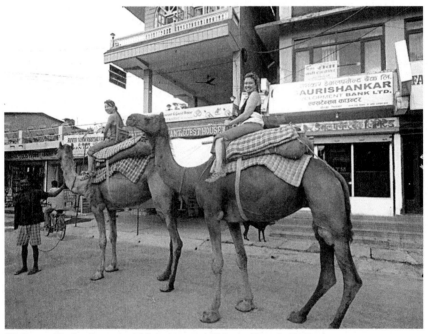

Minling and Terri go for a camel ride in downtown Chitwan. Photo by Eve Ennis.

June 27, 2010 _____

Chitwan was a stark contrast to Narti and the conditions we faced there. It felt like a vacation. I felt a bit guilty that I liked Chitwan, especially because we left Narti early to come to this resort. It's really hard to give up what is comfortable and the pleasures we enjoy in America (a comfortable bed; bathroom with shower, toilet and sink; fan or A/C, delicious meals). I'm definitely living it up over these next few days and enjoying the moment of being here. I guess I still feel a little torn between two worlds. We came to help orphans and now we are living in such nice conditions and indulging. Is it wrong to indulge on this trip?

**Minling Chuang**

We woke up early and practiced yoga with Subash in a large room above the dining hall. The room was spacious, and it was drizzling this morning, so it wasn't nearly as hot as in Narti, but it was humid. We were covered in sweat by the end of 90 minutes. The great thing about practicing every day, often twice a day on this trip, was that my practice was improving so much. I was becoming more flexible, able to do full binds far more easily than I thought I ever could. My body felt great. The other good thing about the regular practices was that it forced the group to be a group. We had to come together to practice as a group even if the day before we'd been arguing and falling apart. Simply aligning our breathing, which happens almost naturally in a large yoga class, was helping to bring us back in harmony, at least for a while.

June 27, 2010

We were staying at a beautiful resort in Chitwan. I roomed with Tingting, and Joyce had her own as there were an odd number of women. When I got to our room the first thing I did was look in the mirror as I had not seen myself in several days. What I saw was quite shocking – so tan!

…I felt myself relax into this day as I felt the worst emotions were over. It seemed everything was back to normal -- although I did not see Jesse around as much.

**Christina Jankus**

After yoga practice, I grabbed a quick shower, followed by a delicious breakfast on the veranda. The highlight of almost every meal on the trip so far, but especially the meals in Chitwan, was the Nepali potatoes. For breakfast they were served home-fry style. I don't know if it was because they were different from the Idaho and Russet potatoes we're used to in the U.S., or if it was because they were organic and fresh from the market, or if it was how they were cooked, but Nepali potatoes are the best damned potatoes I've ever tasted in my life. Marc and I had a long conversation over breakfast in praise of the Nepali potato. Our conclusion: If the government can get its act together, the first thing they should start doing is exporting these potatoes. The country would be rich in no time, we both agreed.

After filling ourselves with potatoes, eggs, bread and butter with jam, and several cups of tea, Jesse gave us the itinerary for the day. A park guide named Hari, who also happened to run the Hotel Parkland, would lead us on a canoe ride down a nearby river that flowed through the heart of Chitwan. Hari promised us a great time, and said if we were very lucky, we might even see some of the famous local wildlife. Excited at the prospect, we gathered in the central gazebo, and Hari led us on a hike down to the river. As we walked through the back streets of the village, we had a good look at how people lived here. Things were far simpler than in Kathmandu, but the conditions were much better than in Narti. Some homes were quite nice, others more rustic or primitive. Most homes had their own chickens, some also had goats, and a few apparently even had their own elephants. The droppings were like bowling balls dotting the road. Given their size, it was easy not to step in them, at least in the daytime.

As we hiked, we saw dozens of farmers out in the rice paddies doing the backbreaking work of planting rice. If you've never seen rice planted before, it's the most labor intensive thing this side of picking cotton. Each rice plant is individually planted in the wet soil, which is itself covered with several inches of water. The plants are tended by hand through the entire growing season, and then picked by hand when ready. The rice is then harvested and dried, and the kernels removed from the husk, which I'm pretty sure in Nepal is also done by hand.

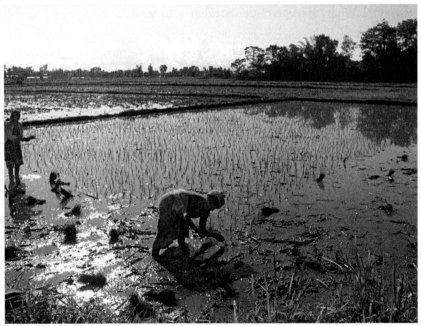

The backbreaking, painstaking, utterly essential work of planting rice in the paddies. Photo by Terri Bahr.

All of Asia is dependent on the harvest, since rice is a daily staple of the diet there. That's over four billion people. A good harvest means good times and full bellies. A bad harvest can mean hunger for millions, and for many starvation or death. Watching the farmers working the fields, I had a sudden feeling of how incredibly important they were, each and every one of them was, not only to their community, but to the whole of Asia.

The hike to the river also gave me a sense of the magnificent beauty of Chitwan. I said a silent thank you to Jesse and Basu for putting this place on the itinerary. When we reached the river, three or four very long, very shallow wooden dugout canoes were waiting for us. Hari was joined by several park associates who guided us all into the canoes docked on the riverbank. It was a bit like walking a tightrope to get to the back of the canoe and take a seat without losing your balance and falling into the river. As we took our seats, each person was no more than a foot in front of the next person. And we were all no more than six inches above the waterline. That's when Hari started to talk about crocodiles.

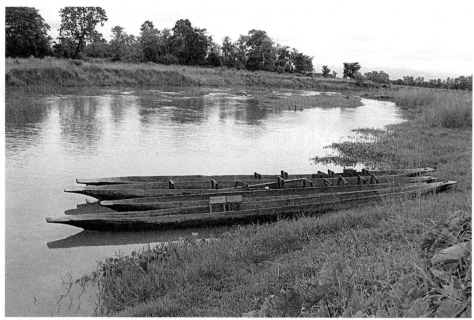

Our canoes await us. And so does one remarkably big pachyderm.

The river, he told us, was full of crocodiles. Don't dangle your hands in the water, he cautioned us. And keep an eye out. The crocs weren't that easy to spot as 99% of their bodies were underwater, keeping cool. Only their eyes and nostrils poked above the surface. Wow, I thought. Sounds like we're going on a Mutual of Omaha's Wild Kingdom expedition with Marlin Perkins. How cool is that!? We were all psyched, excited and a little nervous. Tigers, and rhinos, and crocodiles were out there, and we were actually hoping to see them up close...

June 27, 2010

I love Chitwan! Chitwan is so beautiful and serene!

Today we went on a canoe ride down the river to see crocodiles. We sat in these tiny canoes that fit 8 of us in a row. I was so afraid that we were going to tip over that any sudden move was felt. But, the breathtaking views more than made up for my fears of falling overboard and being eaten by crocodiles. We didn't see many crocodiles. And the ones we did see, they only showed the tips of their heads and their eyes. Maybe they were a little shy.

Minling Chuang

The initial part of the canoe trip was serene. The sound of the water gently lapping past the canoe as we glided across the surface of the river, the warm sun on our faces and the cool morning breeze — it all felt very Zen-like out there in the jungles of Chitwan...

June 27, 2010

This country is like a picture postcard. It is filled with faces, homes, animals, mountains, clouds, valleys, and urban and rural settings. Fantastic! And the other thing about Nepal is the heat! Wow! Every time one steps outside it's more sweat. Crazy hot!

Marc Nathanson

As we made our way downstream, though, things suddenly became very interesting...

June 27, 2010

Being on the river was so relaxing and peaceful. That is until we saw a rhino eating its breakfast next to the river. I've never seen a real rhino in the wild before (and the San Diego Zoo does not count). The rhino was spectacular! It was huge and thanks to binoculars, we could see the many layers of skin it had and the pointy horn.

Minling Chuang

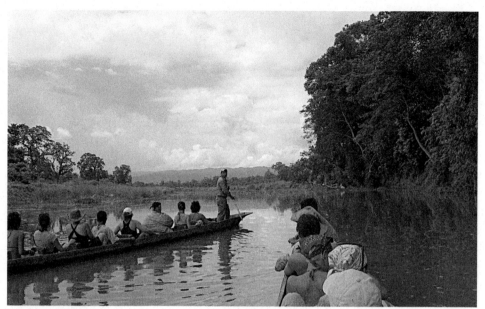
Our guide Hari stops the canoes along the riverbank. He's spotted something on the far shore.

It wasn't only Minling; none of us had ever seen a rhinoceros in the wild before. And here we were looking at one less than a hundred yards away, on the other side of the river. This creature was huge! The size of a Volkswagen bus. Its thick grey skin hung on it like armor on a medieval knight. We had seen water buffalo grazing on the way to the canoes, but this beast made them look small, even dainty, by comparison. As this giant behemoth munched away on the marsh grass that grew along the riverbank, Hari whispered to us to keep very quiet. Rhinos have poor eyesight, but excellent hearing. And they can be very aggressive, Hari warned... If overly agitated, the rhino could charge us and ram our boats, as the water here was shallow enough for it to cross.

June 27, 2010 _____

Wow, could a rhino really ram our boat? I definitely did not want to find out. Neither did one of the boat guides because he climbed a tree and scrambled up the embankment. Was he really that scared? Would the rhino come after us? I told Tingting that if the rhino made his move our exit route would be the same as the boat guide. Every woman (or man) for herself (or himself)!

_____ ***Minling Chuang***

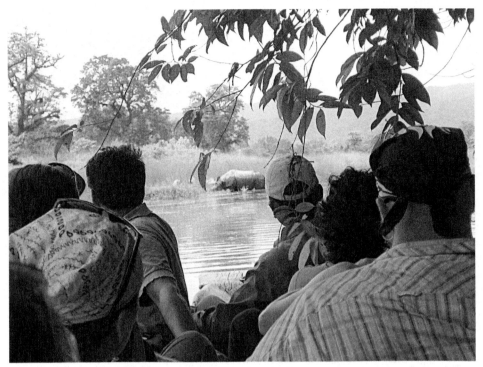

Rhinoceros! Front and Center!

Hari and the other oarsmen backed the canoes upstream a bit and docked them along a mud cliff on the other side of the river. He again motioned to all of us to keep quiet. Of course, this brought out the wisecrackers among us, with Robb leading the way teasing the women. Basu seemed to get a huge kick out of our nervousness, especially when his cell phone rang loudly right then and there. He answered it quietly as the women in the canoes admonished him to keep silent. Their anxiety only grew when one of the park guides suddenly climbed out of the back of one of the canoes, grabbed hold of some dangling tree roots, and scrambled quickly up the side of the dirt cliff where we had nestled the canoe. At first, some of us thought he was scared, but when he returned moments later, we found out that he'd just gone on a little bathroom break. I stifled a laugh so as not get anyone else worked up with my noise.

We quietly snapped pictures and video of the big pachyderm for a good 15 minutes, softly whispering our ooh's and aah's while the rhino made its way slowly through the long grass. At one point, it stood up on the riverbank to find a better spot to eat, and we realized that it was actually twice as big as it had seemed. Like some kind of giant grey iceberg, an iceberg with a horn, more than half of its body had been hidden underwater. After filling up on morning greens, our big grey friend finally lumbered out of the water and disappeared into the jungle.

When the rhino was gone, Hari signaled the oarsmen, and we shoved off from the far bank and headed down river to finish our canoe trip, loudly talking about what we'd just been so privileged to see. We docked about a half-mile downstream, clambered out of the dugouts, and hiked back to where we'd begun our morning sojourn. On the way back, we saw more water buffalo, but they were yesterday's news. All the talk was about the rhino. Seeing that magnificent creature, an endangered species, an animal that harkens back to the era of the dinosaurs, was one of the coolest things I've ever experienced in my life. I was even more elated than before that I had come on this amazing trip.

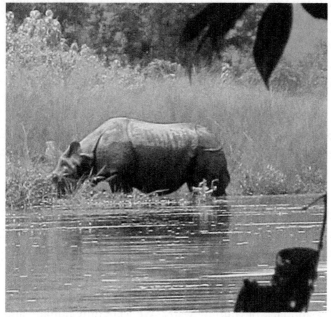

Rhinoceros grazing on elephant grass on the riverbank. Photo by Kathy Hayes.

Back at the Parkland, we grabbed lunch, and then gathered under one of the gazebos for a group meditation. Jesse, who had been very quiet, almost solitary the whole day, finally spoke. He said he needed to get some things off his chest about Narti. He wanted us all to know how disappointed he still was that we left there a day early. He felt like we'd all been selfish, and self-centered, and had not considered the feelings of the girls at Lawajuni, or of Krishna, in making our decision to leave. He told us that we had insulted Krishna and that he was certain that he'd lost a friend in him because of our decision to leave. He said he took full responsibility for all this, as he was the leader of the group, but he just had to get this off his chest. He went on venting for about five minutes, and it was plain to see that he meant every word he was saying.

When he was done, he asked if anyone had anything to say. You bet they did. The one thing I learned about the folks on this trip was that they were not afraid to express themselves. The floodgates opened, and Jesse got an earful. Two ears full. And it was not pretty. He was chastised by various members of the group for being self-righteous, for being unprepared, and for being a poor communicator and a lousy planner, and for not taking the issue of women's safety seriously — an issue that several of the women took very personally and for very personal reasons. The majority of the people on this trip were women and they lambasted Jesse for presuming that he understood more about the plight of girls in the world than they did. The whole thing felt like a volcanic eruption of bile, like the lancing of an angry, festering boil. Though a few people did try to see Jesse's side, suffice it to say, this was not our finest hour as a group. I could only hope that maybe by airing it all out here, in a safe environment, we might learn something as a group, and finally be able to move on.

When the opportunity for me to speak came around, I hesitated. I had no desire to criticize Jesse further. I said that Jesse had found himself in a very difficult position in Narti. We had left abruptly and early, from the place that Krishna and the Lawajuni girls called home. I told Jesse that I hoped that in time, when he returned to Narti, he would be able to sit down and better explain to Krishna what had happened, and to repair that friendship. I also told him that although he had undertaken a very noble task in bringing us here, and that it had been an amazing experience for me personally so far, better planning could have helped on the Narti part of the journey. All the good intentions of taking us there to witness what it was like for the orphans who lived in Lawajuni, no matter how noble, could not combat the intense heat and lack of running water. We were only human, and we weren't used to those extreme conditions. It probably takes months, if not years, to get used to them. Given everything that happened, I thought ultimately that Jesse had made the best decision he could at the time, and I told him he still had my support.

By the time we had all finished speaking, it seemed that the steam had gone out of the conflict. A few folks expressed that this was a good learning experience for the trip as a whole, this being the very first Yoga For Freedom trip, and that the goal should be to improve things for the next time. On that point I think we all agreed. Finally, as a way to get past this whole incident, as a way to gain some catharsis, Jesse asked us to take out our journals and write about what happened in Narti. Most of us took him up on that:

Journaling Exercise:

What Happened At Narti?

June 27, 2010 _____

In Narti I watched people confronted with life, with reality; fear it and run away. Everyone is angry with me for saying it…They were asked to spend two days in tents and live on the grounds of an orphanage. They knew it was coming, I guess it was too hard for them. I shouldn't have asked them to do it. I knew they would have difficulty with this. Most of them are extremely angry that I suggested that they disrespected our hosts.

I feel so alone right now.

_____ *Jesse Bach*

June 27, 2010 _____

What happened in Narti? Tough question… I just listened to Jesse give a talk on disrespecting the people who hosted us. Jesse talked of fear. I had no fear (personal danger). My only reason for wanting to leave a few hours earlier… was [because I was] unable to sleep or even get rest in a tent and on a plastic mat that pulled the fluids from my body. Twice I tried seated meditation to find rest but to no avail… It was totally unintentional. We all gave a lot unselfishly because we wanted to, but the extreme conditions made rest and personal health an issue, not disrespect.

_____ *Robb Blain*

June 27, 2010 _____

I agree that it was important to witness the girls at [Lawajuni], but I also think that we would have had an understanding of them, if we had been brought there. If we had the chance to meet the girls, and had a complete explanation of these girls' lives, prior to arriving there, we could try to understand what they had gone through. An agenda for between lunch and bedtime would help, so we could know what to expect, and what was expected of us.

I felt we were told to stay upstairs after lunch until 4:00 or 5:00, just to "take a rest." Then it just unraveled from there. How could we have known what to expect, or what was expected of us, if no one told us? [Narti] began with no real agenda, or no explanation. I think most of us went into it with no expectation, but it felt like we were just wandering.

We didn't know how safe it was. We didn't know who the "villagers" were when they started arriving. It was hot, with no access to running water. We are all on this trip because we care about helping the girls. I think we helped more in the last two hours we were there, than all of the rest of the time spent. Because we gave it our full attention, and with honest feeling! But when we expressed the feeling that this was too much, and wanted to go, we were told that the girls have suffered, and still are. We can't even suffer for two days. It makes no sense.

Putting the group into that environment, especially without the information of what to expect (or what was expected of us) was not about facing our fears... We did our best with what we were given. I think especially that this is the first trip, and none of us knows what works and what doesn't. That is what it is about, right? Finding out what works to pave the way for the future groups.

Again, we all want to help. That is why we are here. But as the leader of the group, it is Jesse's job to listen and be open to change, if things aren't working. We were extremely uncomfortable there. We shouldn't have been there for two days and nights. It was too much. So when that began to show, we expressed our feelings. I'm sad that Jesse took it personally. It wasn't. It just wasn't working out the way it was planned.

Terri Bahr

___

June 27, 2010

The journaling exercise today was about Narti and what happened there. Jesse clearly is not over the entire situation and started off the journaling exercise by telling us that we disrespected the people for leaving early... I don't know what to think. Do I feel guilty? Yes, of course. I feel so guilty for leaving those girls, especially since I didn't want to leave. Am I going to not enjoy the lovely resort we are so fortunate enough to be in? No. At this point, what's done is done and we can't turn back. We can only reflect and move forward. So I'm going to reflect on what happened.

In my opinion, Narti was when people on the trip hit a wall [of] what they believed they were capable of coping with. It was a situation where people weren't prepared for the extreme conditions they were facing – living inside of a tent under the roasting sun, no running water, a language barrier with the kids.

Were we ill-prepared for this or were we in our own heads and just making up excuses to get out of a place that tested our limits? People started to rally against staying in the village another night when they started to feel uncomfortable and at the outer boundary of their limits. Fear came over people... fear of the unknown. People also didn't want to feel discomfort from a physical standpoint because it wasn't what they signed up for. I really think that people just butt up against their own inner fear and chose to go back to what is comfortable.

What puzzles me is that we came here for the kids. Don't people remember that? Why couldn't people get past their own issues to be with the kids? What really gets me is that people were complaining about not spending enough time with the kids in Kathmandu and when they have this great opportunity to be with the girls at Narti, they bail. Maybe this experience is showing us what we could handle or were willing to handle. They are totally missing that piece and not handling what's coming their way. As the saying goes, "When the going gets tough, the tough get going."

Or maybe what happened in Narti was because people's expectations of the trip were not met. I know I had the trip occurring a certain way in my head, but was open to the idea of things shifting and changing and going with the flow because life often shifts and changes. After writing this, maybe I'm not being as flexible as I thought I was. Maybe it's a test on non-judgment. I don't know what went wrong.

All I know is we left Narti early and I've been judgmental. I guess this is more practice for me to not judge in the moment… It's so hard for me not to judge even though I know that things don't have to always look a certain way and neither way is right or wrong. Intellectually I know that we are all on our own journey and there's not one way a journey should look, but sometimes I don't think about it and I guess I have to keep on reminding myself of this so that the judgment goes away.

I strongly believe that everything happens for a reason and we can learn a lesson in each situation about ourselves. I guess this is my lesson to learn.

Minling Chuang

June 27, 2010

Jesse has asked us to journal about our experience in Narti. What went wrong? He says that we experienced fear and panic. That leaving early equates to our disrespect for the people of Narti.

I feel that what happened in Narti was reality. It is what it is. Jesse often quotes Buddha, who also says that you must accept whatever it is to be free from suffering. Yes, we went. Yes, we left, it is what it is. The only reason people are upset is because they were attached to the experience being something other than what it was. Jesse wanted to stay. He is sad, upset, insulted, and hurt, because we didn't stay. Others wanted to spend time with the children more. We didn't, and they're upset. I think that we were, in no way shape or form, being disrespectful. We HAVE great respect.

Another Buddhist precept is to live without definitions. Once you start to name things, emotions, events…then you reject reality. Nothing is good or bad, IT JUST IS. So…to me, the whole experience is a fantastic lesson in reality.

I also want to acknowledge that I was not experiencing fear OR panic in Narti.

I think it was a mistake to expect us to spend two days there. With the conditions being what they were…I think that getting there in the day and moving on to another location at night would have been more appropriate… None of us ever expected that we're here to "LIVE IN THEIR SHOES." We were here to meet some girls who were saved, visit the orphanage, and see some sights. We were not here to suffer, as they have suffered… We all know that there are people suffering everywhere in this world. We were here to help them… These girls have suffered. There is no doubt about that. Yes, they may still be poor, but they are now better off. Are they not? Living at the orphanage is no piece of cake. However these people are not suffering from the extreme heat. I felt that I could have become extremely sick, because I was sweating so much, no matter how much water I drank. Those girls did not even break a sweat. You cannot equate the experience. You cannot subject people to extreme conditions, without being prepared to help them.

Eve Ennis

June 27, 2010

What Happened in Narti?

I considered drafting this in my other journal first (I brought two journals with me because I knew I'd have a lot of thoughts irrelevant to this trip), but I thought perhaps raw emotion would give a better look into how I see things.

We arrived in Narti. Felt welcomed. Girls (former Kamlari) shy at first, but got along well after a while—understandable. Conditions unfavorable (well duh, most of us are from Cleveland), but not unbearable. Hot. Sweaty. Humid. No bathrooms or running water. Tents. It was camping; nothing more, nothing less (well, camping in Nepal). I understand that it's important for us to witness all of that—what the girls go through. But I also understand that we technically weren't doing anything to better the lives of these girls long-term….

I'm getting bored with this. The entry, I mean. I think the group will be okay as long as we can all learn to just let it go, and as long as Jesse can refrain from isolating himself.

Jaime Furda

June 27, 2010

What happened in Narti?

All hell broke loose. We missed the opportunity to see our situation as rife with possibility… We were not in control; taken away from our familiar surroundings, staying somewhere that felt primitive, scary and foreign… and we didn't understand what was happening and why. Perfect—I imagine that may be how the girls feel when they are taken from their home and put into someone else's, not knowing what to expect; feeling unsafe and not cared for, feeling betrayed by those they love...

So here we were in Narti — not knowing how to interact with these kids, with no toys to use to bridge the language gap, and no info to ground us in what to expect and to understand the importance of our visit. We went in blind, so some people felt we were "idle" there, wasting our time, others needed to understand why we were there, needed to hear more about the Kamlari system, others just wanted a cool room and a soft mattress. I imagine these girls feel the same way — Oh god, can't we go back to what we understand, to what's comfortable and familiar, to what we know as safe?

Our privilege has made us small. Perhaps it is the girls who should have pitied us... But instead these girls sat by our sides holding our hands, sharing their spirits, opening their hearts and homes, also uncertain of why we were there, but happy to see us. Some scared of course, but they didn't stand up and say NO, I'm scared, I'm uncomfortable, I don't trust having strangers at my home, photographing me. Instead they somehow found that space of acceptance and hid while we were there, kept their fears inside and watched ready to try and protect themselves....

So here we are on the other side of all the drama about leaving Narti early. So if Jesse was so strongly feeling it was wrong, why did we leave? He could have told people—Ok leave, here's the local bus schedule, see you in Chitwan. There were many of us who wanted to, or were willing to stay... I likely would have told people to buck up—deal with it and might have given them a stern reminder of what they signed up for... Jesse is a bit more compassionate than I.

...We are here out of love, we have love in our hearts and the Kamlari girls could use love—perfect match. And of course they were so fabulous at giving love to us—so sweet, kind, gentle. So we gave and received as did they and the moments will be of a lifetime for us all.

_____ **Kathy Hayes**

June 27, 2010_____

What happened in Narti?

The major problem is we had to sleep in stifling single and double tents with no escape from the heat. I hated every minute, as I couldn't sleep and was horribly uncomfortable. I wanted to leave and did not want to be there. Jesse wants us to believe we did something wrong because we wanted to leave. But I feel we bonded as well as we made new friends, felt their hearts, gave them ours, and we left. It's over. It was great, and we learned a lot.

We should be talking about how to make it better... I have and will always remember their faces and their story!

_____ **Marc Nathanson**

At breakfast this morning, I sat on a snail and killed it. The snail ended up on the floor smushed to pieces and I ended up with poop-like stains on my board shorts.

Thinking back two nights ago, when the group broke down, there were a lot of poopy pants. People who were selfish and knew it but didn't care. People who thought of themselves as better than and not responsible, so get them the hell out of Narti. People who were small-minded with an incessant need to control the situation and an incurable need to know. People who were angry at being judged and probably knew that their anger was coming from a place of self-judgement. All in all, there were quite a few people who had refused to open their eyes and their hearts and who stubbornly chose to be stuck in their stories because they felt that it was more important for their self-preservation, more important to be comfortable, in an air-conditioned room with hot showers.

Respect—that was what we didn't give them when we left earlier than planned. It wasn't about the presents or the money....

In the morning, after a huge rainstorm overnight, we continued our discussion. I was hoping that the village show the previous night would've changed some people's minds. But no, sadly it did not. It was still about "me vs. them", all about what their own needs were, what they wanted, and they still wanted to leave. I tried my best to contain my own emotions, but I wanted to grab them by the shoulders and shake them until they woke up. Seriously people, how long will you continue to live in your disillusioned world where everything revolves around you and when will you stop being so attached to everything you have, so much so that you've forgotten the greatest gift of life—freedom. You have it, you always have. These children didn't, and they still live at the mercy of the outside world.

_____ ***Tingting Peng***

Jesse has asked us to journal about what happened in Narti. Here is my take on it:

To have alleviated the situation, I believe Jesse should have given us a speech sometime on the hours-long bus ride, just to explain what we were doing in Narti, and what it would be like. There was never an explanation at all. This would have been the perfect place to bring chalk, jacks, bubbles, jump ropes, needle-and-thread, big garbage bags, and actually DO something for the girls, while we were there.

1. Sewing the holes in their clothes
2. Picking up the ever present trash

3. Collecting sticks for firewood

4. Painting a building

5. Helping with a meal

6. Playing organized games with the girls

7. Doing their hair (thank you Kathy and Minling – brilliant idea with the ribbons)

8. Teaching them to count in English, etc…

Some of these were done by individuals who were more adventurous. But for some, the language barrier was just too great, and they didn't know what to do with themselves. It was truly an uncomfortable time, and Jesse did not realize this.

He was in his element, completely and blissfully happy, surrounded by groups of girls who clearly cherish him. This was everything to him, and I think he completely expected us to feel exactly the same way. It didn't even dawn on him that some of us were wholly unprepared for this type of activity—sleeping on the ground, no running water, and filthy toilet. There was nothing planned to do, at all, with no verbal guidance, and nothing printed to follow.

I think it was a huge mistake to bring it up again now. The weirdness was dissipated by the long bus ride to Chitwan, and the excitement of seeing the rhino this morning, but he dragged it up again. Instead of just letting it go… He just doesn't know how to say "I don't know, let's figure it out… together."

_____ *Gabrielle Stickley*

June 27, 2010_____

Asked to journal about what happened yesterday. Yesterday being the day we decided to leave Narti a day early.

I find this extremely difficult because my hand cannot keep up with my thoughts… In addition, my hand is physically shaking from these emotions. I love these girls, I respect these girls, I am proud to have helped these girls. Problem… I'm certain that to continue to help them I can no longer use the "group leader" that introduced us to this journey, as a vehicle, a guide, an inspiration to do so.

I'm borderline panic attack as I sit here in this beautiful, serene environment attempting to journal. I am surrounded by people I know will be in my life, for my life… so much love, yet so much anger for the person that brought us all together, that brought us all here… seems like an oxymoron. So many references are made to Buddha… then the guilt trip about us leaving.

At home, I work out, run, do yoga, eat well…I'm RESPECTED, I'm told the truth.…

Most of this anger stems from my protective nature. I have been approached by a number of people with their concerns… some feel they are being treated unfairly due to living conditions (and he gives himself the best), others feel betrayed as far as misleading info prior to the trip, others feel judged, the list goes on....they come to me and I feel it is my responsibility as their family here, to speak up....to stop this!

That root is the base that needs to be nurtured, respected before we can help ANYONE ELSE.

_____ *Rachel Vincent*

Day 8 of the trip, cont'd

When we finished journaling, we had the afternoon to ourselves. A group of us decided to hike into town for some souvenir shopping. We also heard that there was an internet café there, and as much as I had enjoyed being off the grid, I wanted to email my family back in Ohio and let them know that all was well. We took the short trek into town and spent a good couple of hours shopping and checking email. It was a relaxing way to spend the afternoon, after all the drama of the morning. Then, we wandered back to the hotel. I took a little siesta, then got up around 5 and prepared for yoga. Practice was once again great, and at dinner afterwards the mood seemed to have lightened considerably, though Jesse remained quiet and kept himself pretty separated from the group. A few of us noticed, and we hoped a good night's sleep would put him in a better frame of mind tomorrow.

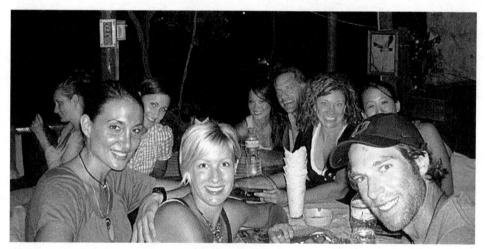

Hanging out at a local restaurant bar in Chitwan. Good times. Photo courtesy of Deanna Lee.

After dinner, Basu took a bunch of us back into town to hang out at one of the local bars, to drink and watch the World Cup on Satellite TV. Basu told us to stay away from the water, and to make sure if we ordered anything to drink that the bottle came sealed. Not because we might get sick, but because the proprietors of some of these places watered down their booze. The bar Basu took us to reminded me of some of the college places where I hung out as an undergrad — full of young people, all drinking, laughing, shouting and flirting. Especially flirting. There were more than a dozen women in our group, and when the young patrons, almost all guys, spotted us coming in, they must have thought they had found themselves at Spring Break in Daytona.

There were a few highlights that night. One was the banana pancakes covered in chocolate sauce that the bar served. You'd think that with all the eating we were doing on this trip, we wouldn't have room for more eating after dinner. But we were burning tons of calories doing yoga, hiking, and just keeping cool, and there was always room for dessert. Tingting, with her bottomless stomach and voracious appetite, put away two forty ounce beers and a huge stack of those pancakes, the latter which she happily shared with the group. They were fantastic. The rest of us had wine and beer, and chatted late into the night amongst ourselves and with the foreigners we met.

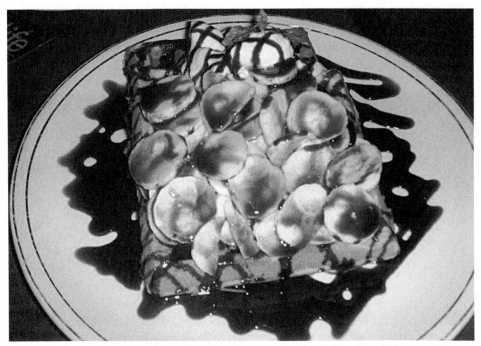

One of Tingting's favorite meals — banana chocolate waffles. Good any time of day. Photo by Tingting Peng.

Around midnight, Basu showed up with Hari in tow. I hadn't even noticed Basu was gone, but he sat down next to me and quietly asked me to get the group together to return to the hotel. He stressed that we all needed to leave together. A tiger had been spotted prowling the outskirts of town. Tigers in these parts were known to attack and kill humans, especially those they found out alone at night. That was a sobering thought, so I quietly passed the word, and we all left together.

It was pitch dark outside as we headed back. If there was a moon out, it was too cloudy to see it. Thankfully, we had flashlights with us to dodge the bowling ball sized elephant droppings on the road, and Basu and Hari to keep an eye out for any stray man-eating tigers. In no time, we were back at the hotel, safe and sound. All in all, it was another great day in our excellent Nepali adventure. I couldn't wait for tomorrow.

June 28, 2010

Day 9 of the Trip

Elephants on Parade

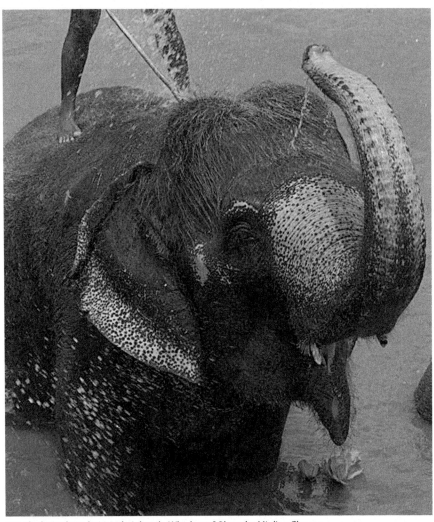

Yes, elephants have hair on their heads. Who knew? Photo by Minling Chuang.

June 28, 2010 _____

Last night we had an amazing practice taught by Deanna and it really showed me that my own judgments can be so limiting. I was wrong to be so harshly critical of those people who wanted to leave Narti. In my own eyes, I had forgotten to see these people as the same as myself.

24 hours after our heated discussion yesterday, we now sit here in the veranda as a whole group again.

_____ *Tingting Peng*

We had our morning yoga practice with Subash once again, followed by breakfast on the veranda. Then it was off to an elephant bath. If you don't know what an elephant bath is, you aren't alone. Neither did I. At first I assumed it was just someone, well, giving an elephant a bath. Maybe with a big hose or a bucket and giant scrub brush. Jesse told us we should wear swimming trunks for this if we really wanted to participate. If we didn't, we could just stand back, watch, and take pictures. I put on my swim trunks. I didn't want to miss out on any part of the adventure.

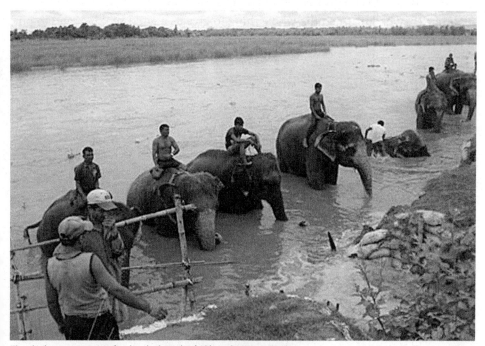

The elephants preparing for the elephant bath. Photo by Jaime Furda.

Jesse and Hari led us on a short hike down to the river, and there I found out exactly what an elephant bath is, or more accurately who's giving the elephant a

247

bath. The answer: the elephant. Of course, once we saw what was going on, it made perfect sense. The elephants and their handlers climbed down the riverbank into the river, and then the elephants, using their trunks, would suck up large amounts of water and hose themselves down, along with anyone who happened to be riding them. When they asked who wanted to volunteer for a bath, several of us jumped right up.

Robb and I were chosen to climb onto one of the bigger elephants together. Before we clambered up on its back, Jesse warned us to keep our mouths shut, and to not drink any of the river water. It had rained hard the previous night, and the water was very muddy, and therefore very full of bacteria. I nodded my understanding, and then Robb and I followed one of the guides down to the riverbank, where he helped us climb onto the back of an elephant that was already in the water. The handler climbed on after us, and the elephant then waded out into deeper water and got to work bathing himself. In seconds I was soaked. And trying not to laugh, so as not to drink any river water. That wasn't so easy, as the whole process was hilarious. At one point, the elephant did a little shimmy and shake and rolled both of us off into the river. I was about to panic, when I saw all the handlers onshore laughing. They had planned the whole thing to give us a good soaking, and to put on a good show for everyone on shore. Mission accomplished.

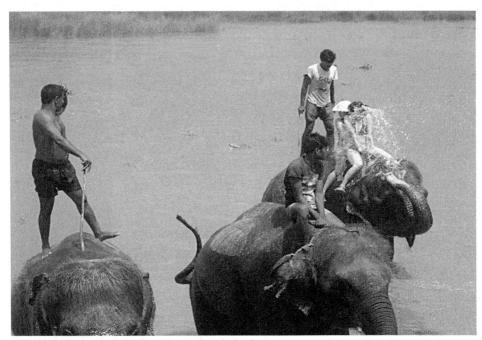

Terri and Minling get the full bath treatment. Photo by Eve Ennis.

The other handlers helped us out of the river, and we watched as a bunch of others in the group got the full elephant bath treatment. It was much funnier watching, though a lot more fun participating. Either way, everyone had a blast…

June 28, 2010

When I signed up for elephant bathing, I thought we were going to the river to help bathe the elephant, but instead they bathed us. We were led to this river and they motioned us to come sit on top of the elephants. With the trainer's instructions, the elephant reached into the water and squirted water back at us. Needless to say, we got soaked. It was very fun though and the elephants are such gentle creatures. Being so close to them was amazing. I actually never knew elephants had a head of hair. It was bristly to the touch.

Minling Chuang

June 28, 2010

Our morning plans included elephant baths. I did not participate [but] I did watch! It was hilarious! The elephant John and Robb were on rolled them off into the river and they couldn't do a damn thing about it!

Christina Jankus

June 28, 2010

…today I went on an elephant when he was bathing himself. Amazing! There's that word again. I wish I had more words to describe all this. I was riding on an elephant's back. It felt so foreign, but safe and so silly, and so very refreshing. Another experience to mirror life: patience and trust, love and hope, and compassion & passion.

Marc Nathanson

Once we were out of the water, Jesse told us to make sure we showered thoroughly when we got back to the hotel. Not because of the smell, which I'm sure would have been reason enough, but to make sure we washed off any bacteria that might infect any cuts we had.

We hiked back to the hotel, and soaped and showered ourselves up nice and clean. I checked myself for cuts and scrapes. I had two nasty blisters on the outside of my big toes, and washed those spots doubly well. I had them because I hadn't listened to Jesse, who told us before the trip to make sure we broke in our hiking sandals if we bought new ones for the trip. Hiking sandals are a must for trekking in Nepal in the summertime, as it's very hot and very wet. Tennis shoes were not a good option in that kind of climate. I had bought my sandals a week before I left, and they were hardly broken in by the time we reached Chitwan. A week of trekking around in them had done the damage.

At lunch I mentioned my blisters, and Christina offered to give me some blister bandages, rubber sticky pads about the size of a half dollar, which turned out to be fantastic. They kept the blisters from being rubbed raw by my footwear. Someone else recommended putting hand sanitizer on the blisters. They said it would dry them right up, and so before bandaging my two big toes, I soaked them with the hand sanitizer. It turned out they were right, and in just a few days, the blisters had dried and healed.

After lunch and tending to my big toes, I joined the group in the gazebo for meditation again. Jesse started to speak, but Marc asked to take over today's meditation. He told Jesse he wanted to do a little emotional exercise with him that he'd learned a while back. Jesse must close his eyes, Marc said. Then everyone in the group must come up, take a seat in front of him, and take his hands in theirs. Then they had to tell Jesse why they loved him.

Some people in the group, Jesse included, were a bit taken aback. Jesse, to his credit, went with the flow. And to the group's credit, everyone eventually took their seat in front of Jesse and told him why they loved him...

June 28, 2010_____

We were in a very negative place following the stuff in Narti, and I decided we needed to change the dynamics. So, we did a "What do I love about you" for Jesse. It was really powerful for the group and Jesse, and brought us all together again.

_____*Marc Nathanson*

June 28, 2010_____

Then there was meditation. Thankfully Marc took over... they [had] started to become bitch sessions. [He] asked us each to tell Jesse why we love him. I told Jesse that I love him for having as much compassion as he has passion and for making me feel again. I cried more in these past few days than I had in months – maybe years.

When Tingting and I got back to the room we noticed a cricket being overtaken by a small army of ants. For some reason I was fascinated watching the scene — maybe to distract me from my tears. Upon returning from lunch I noticed that the cricket and the ants were completely gone —not a trace of them any-where. I guess in the grand scheme of things size does not always matter.

_____ *Christina Jankus*

Some people choked up talking to Jesse, a few cried. Everyone was riveted watching it all unfold. People told Jesse they loved him for putting the trip together, for being brave, open, caring, compassionate, selfless and kind. We told him we loved him for his service to the children of NOH and for the work he'd done throughout Nepal. We told Jesse how much we appreciated him, and how unique he was in the world. As each of us spoke, one right after the other, Jesse heaved enormous sighs, fighting back his own tears at this unexpected outpouring of love directed toward him. The whole thing lasted less than half an hour, but it was incredibly emotional, and very cathartic, not just for Jesse, but I believe for all of us. Afterwards, I went up to Marc and thanked him for doing what he did. I love you man, I said, and gave him a big bear hug. By the time we were done, everyone, including Jesse, seemed to be in a much better place than we had been at any time on the trip so far. Maybe the Beatles were right; maybe all you really do need is love. I was hopeful that we had now been through the worst of things as a group, and that we had all grown from the experience.

This emotional exercise had encouraged everyone in the group to return to a place of love, and it encouraged Jesse to forgive himself and others for what happened in Narti and what had been said about it. It helped us all get back on track, back to our journey from me from we. Time would tell if this harmony would last. We still had almost a week left on the trip…

June 28, 2010_____

…Jesse seems to be coming around after we all told him how much we loved him. Hopefully, he's not going to remain secluded from the rest of the group. He is the leader of this trip. While I understand he has certain expectations, I hope he understands that things don't always turn out exactly how we thought, planned, hoped.

_____ *Minling Chuang*

The storm seems to be calming, so much expectation. 19 different people from different backgrounds, different experiences with different expectations on one journey. All with different levels of commitment to yoga, to the group, to the cause. It's quite a mix to manage. Why should no one be disappointed or unhappy momentarily? It's OK.

_____ *__Kathy Hayes__*

Before we adjourned from the gazebo, Jesse gave us another journaling exercise, which he told us he would like us to do before we went off on our afternoon excursion. This time, he asked us all to think about what we'd gained and what we'd lost on this trip so far, and then to write something on the theme of impermanence...

Journaling Exercise:

What does impermanence mean to you?

June 28, 2010_____

Impermanence

I didn't mean what I wrote yesterday, I was angry and hurt.

I am totally glad I brought everyone and they have seen a small slice of the world, a small piece of reality.

I am glad everything unfolded like it did. I only wish I could be a better leader, one that they deserve. Strong like Johnny Kest or compassionate like Sean Corn or amazing like Tami Schneider, my [yoga] teacher.

This has been the hardest thing I've ever done.

_____ *Jesse Bach*

June 28, 2010_____

Impermanence…

The wind, everyone feels the wind, everyone is affected by the wind. The wind refreshes a warm body. The wind devilishly extinguishes a candle. The wind can do tremendous devastation. Yet, the same wind can supply power and life to an entire city. This trip has been the wind. This trip has changed my life. I have not only witnessed the wind's impermanence to the lives of children by the smiles that were shown at the presence of a handshake or a kind word not the giving of a cell phone, a computer or an automobile. A smile for a piece of rubber for a bracelet, we were the wind and they were the wind. I witnessed direct change but mostly I witnessed the crossover from fear to love. I am thoroughly convinced that in the human world fear is the absence of love and when you replace fear with love, miracles occur.

_____ *Robb Blain*

June 28, 2010_____

Journaling exercise: Impermanence

To me, this means the ebb & flow of life. Nothing ever stays the same as we drift through life. Can anything be permanent? I think in some ways we'd like things to be permanent so that we feel safe and secure, but impermanence is what makes life interesting and allows us to grow. Learning new things and having new perspectives is what I think life and "growing up" is all about.

Living in Narti and at the Korean monastery showed me how little we need to live on to survive. All these material things are so unnecessary. These "permanent" fixtures, material things are not things we need to survive; yet we hold onto these things. Is it because we fear the unknown of not having these material things as safety nets?

In Narti I saw people living on, what I would perceive, very little. But seeing the girls' happy faces and the joy in the villagers' eyes when they put on the show, made me think that all we need is love and laughter. They didn't have much, but at the same time they didn't need much either. But could I quit my job and live on nothing or very little? Boy is that a scary thought. Not sure if I could do it.

Minling Chuang

Impermanence

Impermanence is what makes life so beautiful, and challenging—unless you embrace it. I have been able to. Many people are terrified of change—of impermanence. But when you realize that just as positive good things don't last forever, neither do the terrible rotten horrible things. They come and go just as easily...

Eve Ennis

What I've Gained and Lost on This Trip

First and foremost, I've definitely lost track of the days. I've lost my fear of trying new things (especially when it comes to food), almost my fear of heights through practice on rooftops, and, quite unfortunately, my umbrella. I'm sure I've lost more than just that, but what I've lost pales in comparison to what I've gained.

I've gained some friendships that will last forever (not only with the others in the group to whom I've gotten relatively close, but also with Asmita, Dhiraj…all the kids); I've gained the ability to see my own personal strength without harsh judgment; I've gained a sister through meeting and getting to know Rachel; I've gained an appreciation for things I might never understand; I've gained the ability to better adapt to a completely alien culture and environment.

I'm sure I've gained more than just that, too, but I'm finding it to be very difficult to concentrate with this large ant (is that an ant?) parading around my feet.

Jaime Furda

June 28, 2010 _____

"Impermanence"

What I have learned in my life is that there is constant change, that even the darkest longest storm will eventually be followed by the brightest warmest sun. I have watched people I love come and go and come again. I have had arguments that in the moment seemed so valid yet in the end were all trivial, fallen in and out of love, had moments that felt like eternity but now seem so far away, old ideas that have been replaced by new beliefs. I have learned to embrace change, learned to overcome the fear of the ending of things to know that what follows is what is necessary, and what has happened is what was necessary... The only thing that is eternal is this cycle of change. And us, we are infinite.

_____ ***Deanna Lee***

June 28, 2010 _____

Day 9 – Impermanence

Impermanence is really freedom. Because if you find yourself in a bad situation, and if you realize it will soon be over, that makes it easier to bear. Forgetting that life is impermanent makes for sadness and suffering.

I am not sure what to do about all this. I feel like I have found my strength in a way that I have never allowed myself to feel. I can manage well. I am not afraid.

I have got to be true to myself.

_____ ***Gabrielle Stickley***

June 28, 2010 _____

Gained & Lost??

Meditation led by Marc. Marc put Jesse in the middle and we went around, each holding his hands and telling him a reason we love him. This was a result of yesterday's journaling session since we hashed out quite a bit (to put it very mildly). I definitely was extremely verbal. I was speaking for so many and couldn't take their/my frustration, pain, anger anymore.

So... gained:

A deeper respect for my mom's ability to accept, not judge. Her grace to forgive and love unconditionally regardless of the way she may feel towards someone or what has happened between them. Although I'm skeptical... I was raised by people that find peace through acceptance, love and the beautiful, powerful ability to LET GO. What occurs here does not define me; but if allowed, the negativity could poison a being I've grown so proud to represent:

MYSELF

Most importantly — I've gained lifelong friends. People I will care for, love and share my life with. I am so, so very grateful for that gain.

Also… the undoubtedly irreplaceable gain of experiencing compassion, acceptance, and love without judgment from incredible children who have hope when it would seem most impossible. Perhaps seeing my mother's strengths mirrored in their spirits… They helped to remind me of the valuable lessons she instilled and lives by.

Lost: Usually taken negatively…

I will admit I've unfortunately lost trust in Jesse, although I do accept him and am trying to work towards forgiving him.

However, a positive loss: I lost the attachment I had to people, emotions I had back home to come here for an open experience and I've had just that. Although the people in my life are very much in my heart and I give thanks for them every day…I've lost the attachment to the situations and relationships I am uncertain of…the desire to try to control their outcome.

_____ *Rachel Vincent*

June 28, 2010 _____

On Impermanence

Our bus driver on this trip is named Buddha. Buddha Saktia. He's a 5 foot 6 inch tall fireplug of a guy with tattoos of the English word "Buddha" on his left forearm and a huge spider web on his right shoulder, among others. If he were in LA, you might at first mistake him for a gang banger. Or at least an ex-banger. But then you notice the Buddhist pendant around his neck, and the soft Zen-like smile he always wears on his face. This guy is cool personified, and he isn't even trying. His strong back, shoulders and arms serve him well in his job. We've come to believe on this trip that he was the best bus driver in Nepal, if not the world. If you've driven on the roads of Nepal, or any other traffic crazy developing country, you will understand that this is a very high compliment indeed. He is that good.

Several days ago we took a 10 and ½ hour bus ride from Kathmandu to Lumbini. The trip started out with joy and camaraderie — singing, laughing, music, our own little caravan of love. As the hours rolled by, fatigue began to slowly set in. Bathroom breaks became less and less pleasant, and after a brief but wonderful lunch at the riverside restaurant, Blue Heaven, the afternoon bus ride turned to evening and the jostling and the bouncing of the bus ride slowly but inexorably turned to bone rattling, teeth jarring, back aching, hamstring cramping pain.

Humor gave way to silence, gave way to bitching and moaning. Where are we? How long until we get there? Is this bus ride ever going to end? By the time we stopped at the Siddhartha Hotel, 10 hours or so into the ride, we hated that bus. The seats, the loud music, then the silence, the cramped, trapped feeling of being in one confined space for too long, the air conditioning shutting off every time we climbed another hill — that bus became a symbol of all our misery. It was a vessel for all our frustrations, our gripes, complaints and whining. We truly hated that fucking bus. I said out loud that I'd like to light a match and torch it. Set it on fire and happily watch it burn.

Several days later, as we left Narti, of which much has been written; having suffered the hardships of intense, nearly unbearable heat, unpleasant smells and primitive outhouses, sweat that became one with your body, your clothes, your skin, external hardships that tested each of us in powerful and uniquely individual ways, and emotional group turmoil that came on like a sudden summer storm, we all got back on the bus.

The first little breath of cool air from the bus's A/C brought us sweet relief. The trip from Narti to Chitwan was about 6 hours long. But the love we felt for that bus, our shelter, our comfort, our ship in the night, was every bit as strong, every bit as heartfelt, as the hate we felt for that exact same bus just two or three days before. Buddha was back behind the wheel, and everything was right again with the world.

_____ *John Vourlis*

Day 9 of the Trip, cont'd

After journaling and lunch, we went on another fantastic elephant adventure. This time it was a safari. Hari led us to a spot near the entrance to Chitwan National Park where they offered elephant rides through the jungle. Four of us at a time would climb up a ladder to an observation deck, and then walk from the deck right onto the back of an elephant. Each elephant had a "saddle" on his back. The saddle was sort of like the gondola on a hot air balloon, except instead of sides, it had open sections like a fence which you swung your legs through and a top where you could rest your arms. Each person took a corner of the gondola, and the elephant handler rode on the neck of the big grey beast. These elephants seemed bigger than the ones we'd taken baths on in the morning, and they seemed to have no problem hauling around four full grown adults on their backs, five if you counted their handlers.

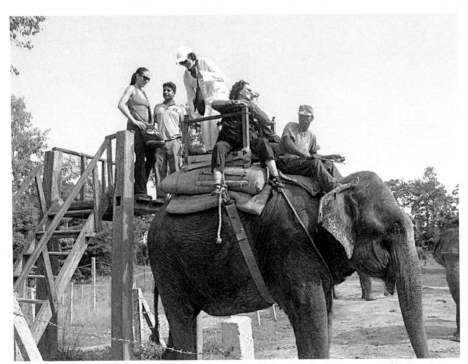

Boarding our elephants for the jungle trek through Chitwan National Park. Photo courtesy of Deanna Lee.

When we were all aboard, we set off into the jungle in search of wildlife. As we moved out of the bright sun of the embarkation area and into the dark, shadowy forest, things quickly grew interesting, when we found ourselves at the edge of a giant watering hole in the middle of the trees, right smack in the middle of which stood another rhinoceros. This rhino seemed even bigger than the one we saw while canoeing. And it was definitely closer. A lot closer. We couldn't have been more than twenty feet away and of course ten or twelve feet up from it. Rhinos have notoriously poor eyesight, so the big guy hadn't realized we were there until we were practically on top of him. When he did spot us, he looked up in our direction and gave a series of short angry snorts. He clearly wasn't happy having his afternoon pool party interrupted.

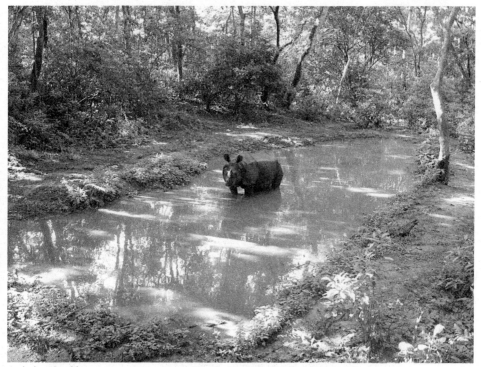

And what should we spy, not 10 minutes into our jungle trek, but another rhino!

What was also evident immediately was that this rhino had a great deal of respect for the elephants. Though obviously not happy with our presence there, he made no attempt to charge us, or even take an aggressive posture. For a while he just tried to ignore us, and went back to wading in the pool. But there were too many elephants for his liking, all watching him bathe. Exasperated, he rose up out of the muddy water, snorted loudly at us one more time, just to get his point across, and

259

then lumbered out of the pool and into the jungle. We all sat there with our mouths open. Spotting one rhino, a hundred yards across the river, had been awesome. Seeing a second one, not more than 20 feet away, had been utterly astounding.

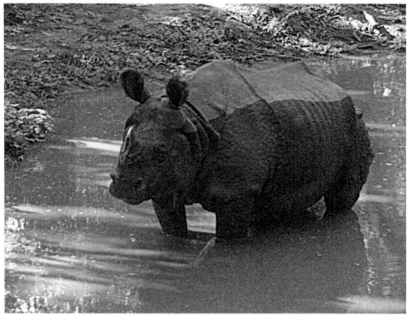

A rather unhappy rhino, as we disturbed his morning bath in his favorite watering hole. Photo by Joyce Fijalkovich.

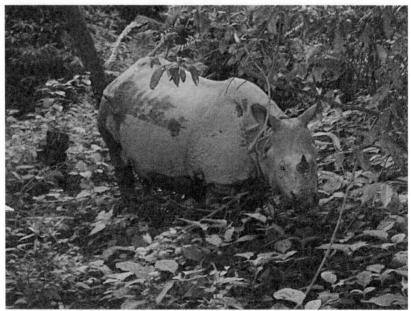

This may have been a third rhino, perhaps a female, in the jungle not far from where we saw our second rhino leaving his watering hole. Photo by Tingting Peng.

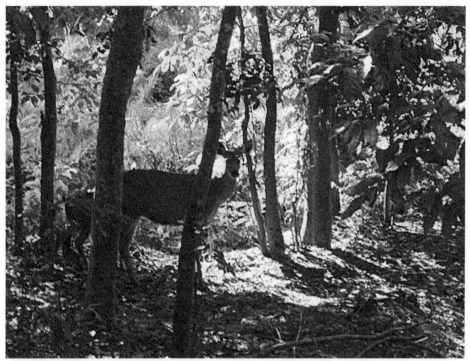

Asian deer, well camouflaged in the dappled light of the late morning jungle. Photo by Jaime Furda.

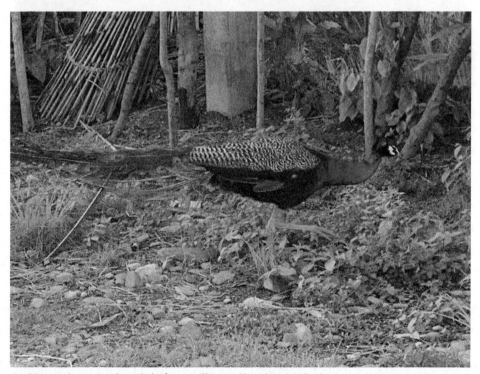

A wild peacock strutting through the forest at Chitwan. Photo by Jaime Furda.

The rest of the time we spent out in the jungle, we kept a sharp lookout for other animals. We saw some well-camouflaged Asian deer, and a large warthog, along with all kinds of spiders, butterflies and several different kinds of birds. We had been told there was a slight chance we might see a tiger, but we never did. I didn't feel too bad about that, though. The rhino had been fantastic enough for me. Eventually, we left the forest for more open jungle savannah. While the morning elephant bath had been like something out of *The Jungle Book*, this afternoon safari, once we'd seen our second rhino, took on a more *Passage to India* vibe.

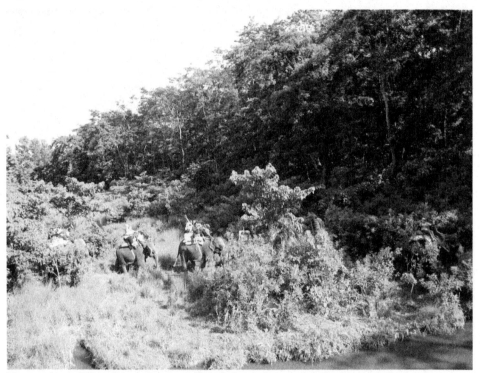

Like a scene out of A Passage to India, we trek through the jungle on elephant-back.

It was very warm and sunny, and hats and sunglasses were the order of the day. We even saw a group of Japanese ladies riding an elephant, each with an open parasol to provide some shade. Several times on our safari, especially when we were out in the grasslands, the elephants would stop and graze. The handlers didn't seem too happy about these random, leisurely rest stops, but when an elephant decides it's time to eat, even its handler has to respect that. The elephants had a fascinating way of eating, too. They'd wrap their enormous trunks around and around a tall clump of succulent elephant grass and pull it out of the ground, dirt and all. Then they would whack the roots against their front legs, knocking all the dirt off, before stuffing the grass neatly into their huge mouths and chowing down. It was hilarious watching them do this over and over again. Eventually, the handlers would grow impatient and yell at the beasts, and give them a good whack on the side like a jockey on a thoroughbred to get the caravan moving again. These guys didn't use a whip, though. They all carried large steel bull hooks that they used to guide the animals.

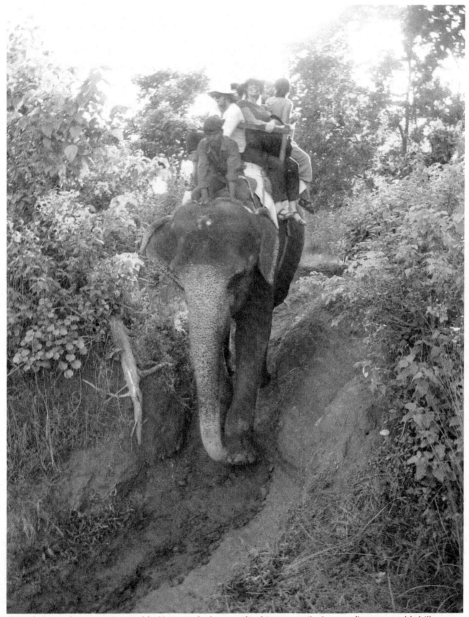

These behemoths were quite nimble. Here an elephant makes his way easily down a slippery, muddy hill.

At first this seemed a rather cruel thing to us, as they would whack the sides of the beast with what amounted to a crowbar. The hooked end they would use to pull the animal by the ear or mouth in the direction they wanted to turn. Despite our concern for the animals, Hari assured us that the elephants were in no way being harmed. They were after all incredibly thick skinned, as you could immediately tell when you climbed up on them. Their hide was rubbery, hard, and we could see no marks on the animals from the bull hooks.

Once their appetites had been satiated, at least temporarily, the elephants would get back to work, hauling us around. As we began to circle back into jungle from the savannah, we came to the edge of a river, undoubtedly the same river we'd 'bathed' in that morning. We had to cross it to get to the other side and back to base camp. This should be interesting, I thought to myself. The elephants seemed to know the way, lumbering down a very steep embankment along the trail and right into the water.

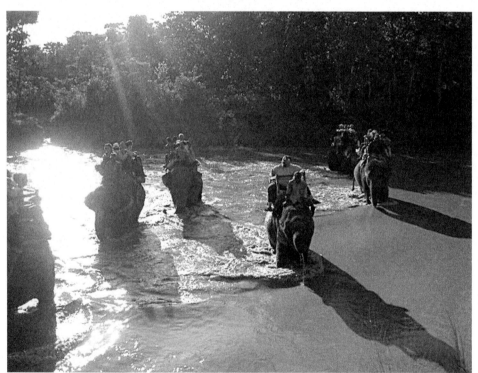

Why does an elephant cross the river? To get to the other side, of course. Hopefully with us still onboard. Photo by Jaime Furda.

Amazingly, elephants can swim. In fact, they are apparently excellent swimmers. It turned out that was a good thing, as the river had risen considerably from the overnight rain, and swimming across was the only option. It was amazing finding ourselves riding on the back of a swimming elephant. For a moment we were worried the poor beast we were riding might drown, as its head was more than half submerged in the river. This certainly would've sucked for us as well, since we'd be left up to our eyeballs in deep water too. But then, just as comedy was veering toward something a bit less humorous, up went the elephant's trunk like a periscope, providing the animal with all the fresh air it needed to breathe on the swim across. Our foursome was saved, but everyone else wasn't quite in the clear yet…

Now, I've already mentioned that Jesse was a big dude. Because of this, he'd been given his own elephant to ride on the safari. But since he was the only one riding it, he had also been given the smallest elephant to ride. Halfway across the river, the poor little guy began drifting downstream, as the current from the heavy rainfall had become pretty swift, and being smaller than the other elephants his shorter legs couldn't find the river bottom in the now deeper river. Like a VW bus caught in a flood, downstream went Jesse, the elephant and its handler. The handler seemed to panic for a moment when he and Jesse found themselves hip deep in the flowing water. He started shouting at the elephant.

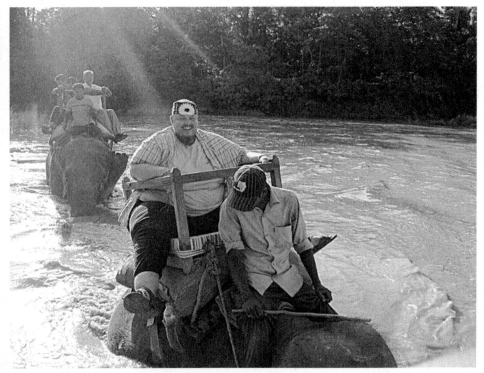

Despite some midstream drama, Jesse and his trusty little steed make it across. Photo by Kathy Hayes.

We were behind Jesse and watching the whole thing, simultaneously laughing and worrying what would happen to Jesse and his trusty little steed if they continued unabated downstream. We asked our guide if everything was okay, and he said, between laughs, not to worry. Elephants, even smaller ones with Jesse on their back and a handler shouting in their ear, can still swim amazingly well. Jesse's little elephant must have dog paddled, or elephant paddled in this case, like crazy under the water because in a minute or so, he had made it to the other side and clambered up the far embankment taking Jesse safely with him, pants a little soggy but otherwise just fine.

The elephant trek ended where it began. Once we were back, we got to feed the elephants a few bananas as reward for their hard work lugging us around the jungle all day. For a few rupees you got a banana and you either handed it to the elephant, who would take it with his trunk, or if you were braver, stuck it in the elephant's mouth, and let him take it from you that way. Either way they got their reward; I swear those elephants had smiles on their faces as we fed them banana after banana. Whether it was because we were finally off their backs, or because they really liked bananas, I couldn't say.

June 29, 2010

Day 10 of the Trip

A Walk in the Park

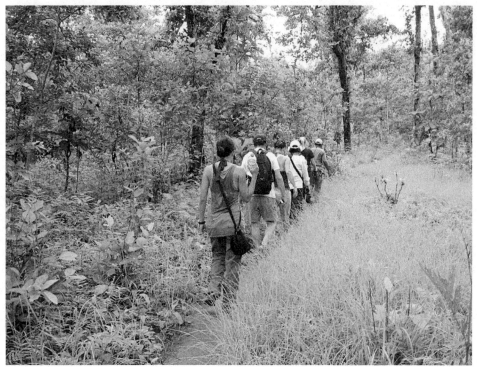

This time the brave adventurers trek the jungle on foot.

By now we were getting pretty comfortable at Chitwan. We practiced yoga in the morning, had another great breakfast, and then a bunch of us, led by Hari and Basu, went on a nature hike through the jungle. On the way we stopped at an elephant breeding facility. There were some huge bulls there with enormous tusks. Hari told us not to make direct eye contact with them, as getting in a stare down made the bulls feel threatened and become angry and aggressive. So mad that they might pull their chain loose and come after you. I kept my sunglasses on, not wanting to offend or antagonize anyone. The highlight of this stop was the twin baby elephants. Twin births are rare in the elephant world, so we were privileged to see these little guys lounging in the hay at their mother's feet. At one point one of them got up to suckle, drawing some "aww, how cute's" from the crowd.

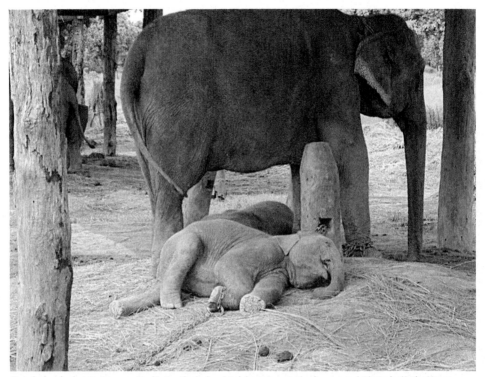

Twin baby elephants. A true rarity. Notice the baby-sized droppings in the foreground. Photo by Kathy Hayes.

From there we trekked off into the forest for a couple of hours. We spotted some cool birds, and far off in the distance, behind a tall wooden fence, we watched elephants out foraging in the wild. Apparently, they were allowed to do a little bit of freestyle munching by the breeding facility, to keep them from becoming too domesticated. Seeing them in their natural habitat out there, I was impressed even more by how big they really were. And lucky for us, how far away...

We also saw some water buffalo grazing in the fields, and some amazing bugs, including a giant millipede several inches long curled up in a ball near the hiking path, a pile of red centipedes that must have numbered in the dozens, and several varieties of spiders that spun huge webs, though none as impressive as our friend at The Grand Norling Hotel. We also encountered termite mounds that were taller than Joyce...

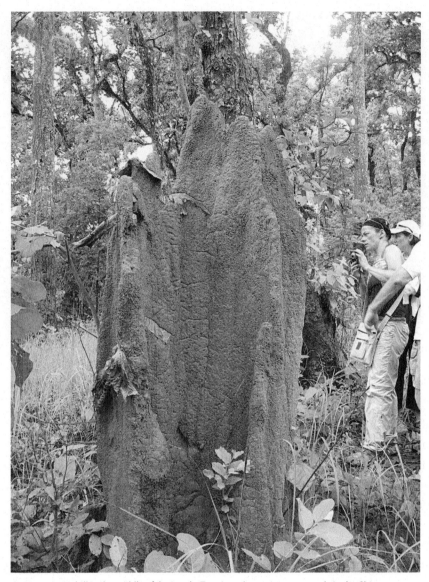

A giant termite hill in the middle of the jungle. Termites play an important role in the Chitwan ecosystem by recycling fallen trees, branches, and leaves into rich nutrients for the soil (source: http://en.wikipedia.org/wiki/Termite).

One of the cooler plants we encountered was the strangler vine. These vines grow up and around weak trees in the forest, wrapping themselves tighter and tighter around them until they almost become one with the tree. And they can move from tree to tree as well, forming bridges, which, if you are Basu, or Subash or Hari or David, you can scramble up and swing and climb on like a kid playing on the local park swing set.

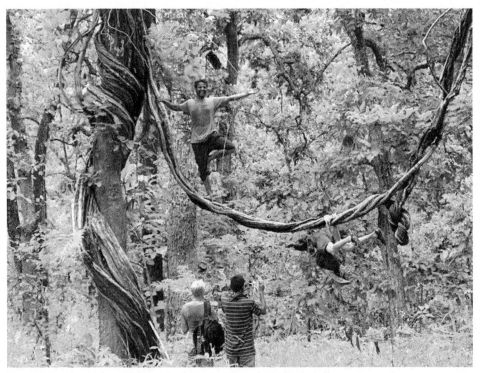

Basu and David monkey around on strangler vines. Photo by Kathy Hayes.

By the time we returned from the jungle hike, I was wiped out. Even in the morning, a two or three hour hike through the jungle is a hot sweaty enterprise. Luckily it was just about time for lunch. Jesse had scheduled a long afternoon bike ride to a nearby lake for anyone who wanted to go, but I begged off. After lunch, a few people ended up going, though, and they had quite a good time....

June 29, 2010

... After lunch, Kathy, Rob, Joyce, Tingting, Hari and I set out on a bike ride. The ride was 17 km to the destination and back. We had these old rickety bikes. From the moment I got on the bike, I wasn't sure if I was going to make it to the destination and back. The paved roads were fine, but once we got on the gravel, you could feel every rock as I bobbed up and down. Rob and Hari also took a nasty spill at 3 km when making a turn. This does not look good. At 6 km, I decided I wanted to turn back around. This was my breaking point and I knew I had to make a choice to turn around now or to go all the way to the end. There was no way I was going to make it there and back so I told the group I wanted to turn around. Everyone objected because they were afraid that I would get lost since we made so many turns up to this point. Luckily, I have a great memory for direction and paid attention to all the landmarks. So I headed back to Hotel Parkland.

The ride back was so beautiful. I was able to go at my own pace and enjoy the views of Chitwan. It was also so peaceful to go through the countryside by myself. I also have to say it was liberating because I was doing it by myself. I was going so fast before and making sure I stayed with the group that I didn't pay attention to the people and the views. Now, alone on the bike, I saw the beauty of each person I passed and the landscape. It's so surreal that I'm even here.

Minling Chuang

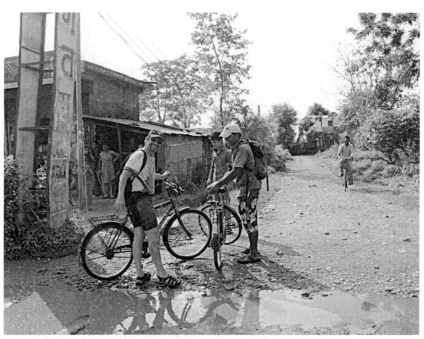

Robb takes an unscheduled pit stop on the long, very bumpy bike ride around Chitwan… Photo by Kathy Hayes.

While the bikers were off doing their thing, the rest of us hung around the hotel. Basu and Subash climbed several mango trees in the courtyard and came down with a feast of ripe fruit. We cut it up and ate it for dessert. It was juicy, tangy, sweet and absolutely delicious. Afterwards, I took the opportunity to catch up on some journaling and reading. I parked myself in a chair on the little patio outside our room and opened up a copy of the Bhagavad Gita translated by the great British author Christopher Isherwood that I'd brought along on the trip. As I sat there reading and enjoying the afternoon shade, Subash walked by and asked what book it was that I was holding. I showed him the cover, and he got very excited, and asked if he could check it out sometime, as he was looking for a good English translation of the Gita. I gave it to him right then and there, and told him to enjoy it. I was go-ing inside for a short nap. He told me he'd have it back to me by dinner.

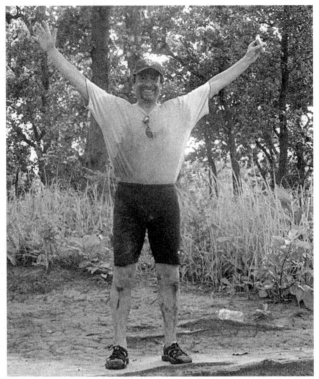

...and shows off the bloody knees and muddy pants he got after a nice tumble. Photo by Joyce Fijalkovich.

The bikers didn't all get back to the Parkland until around dinner time, when they filled us in on the bike trip and showed off the scrapes they acquired from wiping out. It sounded like they had fun, but I was just as happy to not have gone. I was just digging hanging out and doing nothing. It was then I realized I hadn't felt able to do that in a long long time, since Christmas vacation maybe even longer. I had been working, writing non-stop, right up to the time we left for Nepal, and only now was I finally just relaxing. And man was it a great feeling. I have got to do this more often, I thought to myself.

That evening, yoga practice was led by Christina Jankus. She had a warm, soothing style of talking as she led us through practice, and she paced the class perfectly. It turned out to be one of the best sessions that we had during the whole trip. Chris was also remarkably insightful in discussing our experiences so far on this trip. When her session was over, we all were buzzing...

I taught the evening yoga practice. I had brought a book with me to read – The Yoga Sutras. While everyone was in savasana I spoke about right knowledge as I learned while reading the sutras. I explained that someone can tell you when you go to Nepal you will see abject poverty with animals as well as people eating from trash in the streets, but you don't know it until you experience it and see it with your own eyes. I reminded everyone that Jesse charged us with the task of spreading the message to help eradicate the Kamlari system and now we know what we need to do.

I was pleased that several YFFs like my style and my words spoken. Recently I have been having doubts about my abilities as a yoga teacher. I floated on air until at dinner a grasshopper the size of a small potato as described by Eve landed on my shoulder. Oh my! What a commotion I caused! Ha-ha!

Christina Jankus

David and I both complimented Chris afterwards, as did many of the others. Then it was off to shower, and to the dining hall for chow. At dinner, Hari stopped by to ask us all to join him afterwards in the parking lot area for a special presentation. Local Tharu villagers were coming to put on a traditional dance performance for us. We were excited, as traditional dancing had been one of the highlights of our Narti stop as well. And once again, we weren't disappointed by the show...

The traditional Tharu stick dance is performed by young village men and women who chant rhyming songs and play drums as dancers move in a circle whipping large bamboo sticks around their heads and bodies, smacking them together like Bruce Lee fighting in a Kung Fu movie. The clashing of sticks is more than symbolic. It illustrates how the Tharu actually scare tigers and other wild animals away from their homes and their farm land by banging sticks together. I can't say if it's an effective deterrent in real life, but it all looked pretty fierce to me as I watched the performance.

Late in the evening the villagers came to dance the stick dance and traditional dances. It was AWESOME! It was like the Blue Man Group and STOMP melded together! They welcomed us to join in and dance with them. Of course I did! I love dancing!

Christina Jankus

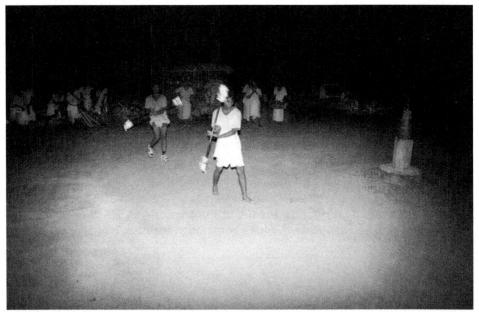

The Tharu dancers arrive, sticks blazing. Photo by Minling Chuang.

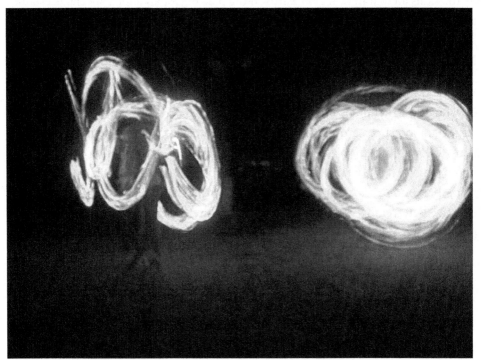

The whirling, twirling, flaming sticks of the Tharu fire dancers. Photo by Jaime Furda.

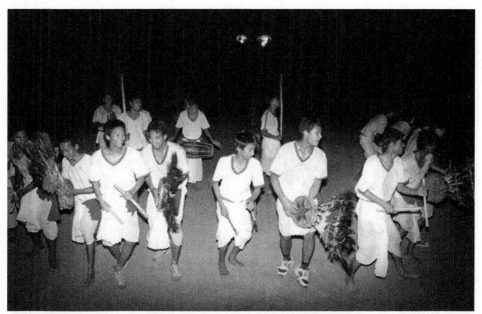

The Tharu villagers perform a traditional stick dance for us. Photo by Minling Chuang.

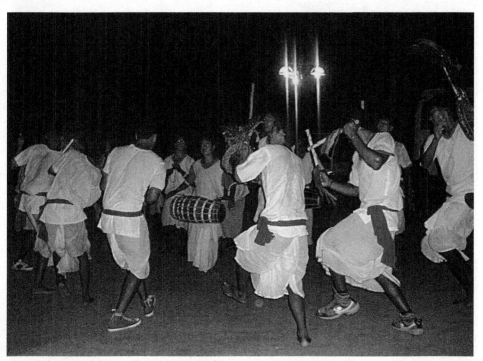

The stick dancers in full swing. Photo by Jaime Furda.

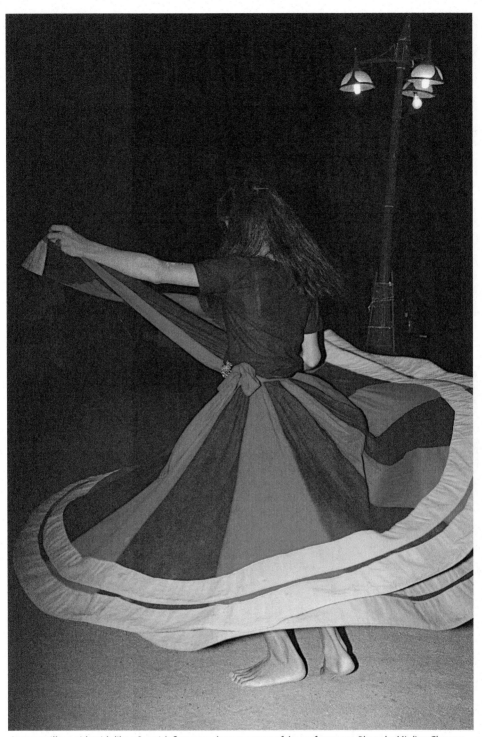

A young village girl swirls like a Spanish flamenco dancer as part of the performance. Photo by Minling Chuang.

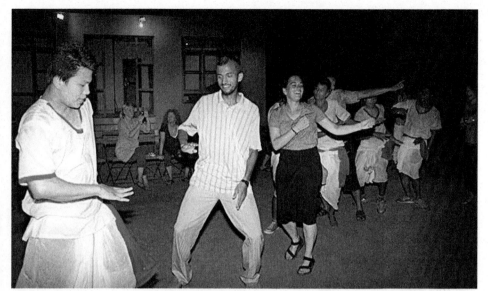

Subash and Gabby join the dance. Photo by Minling Chuang.

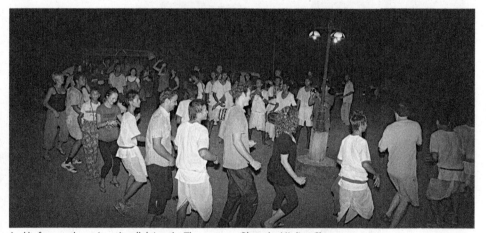

And before you know it, we're all doing the Tharu conga. Photo by Minling Chuang.

We gave the villagers a standing ovation as they finished their performance and retreated back into the night. Afterwards, having built up a serious thirst from all that dancing, we went into town and hit the local bars again, to partake in some more beer, wine, and banana chocolate pancakes. When we got there, a World Cup match was on the satellite TV, and a large contingent of Japanese travelers were already seated watching Japan play Paraguay in the quarter-finals. Unfortunately for them, Japan lost. Despite the defeat, and the language barriers, we all had a blast late into the evening. I heartily recommend the bar scene in Chitwan to anyone looking for a good time. Just remember to always bring your own toilet paper…

On this trip so far, I've done my best to stay clean, by watching where I walk, and diligently showering and hand-washing my clothes, but really what is up with my need to be clean?!

_____ ***Tingting Peng***

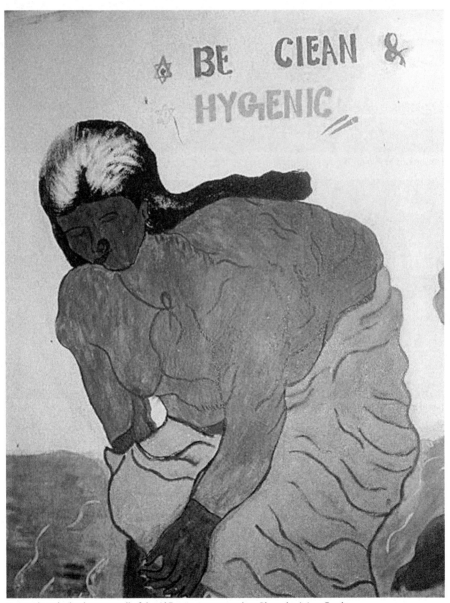

A mural on the bathroom wall of the Al Fresco restaurant bar. Photo by Jaime Furda.

June 30, 2010

Day 11 of the Trip

Namo Buddha

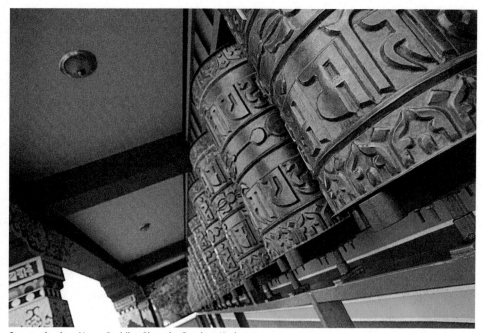

Prayer wheels at Namo Buddha. Photo by Candace Koslen.

After morning yoga, we had breakfast and then said our goodbyes to Hari and the staff at the Hotel Parkland. We had an absolutely amazing time in Chitwan and leaving was very bittersweet, especially since we knew we only had three days left in Nepal. The bus ride back to our next stop was scheduled to be 5 or 6 hours, but the group was re-charged and renewed after relaxing in Chitwan the last few days, so no one was complaining. We were on our way to Thrangu Tashi Yangtse Monastery, located at the sacred Buddhist pilgrimage site of Namo Buddha, Nepal, about a

40km drive southeast of Kathmandu, where we were going to pick up Candy, Marni and Jennette to join us. We were all excited about seeing our volunteer friends again and trading stories of our adventures in Nepal.

June 30, 2010_____

The bus ride to the Namo Buddha Monastery was mostly uneventful. I spotted a rainbow and pointed it out to everyone. It seemed like a positive omen. On a bathroom break I got the best compliment from Rachel. She said, "Mmm... You smell good."

_____ *Christina Jankus*

The trip to Kathmandu took a lot longer than expected, however. Traffic on the road back was heavy, and there were a few accidents on the mountainside that turned the two-lane road into a one lane parking lot in several places, slowing us down even more. At one point, we saw a flat-bed tow truck pass us hauling a smashed bus. Apparently the bus had collided with a semi-truck that morning. As it passed we could see the destruction – the front of the bus had been completely torn open, the twisted metal hole revealing the inside of the front cabin. It was hard to imagine that no one had been hurt in the accident. I said another silent thank you to Buddha, our driver, for having kept us safe throughout the trip.

Around noon or one o'clock, we stopped at the Blue Heaven Restaurant again, and had another excellent lunch, then got back on the road. We finally made it to Kathmandu 3 or 4 hours later. It was still light when we stopped to pick up Candy, Marni and Jennette. Once the women boarded the bus, however, we found ourselves stuck in Kathmandu traffic yet again. By now, we were all feeling annoyed with the starting and stopping, and it began to show. David seemed to get hit with claustrophobia, or maybe just a major bout of frustration at being stuck in an un-moving bus again...

June 30, 2010_____

We picked up Jennette, Candy and Marni to come with us to the monastery. Then David jumped off the bus to move on to Thamel. Oh no! It's happening again!

_____ *Christina Jankus*

David is a very free spirit, very much of a solo flyer, I came to learn on the trip, and now he decided that he'd had enough of the group activity and wanted to get off the bus right here, right now in Kathmandu. He said he didn't want to go to Namo Buddha, that he wanted to be closer to the kids. That didn't go over well with some folks. The mention of the kids set off another intense debate about what we were really doing here in Nepal. Should we really be doing so many touristy things? Shouldn't we be spending as much time as we could with the NOH kids? The debate was on the verge of getting really heated again. The newcomers on the bus were confused by David's actions, and by the sudden tension that had welled up in the group as the bus sat idling in traffic. They hadn't been with us in Narti, and so they were taken aback by all the emotional drama…

June 30, 2010 _____

… we were psyched to meet up with all of [those guys] and have this trip. And then we got on the bus and it was like "whoa." Seeing David… looking totally freaked out, …just looking at him and thinking, "Oh… he is freaking out." And thinking, "You don't get to just bolt." But at the same time feeling, well everybody gets to choose every part of the way what you're going to be a part of, just like sometimes in a class, the teacher calls out "handstand" and you can opt in or you can opt out. And who are you gonna be all the way there?

So here we were on this bus, and what I notice is all the people that had been on this amazing tour to some very beautiful places, it sounded like, and also some pretty hot and sticky places. It was like the yoga of living on a bus together. Forget just being in a hot room and practicing yoga for 90 minutes where you have to do a hundred sun salutations or 108 sun salutations or whatever it is, but put yourself in a bus with 20 other people and figure out how to get along; that's the yoga.

_____***Marni Task***

Jesse was so worn down by all the fractious debates that he didn't fight it, and let David get off the bus to do his own thing. Dave waved goodbye to all of us, and said he'd meet up with us in Thamel. Then, with our three volunteers on board, and David off, we resumed our ride to Namo Buddha. But all was not well. You could see the disappointment in the faces of some in our group. It felt like things might fall apart again, just as we'd finally become whole. I just shook my head. To each his own, I thought. I liked David, and if he really wanted to take off by himself for a bit, who was I to stop him? He seemed streetwise enough to take care of himself. I settled back in my seat, hoping for a quiet, uneventful rest of the ride.

We were told that Namo Buddha was right outside of Kathmandu and it wouldn't be long before we'd be there. That was enough to get everyone else settled down for the time being. But the ride to Namo Buddha was really only just beginning. Like that first long hill up to the highest point on a roller coaster, the hill right before the death defying, scream-inducing free fall down, we hadn't even really begun the ride, at least psychologically.

Buddha eventually navigated us out of city traffic and we began our ascent out of the Kathmandu Valley and into the surrounding mountains just before dusk. It was a slow but pleasant climb at first. The scenery was spectacular, hills and mountains covered in pine trees that reminded me of drives I'd taken around Yellowstone or the Samarian Gorge in Crete. As we rose in altitude, the temperature was more and more pleasant. I was actually getting excited thinking we'd be spending some time outdoors in 'normal' weather.

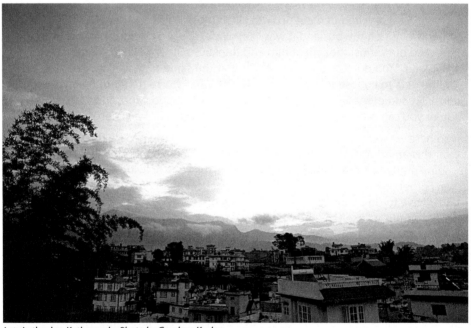

Late in the day, Kathmandu. Photo by Candace Koslen.

When we turned onto the final road up to the Monastery, night had fallen. We had no idea how far up we still had to go, and after 9 hours on the bus, people were once again really tired. Like Homer talking to Bart and Lisa on The Simpsons, Basu frequently assured us that we were almost there. Just a little further, he'd say. Just a little further. As we climbed higher and higher, the road became narrower and narrower, until finally we found ourselves on a one-lane rocky, uneven dirt road with the mountain on one side of us and a very steep cliff on the other. The bus's headlights were shining out into the blackness of the forest, illuminating the trees in front of us in harsh black and white shadows. As we continued lumbering uphill, every new bump, dip and jolt elicited louder "ooh's" and "whoa's." It looked and sounded like we'd stumbled into *The Blair Witch Project* or something. With every twist and turn, and every sudden unexpected jolt, more people got scared. After one especially violent and sudden lurch sideways toward the cliff, several people became seriously frightened thinking that the bus might actually tip over and go tumbling down the side of the mountain. It looked, and felt, like we were driving right along the edge of the cliff, which, along with the harsh shadows, the panicked voices, the sudden bumps and the unexpected jolts, unnerved everyone.

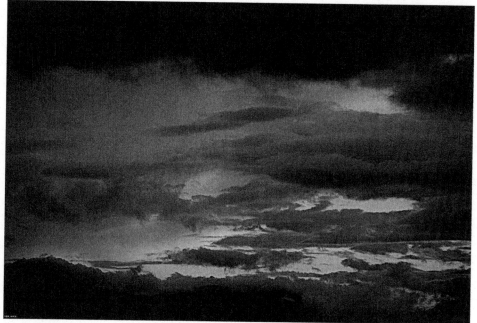

Sunset, Kathmandu. Photo Candace Koslen

And what none of us had known before, probably not even Jesse, was that there were at least two people on board with very serious acrophobia — a terrifying fear of heights. Jaime and Marc were not doing well at all. Marc asked for the bus to stop so he could get off. Both he and Jaime were close to hyperventilating, and some of the people around them, like Deanna and Rachel, were being adversely affected by their growing panic attacks and getting freaked out themselves. Marni tried to calm Jaime with some yoga breathing, with only slight success. At this point, the fear was infecting the entire back of the bus so much so that at one point Rachel threatened to jump out a window if they didn't stop the bus to let people walk the rest of the way. We were in the middle of nowhere and it was very dark, Jesse said, it wasn't safe to get off now. His response did not sit well with the people who were freaking out; it only infuriated them. They started venting their anger at him again...

As we started to go up this mountain it was really dark, night, and I said to myself, there are a lot of issues happening. But they're the same issues that I had been dealing with during the week as all my buttons got pushed, but issues nonetheless. As a yoga teacher, I tried to remember this, and of course, because I'm also a yoga student and I'm a human being first before I'm anything, I forget all of my yogic lessons often. And so as I watched people start freaking out on this bus, I was in my mind thinking "Where's the yoga?" We have almost, I can't even remember how many yoga teachers on the bus. There were definitely at least 15 yoga students, dedicated yoga students, and what I noticed was how our yoga practice went out the window.

So I just sat there and I was like, oh my god, things are escalating, it's like there's a fire, and people are just pouring gasoline on the fire as we went up this mountain, and peoples' issues like fear of heights started coming up, and I was afraid of heights, too, but I just wasn't looking out the window. I was having total faith in our driver... One of the people on the bus started hyperventilating now and freaking out and... I was thinking, "Oh my god, now someone's gonna pass out on the bus, and it's gonna be crazy," and I literally leapt out of my seat, grabbed this person, and started doing ujjayi breathing and said, "Breathe with me now." And it sounded like her breathing slowed down, she seemed to calm down. I don't know how she felt about it, I don't know if she hates my guts, but it was definitely something where I thought, Oh my god, this is why we do yoga. When someone's having a panic attack, the recipe is ujjayi breathing. That's the prescription. Not Prozac, not anything, the yogi's say ujjayi breathing and you'll slow your heart rate down, you'll slow your nervous system down, and your fears will subside and all that stuff will happen.

*Marni Task*

What I can see now, in hindsight, and what I couldn't see then because I'd been too deep in the middle of it, is that we were being stalked by a beast this whole trip. That beast was fear. Fear stalks from the shadows, watching, waiting for the right moment to strike, to take down its prey. Often we know that it's there. We can see it, smell it, feel it. Other times we don't; it's too far back, too well hidden in the shadows. Whether it's in our heads, or actually out there, the beast is real. Real and powerful, and when it's on the hunt, it doesn't give up its prey easily. It's unrelenting.

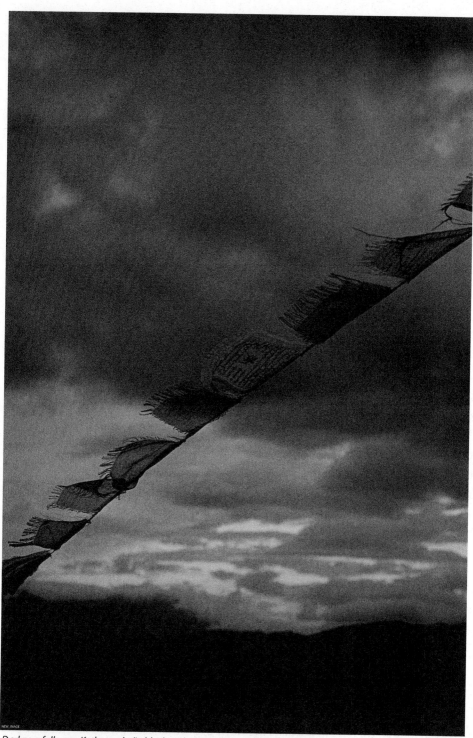

Darkness falls over Kathmandu (in black and white). Photo by Candace Koslen.

Fear had made several moves for us on this trip. Some were tentative probes, like the spider in the tree at Norling, or the plane ride to Everest that had spooked Kathy. And some of its strikes had drawn blood, like in Narti. But each time we'd managed to beat it back, like the Tharu stick dancers in Chitwan who used their clashing bamboo sticks to scare off wild beasts in the night. We hadn't let fear destroy us, we'd regrouped, circled our wagons, huddled together like bison on the Great Plains sticking together when the wolves come for them because there is strength in the group. Until now, we had kept fear at bay. But right then and there, on that Blair Witch bus ride up the mountain, fear pounced. And it was tearing into the group with a real zeal, turning our hard fought "we" back into a bunch of frightened "me's".

At this point Basu spoke up. It's rare that you see Nepali people get demonstrably, genuinely angry. At least I hadn't really seen it. They are used to such a chaotic living situation, I think, that it takes a lot to get under their skin. But Basu must have reached that point, and he told everyone in a loud firm voice to calm down. No one would be allowed off the bus, he said, as this was a wilderness area and it was not safe to be outside at night. You could stumble off the road, get lost, and get hurt, or worse run into a wild animal like a tiger. Getting off here was not an option. He assured us that we were safe, and that he and Buddha had made this drive many times before without incident. He asked, almost pleaded, for patience. Perhaps it was because of Basu, who everyone universally loved and respected, or perhaps because we soon found ourselves on a wider flatter road near the summit, but things finally settled down a little, and after 2 hours driving up the mountainside, we arrived at Namo Buddha, physically exhausted and emotionally frazzled. We got off the bus, and took a look around....

Namo Buddha looked beautiful in the late twilight. Like a real life version of Shangri-La, the Thrangu Tashi Yangtse Monastery sat perched on the mountain top we'd just climbed, looking out over the countryside below. The views were incredible, as was the cool fresh clean evening air. Breathing it in was intoxicating, absolutely refreshing to body and soul. And having our feet on the ground again was helping. At least some of us...

June 30, 2010 _____

Even though we were in the dark, the views of the monastery were spectacular. I've never seen a place more beautiful than this. However, other people's excitement was overshadowed by the experience of the ride up to the monastery....

It was a long day and I could understand their fears. It didn't help that we saw accidents on our ride to Kathmandu and we were going up the mountain at night. I can't believe that we just left Chitwan this morning. It seemed like a lifetime ago we were in Chitwan doing dancing meditation. I'm just glad we made it safely and we could go to bed. This day has been exhausting.

Minling Chuang

June 30, 2010

Buddha, our awesome bus driver, had to navigate to the top of one of the mountains to get to the monastery. It was dark and all you could see was the drop off the mountain. Thankfully I am not afraid of heights. Unfortunately some group members are afraid of heights and experienced great panic and distress with the drive to the top of the mountain.

When we finally got off the bus we found that the temperature had dropped around 30 degrees. The air was so crisp. It was good sleeping weather!

Christina Jankus

June 30, 2010

The ride up the hill of the Himalayas in the dark was frightening to say the least and we were shaken up when we got to the top. [There] was a moment in the trip where I felt totally unsafe and scared, and I wasn't alone. Rachel, Tingting, Jaime and I were in the back row and we were all crowded up against each other so tight I think I was pretty much sitting on Tingting, lol. [It] was worth the scary ride though… [for] the stillness and crisp clean air of the mountains.

Deanna Lee

Unlike the Korean Monastery at Lumbini, the monastery here was completely finished, a working, fully staffed, Tibetan Buddhist sanctuary. The colorful temples and other buildings that made up the monastery are a renowned pilgrimage site for Buddhists from around the world. The monastery itself is built on the site where legend has it that Lord Buddha gave his life to feed a starving tigress and her cubs. This sacrifice holds special meaning to all Buddhists. The area around the monastery took its name, ironically enough, because in the distant past people found it difficult to travel through the region for fear of all the wild animals, so they developed the practice of reciting "Namo Buddhaya" ("I take refuge in the Buddha") to dispel their anxiety. To this day, the local inhabitants call the area Namo Buddha.[13]

---

[13] Sources: www.wikipedia.com, www.namo-buddha.org

Most people were just relieved to be off the bus, and back on solid ground. That was certainly the case for me. I was already tuning in quickly to the peace and quiet I felt here. But others had not entirely recovered from the ride...

July 1, 2010

The trip was long for all of us, and emotions were raw. One of us left the group, and that was hard on many levels. Part of me was relieved, and yet part of me was sad. Then came the mountains. It was dark, and the road was bumpy. The road itself was along a cliff, and I was consumed with fear. I do not want to die here. I feel this amazing urge to do more in my life. I have much to do, many to serve, and many to love. I do not want to fall off of a cliff. We did make it. Not sure if it was just plain fear or the fear of heights, but I'm here. And tomorrow I will have to deal with it all over again. I am trying to stay in the present. Tough stuff for me...

Marc Nathanson

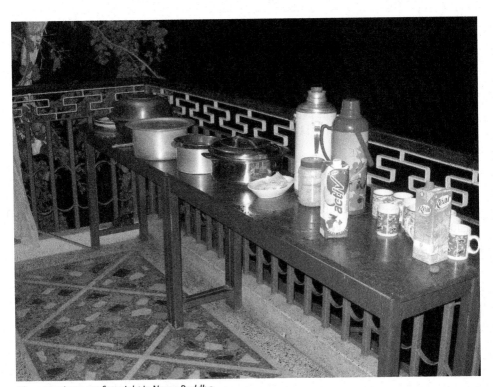

Dinner awaits us our first night in Namo Buddha.

After getting our things squared away in our rooms, we had dinner in a dining area on the second floor of one of the buildings at the base of the monastery. The food was once again simple, fresh, hot and delicious. A few of the monks joined us for the meal. There wasn't much conversation, though. Unfortunately, the ride up had split the fissures in the group wide open again.

June 30, 2010_____

The peaceful serenity of the mountains and crisp cool air are a fair trade-off with the harrowing bus ride we took to get here.

People freaked out ... because the bus ride had been too long, too cramped, and too hot. Then when we got closer to the monastery, people REALLY freaked out because it was pitch black on the windy dirt road in the middle of the mountains. Without their stories, it would've been just another bus ride... I went for a walk around the grounds after dinner. It was one of the greatest moments of solitude I'd felt since the trip started. If only people could just breathe and look up (rather than down) they too would get to see the beauty and magnificence here, the temples, the amazing mountain view, all of the prayer wheels, the energy here is one of purity, devotion, and austerity and strength. If only they could breathe it all in.

I am tired of the drama, talking behind people's back, the DRAMA.

Sitting back now, two more days including one day of silence, I am sincerely looking forward to it....

_____ *Tingting Peng*

July 1, 2010

Day 12 of the Trip

Day of Silence

Do not speak - unless it improves on silence. ~ Buddhist Saying

We were starting the morning with our usual yoga practice, this time on the large concrete walkway leading up to the main temple. Several people were late, and we delayed the start, quietly waiting for them to arrive.

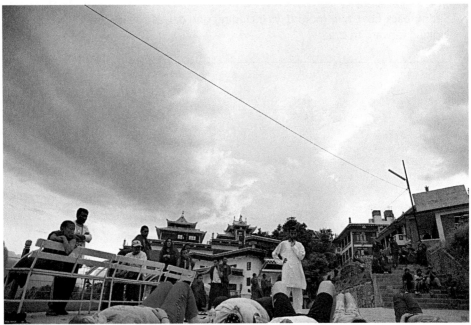

Morning savasana at the monastery as the monks look on with curiosity. Since it was founded in 1978 the monastery has grown such that today it is home to more than 250 monks along with various caretakers and their families. Photo by Candace Koslen.

When they didn't show we began without them. As we were going through the first warm-up poses, we found ourselves surrounded by a large group of curious monks who had just exited the temple from morning prayers. They were obviously surprised to see a dozen or more westerners doing yoga in their front yard. As they observed us, stretching and straining, in our lululemon yoga pants, t-shirts and Nike running shorts, we wondered out loud what they must think about us doing yoga out here on their driveway.

When practice was over, the monks drifted off to breakfast, their curiosity quickly satisfied. Jesse then began to describe the day ahead of us. The plan for today, he said, was to practice silent meditation for eight hours. Silence, however, was the last thing on some people's minds this morning.

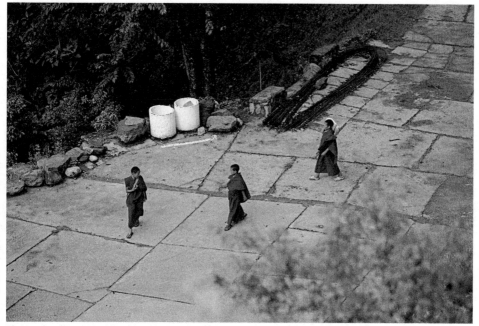

The monks of Namo Buddha. Photo by Candace Koslen.

The conversation turned to our mission here. Several people were disappointed that we weren't doing more with the kids. There was a lot of residual guilt coming out about our inability to really do something constructive for the children of NOH and for the overall situation in Nepal. You could hear the frustration in people's voices and things started to heat up once again. Then Candy, Marni and Jennette spoke up. This was the first time they'd been a party to our discussions, and they felt like they could offer another perspective.

Just as it felt right at the end of yoga practice that morning to listen to their stories, it feels like a good time now to circle back and see what this Yoga For Freedom journey was like for Candy, Marni and Jennette up to this point. For me, their perspective was invaluable in trying to come to grips with all that I had experienced in Nepal so far. Their story stands in stark contrast in many ways to the experiences we had, on the one hand. But it also affirms many of the underlying emotions we were all feeling at the time about Nepal, on the other. So here, in the chapter that follows, in their own words, without any embellishments from me, is the story of our three volunteers from their arrival in Kathmandu right up to the day of silent meditation at Namo Buddha…

The Volunteers' Journey

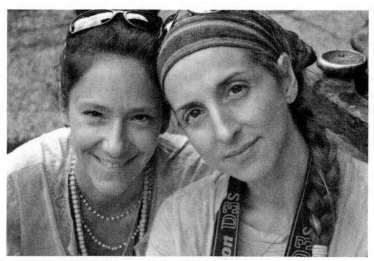

Marni Task and Candace Koslen. Photo by Jennette Zimmerman.

June 21, 2010

Landing at the airport [I was] thinking it was gonna be so intense right off the bat, but the airport was so pristine, so clean and beautiful, and everyone was really nice. And I was really scared and made sure I remembered to say "namaskar da zhu, namaskar da zhu," but everybody was super friendly and super nice. And then we get out of the airport and Jesse picks us up, and we go back to the volunteer house. Our bed is hilarious; Jennette and I share a bed; our little bed is too small for the mattress so it's up on a diagonal. That is hilarious to me.

Marni Task

June 22, 2010

Arrived in Kathmandu... we went straight to volunteer house. Carola showed us around all of the kids' houses... Sanctuary, Imagine, Boys' house, and Papa's house. We picked up the kids for tiffen and walked the kids back to school. Napped, overslept... (Jennette no longer in charge of alarm... haha)

Jennette Zimmerman

Everest flight [with the whole YFF group], then the first trip to Bal Mandir orphanage...

Sure, I packed my headlamp, check. Flip flops, camera, check, check.... but prepared?!... I walked right up the gates of hell, yoga mat rolled up under my arm, and knocked....

The government orphanages are corrupt and the conditions so intense, that I vomited in my mouth. Marni twice. While (many) administrative types sip tea in the offices, a few exhausted ditti's tend to an amazing amount of babies. The structure of Bal Mandir is grand, painted in bold colors of green and blue. You walk up a massive staircase with paint all chipping away and the smell of piss and shit and formaldehyde penetrate the air. There is a sign prohibiting photographs and the rooms where the babies are kept have to be unlocked by key. The hallway is dark, and damp. The first door on the right has older toddlers, running around in cloth diapers, or no diapers, dirty shirt, snotty nose. But they are happy to see us... so I just run in and immediately swoop two of them into my arms and I am kissing them and trying not cry, and laughing, and hugging them like crazy.

There are a few older kids with cerebral palsy in this room as well who are just lying on the floor. They are happy to see us too. They start clapping their hands and squealing like crazy. I kiss them too and rub their third eye with my thumb. I tell them I see them and that I am happy they are so happy. The babies find a water bottle that I start letting them drink from. They made a mess with it, which made it more fun and they started following me around the room pulling on my skirt for more. I left the water bottle with the ditti and went into the infant room, most of me anyway. At least 30 infants. The smell takes your breath away and the next time we visit we rub Marni's oil under our noses to filter the smell. 15 babies on a mattress... feeding themselves bottles, half of them pooped, half of them sick. All of them dirty. We just jumped in and started changing diapers, feeding babies, holding them, singing, kissing them, crying. I fell in love with a baby girl in that room. I fell in love with innocence on that day, even in the face of suffering.

On our next visit we are now privy to the 2nd room in the orphanage for younger toddlers. Other volunteers explained that these babes were the worst off as they were not being fed. They are given exclusively milk, 2 bottles a day. So we brought baby cereal with us, spoons from the VH, and Jordan. It's amazing how effortlessly people truly can connect. The water is boiling. Candy is mixing a huge batch of baby cereal, I pour the bath. We all get a bowl and spoon and before you know it, we each have a group of little birdies eating as fast as they can get it down. One by one in a little assembly line we bathe every single baby, and give them clean clothes, (even when the dittis tell us not to,) and a massage with Marni's indu lotion. We all sit in the playpen area blocked off by the windows and play with the babies. Everyone is getting held, some are dozing off in our arms. We sang baba hanuman, and devakinanda, as the babies danced and swayed, and ran up to us for hugs. (This is one of my most favorite memories, because it was the most bitter and the most sweet.)

I cried... Marni cried. Candy cried too.

Jennette Zimmerman

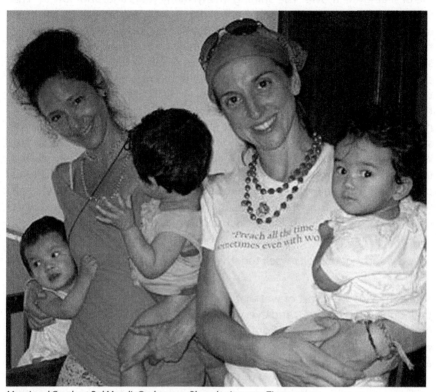

Marni and Candy at Bal Mandir Orphanage. Photo by Jennette Zimmerman.

June 23, 2010

Bal Mandir – Baby Orphanage

We have gone three days to this place...the last day was the hardest. To say goodbye was difficult. The first two days we spent feeding and bathing the toddlers. They do not eat solids so well, mostly formula. I held the sweetest girl. She just wanted to be held. I am not sure if two of the babies will make it. They look so far gone, malnourished.

The last day we spent in the newborn room. One baby was so small and still had the umbilical cord. They were so dirty... We cleaned them and fed them to the best of our ability. But mostly we sat and just held them – looked into their eyes.

Candy Koslen

Going to Bal Mandir, the government orphanage that we hung out at a few times, the thing that hit me the most, again in terms of my senses was the smell. You walk into Bal Mandir and it looks like a giant building, reminded me of seeing the movie "The Shining" many, many years ago, and how in "The Shining" it used to be this gorgeous building, with marble and big columns and now it's just dilapidated. The sign for Bal Mandir looked like it was almost falling off, very makeshift and painted. It was not a neon sign or some professional sign, if you will. Walking in you find this deserted building. Giant rooms that looked like palatial living rooms, but with old furniture in there and not that much of it. It's like calling down the hall—"Hello? Hello? Hello? Is anybody there? There was this winding staircase, and I would not want to go there at night, it would definitely freak me out at night. Then seeing all these people sitting in their offices just sort of hanging out and pushing papers. And I just wondered if they ever go down the hall to play with the kids. I finally walked into one of the rooms… and tears began rolling down my eyes as I picked up one of the kids. I felt like I wasn't gonna be able to do it. I had to pass this kid off to Candy 'cause I thought I was gonna throw up…. But I calmed down and I just told myself, "Just suck it up, Marni, suck it up." And then I slowly just got over it, I guess. I really didn't think I was gonna cry telling this story…

Anyway, sorry, gotta pull myself together as I'm trying to figure out what to say next.

So, all the kids were sort of wet diapered and it's not like they're Pampers, so their urine is now on you. And everybody's shirts are soiled, and in the far right near the windows, far away from the door, I mean it's not a very big room, it was a 20 by 20 room maybe or 20 by 30 or 40, not huge, and there's probably about ten old, wooden cribs with soiled mattresses. There was one baby who was either blind and deaf or just deaf, I don't know, sort of rocking herself side to side in the crib, probably trying to be stimulated or something. Near the windows, of course there are bars on the windows, there were about 4 or 5 or 6 kids who probably had cerebral palsy or autism or something like that and they were lying on the ground, and they were not young children, 'cause this was the toddler room. They were probably 8, 9, 10, 12 years old, with diapers on, with dried saliva, dried eye stuff in their eyes. And I said to myself, "Oh my god, what am I gonna do now? How am I gonna deal with these kids?" And actually, Jennette was really amazing with them. She was totally interacting with them and making them laugh. And so I went over and tried to play with them too, while I had one baby, a toddler, in my arms. So that was that room.

We changed a bunch of diapers and all sorts of stuff and just played with the kids and they were super cute, and they were probably 2- to 3-year-olds. And then we went to the baby room. We went there a few times. There were brand new babies— two weeks old—there were babies 3 months or 6 months old and just so sweet. It was a little funky. You walked into this very long room and there were cribs lined up. Kind of like that book that cute little kids' book Madeline where she's this little French girl—I can't remember if she's an orphan or if she's going to a school— there's all these teeny-weeny cribs. But then there's also a small square room that has bars on the windows and these mattresses on the floor, and there are cribs gating and blocking the kids in near the window. It's like their play area. We sat in there and played with them and held the babies and rocked the babies and changed diapers and did all that.

Marni Task

June 24, 2010

Volunteer House

My bed is by the window. I feel the breeze at night, and hear the dogs barking… they bark… all… night… long. It's funny how their howls are starting to comfort me.

Did some yoga on the rooftop and took pictures of the sunrise. Love the flags against the sky, as the light filters through the clouds.

Candy Koslen

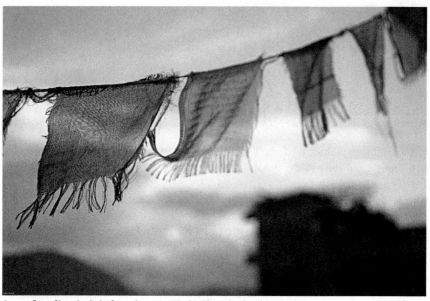

Prayer flags filter the light from the morning sky. Photo by Candace Koslen.

June 24, 2010

Nepal is fascinating, and scary, and lovely, and chaotic and dirty and dark and colorful and glorious, and spiritual... Nepal is all of it, and Kathmandu is all of it on crack. It's gotta be one of the craziest places on earth and in my clumsy attempt to describe Kathmandu, I'll start with a metaphor... If I handed you a glass of water and told you whether or not it was hot or cold, you would certainly know what that means. You have enough in your own memory to know what hot or cold is... but if instead I handed you the glass of water and had you taste it, your understanding of its temperature would take on many new dimensions. When you taste it, you know. You know how hot or cool, you know the texture, the taste, you know how it feels in your mouth, on your tongue, down your throat, into your belly. Feeling it all the way down. Kathmandu is the water.

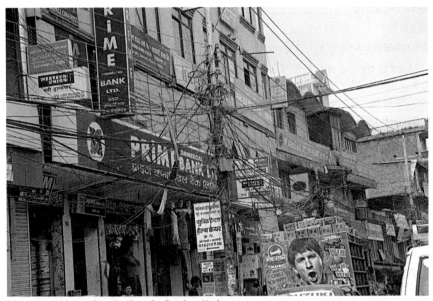

Electricity, Kathmandu style. Photo by Candace Koslen.

I can try and explain it, and you'll get the idea, but without tasting for yourself, you really can't fully know what Kathmandu will awaken in you. Statistically, and for a visual, Kathmandu is crowded. Very, very crowded. It's also poor. Very, very poor. Many people residing in homes that are the exact equivalent to being homeless in the United States. Entire families sleeping in little shacks of tin, or cardboard, and lumber, plastic tarps for roofs, held up by sticks. Living conditions of this standard are completely normal. People will sorta gather outside in front of their "box" and happily chat while the street dogs and barefoot little filthy children play with trash freely within an inch of a major road with buses and micros and motorcycles zipping thru at crazy speeds. The older kids may be selling trinkets or begging or both. A haircut is performed on a wooden chair with a mirror nailed to a tree next to the highway, as is most commerce in Kathmandu. Amidst the hundreds of colorful Kirta wearing women busting their asses doing work such as carrying 100 pound bags of rock up flights of stairs on their heads for new construction, you may also find them digging up the road... by hand... before dawn... You will also find the women of Kathmandu selling goods, running shops, cooking, begging, teaching, tending to the children and most everything else. The men had a lot of sipping tea, smokin' smokes, and hanging out going on. Of course my experience is limited. Additionally, and not to pick on the fellas, but these are also (sometimes) the fathers and step-fathers who sell their daughters to pay off debt. These are also the landlords that take these children as their payment. It's a helpless situation for the women and children of Nepal, who are at the mercy of the more respected male. Extreme poverty and destitution are the criminals here. Complete desperation leads to moral decay, and pretty much everything is corrupt. From the government to the orphanages, from what I've heard.

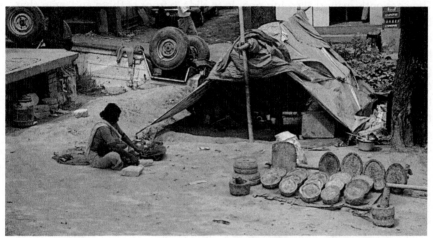

Just one example of what it means to live in poverty in Kathmandu. Photo by Candace Koslen.

This city is on fire. The poverty is staggering. Unspeakable. I passed an infant on a sidewalk with a toddler, both filthy, hundreds of people stomping thru and some would throw a coin or two at them. I saw a boy with no arms and no legs rolling around on the sidewalk, for money. I immediately began wondering if someone had done that to him, so he would make more money begging for them. And then I kept walking... but I think he walks with me now. I saw boys my son's age huffing sealant until they were so gone that their eyes rolled back into their heads and they started thrashing about on the sidewalk. (Children who have lost all hope for life will rock your soul.)

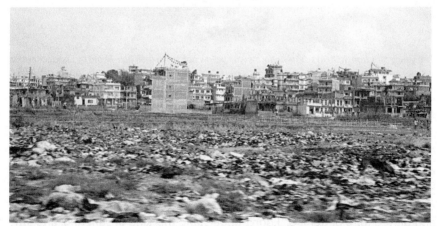

A dog searches for food in the garbage strewn on the outskirts of Kathmandu. Photo by Candace Koslen.

I saw Thamel, the tourist, trekking district after midnight and all that went thru my head was "I sure hope I don't get raped... cause that could totally happen right now." I saw HUGE bulls strolling in and out of darting traffic with everyone treating them with the utmost respect. I saw a goat get slaughtered while we were walking home one day, (Marni said a blessing.) I saw at least 30 cars, and 50 motorcycles sit in 105 degree weather, in black smog for over 30 minutes, and no one lost their temper. No one so much as gave a look of frustration. They patiently waited allowing people to slide in front of them and even chatted and smiled. I saw an entire row of Buddhist monks stand from their morning prayers to pull the rug out from underneath them so that their guests, who had wandered in off the street, could meditate more comfortably. (They also gave us their food :) I saw a mattress of babies covered in flies. I saw the sunset over the [Himalayan] mountains from the rooftop. I saw a train of young girls braiding each other's hair with yellow ribbons. I saw a man kiss 150 children on their way into school. (All his, and he does it every day :) I saw all of my friends cry, and they saw me cry. (much more than I saw them, but still.)

_____ **_Jennette Zimmerman_**

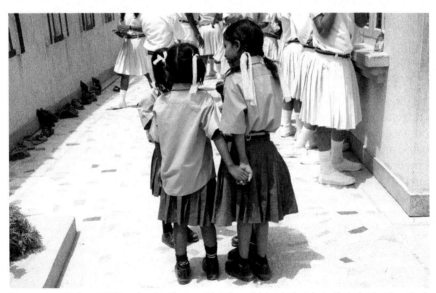

Two young girls from NOH in school uniforms with yellow ribbons in their hair. Photo by Candace Koslen.

June 24, 2010_____

Durbar Square

Center of Kathmandu… The hardest walk of my life, on the sidewalk toward a boy with no arms or legs, that rolls around for rupees… The handicapped and elderly also line the streets here. It's so very sad. I cried behind my sunglasses, and prayed for a better life. I don't understand this kind of suffering, and am grateful that I don't have to see it every day. Is it wrong to say that? I wanted to pick up that child and take him somewhere else. Why didn't I? Could I have done something other than keep on walking?

Candy Koslen

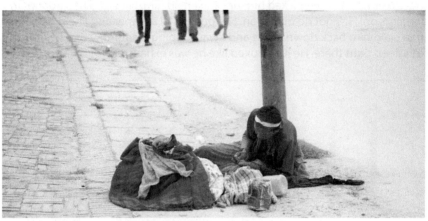

Living on the streets in Kathmandu. Photo by Candace Koslen.

June 25, 2010

We went back to Bal Mandir, to the government orphanage — we had heard about another room that we didn't see — kind of the 12-month to the 2-year-old room, and that room had some kids that were completely malnourished. They had the big bellies. We finally got to that room a few days later, and we brought rice cereal with us and fed all the kids and bathed them all. And we ended up chanting and clapping, "hari Krishna, hari Krishna" or "jay si ram jay jay han an" and then "sitaram sitaram, jay jay sitaram". I found a little bag of Legos and gave every kid a little Lego and one was banging it against the wall, and we were making music together. They were just so huggable and so cute.

There was one kid in the room that we had been warned about by our friend Colt, who was another volunteer who had been there. Colt said, "Somebody's gotta make sure to hang out with this kid." And you know, what he had said to us was that this little kid was a little out of it and not progressing in terms of his age and interaction with people. So I kept looking for this kid, but I didn't see him, I didn't notice a kid like this. And then all of a sudden, a few kids were brought into the room. I don't know where he had been, maybe because he's in a transitional age, like 19 months or 22 months, not two years old, they're starting to gradually put him into the other room with the older kids, but he's still with the younger kids, that kind of thing. So, he comes into the room, and I notice this adorable little boy who has this blank stare on his face. If you smile at him, he doesn't smile [back]. He just stands there, but he somehow found a Lego — this little orange Lego, I think it was — and he hung out in the corner, and I felt sort of shy, as I said, I'm meeting all these new people and you keep

301

waiting for someone to come up to you and say "Hi!" But you're the grown up! So I go up to this little kid and smile at him, but he doesn't seem to be at all responsive. But I said to myself, "alright, well, fuck it, I guess I'm just gonna pick him up." And I picked him up and he totally glommed onto me and just relaxed into my arms. And still no response. I tossed him into the air a few times, no smile. Nothing. When I picked him up, and I held him, I realized he's got no underpants on! He's got no diaper on. So I put him in a diaper and I held him. And then I laid him back down again and I was rubbing his tummy and he literally fell asleep right there. He just looked like he was exhausted.

_____Marni Task

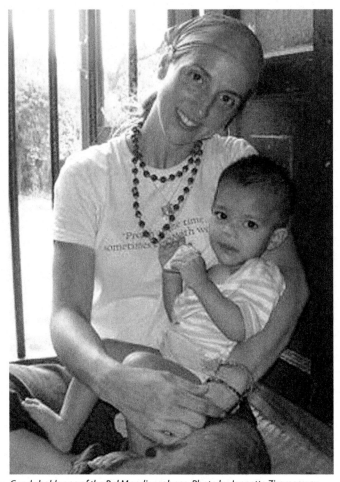

Candy holds one of the Bal Mandir orphans. Photo by Jennette Zimmerman.

June 25, 2010_____

Nepal Orphans Home is a Diamond in the rough of Kathmandu. It is a safe haven for children who know suffering. The education and love given to the children of NOH is unparalleled. The children are beautiful and grateful and hopeful and full of love. There are no material possessions that these children would trade for the love of their sisters and papa. All of the children help each other with homework. They braid each other's hair and tell each other how much they love each other. They are curious and happy, they are connected to God, and without Papa's house they don't stand a chance. Kathmandu is hell on earth for orphaned children. They will simply get swallowed up into the sadness, and suffering, and lack. Falling away into addiction, and poverty, and despair. Nepal Orphans Home provides actual hope and possibility to children that are literally as good as dead if left to the demise of child slavery. Moreover, these children will be powerful citizens of Nepal; Michael is raising a generation of leaders. They have the best shot at making real change for the people of Nepal, these children are the future.

*_____ **Jennette Zimmerman***

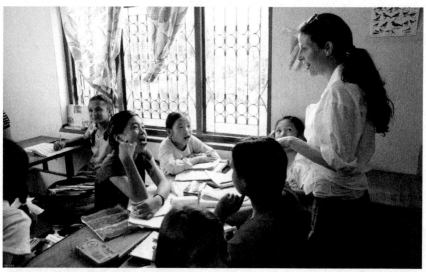

Jennette teaches school at NOH. Photo by Candace Koslen.

June 25, 2010 _____

The Bridge School

School's closed for vacation – not sure if we will make it. It's my understanding that the people here made the school. This is remarkable, because it's under a bridge in the middle of a garbage dump. The people of Nepal want to rise above – I hope I get to go. This would be an example of the strength of these people. This is the hope, the love that they share for a better future…for the children… I helped a boy with his homework, and watched him play basketball. He asked if he could call me "mom."

*_____ **Candy Koslen***

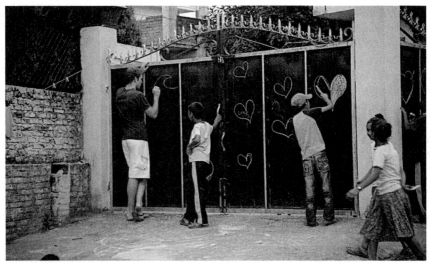

Volunteer Jake Hickey, left, joins in the chalk drawing at NOH. Photo by Candace Koslen.

June 26, 2010 _____

I watched the kids cut the grass at Papa's house. Then all day play day at Papa's!!! Frisbee, notes, rainbow parachute, jam session, and all of the June birthdays were celebrated! Tried to get a massage.... Marni and I got a Thai massage at the nature club; we ate spicy masala chips waiting forever... Candy got her kirta made. (Thai massage on a mattress on the floor... interesting.) Came back to [Volunteer house], Jordan took us up to the rooftop and we meditated while he did some energy work on Marni.

_____ ***Jennette Zimmerman***

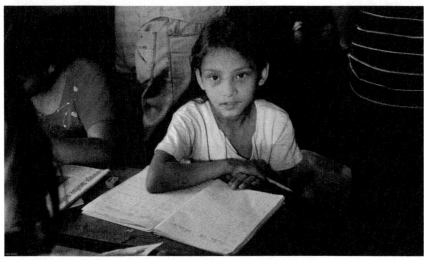

The kids take their homework very seriously at NOH. Photos by Candace Koslen.

June 26, 2010 _____

Sanctuary House

{The girls] put together a Disney puzzle with me this morning… it felt like heaven on earth…such contentment in all their actions. [They are] so sweet and gentle. [Their] smiles melt my heart. [They] have such depth. You can see it in their eyes. They speak volumes without a single word being spoken. [One girl] is very quiet and quite serious… but loves music and to sing.

_____ *Candy Koslen*

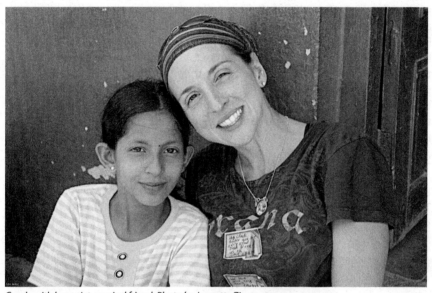

Candy with her quiet, musical friend. Photo by Jennette Zimmerman.

June 26, 2010 _____

Of course we want to take all the kids home with us, but we can't take any of them 'cause of the way the government is run here, and because there's no paper trail and because of the black market and because of the Kamlari system and the human trafficking system. Some of the kids are stolen from families that still want their kids. And then somehow they wind up in the system. Some of these kids could have been brought and just dropped off at the orphanage, but they don't know who the parents are. And so because they don't know who the parents are, they can't place the kid 'cause there's no paper trail. So it's this totally whacked out, crazy system…

I loved going to see the kids, but I noticed I was a little shy meeting all these new people. And really struggling and really really wanting to learn their names, every single one of them because first of all, I wanted to get to know them, but also I feel like there's something important about knowing someone's name and, so it was really daunting to me. I don't know, sort of, not sad to me, but it was just hard. I really wanted to learn their names, and I know there's some that I really know well now by name, and there are some that I don't, and there's this guilt around it.

The kids in Nepal Orphans Home are incredibly beautiful, so happy, so appreciative, so smart—that really struck me.

... I tried to learn their names but couldn't get them and so I finally asked Shivani, she is the person in charge of the volunteers at the volunteer house at NOH, to take me to a stationary store for name tags, or sticky labels. But ahhhhhhhh yes, we are in Nepal so finding Avery sticker labels or any labels at all was not easy. We went to a teeny, tiny store on our street in Dhapasi Heights. It was packed floor to ceiling with stuff. The stuff had dust/dirt all over it, but Shivani asked the owner about name tags/stickers. The man had several kinds; Power Ranger ones, Spiderman, sailboat name tags (he had a lot of these), a few other funky ones. They were definitely stickers, but I had hoped for plain ones that they could color and decorate. So I took them with me to the big Saturday party at Papa's house. Every Saturday is a big "family" get together for all of the houses at NOH. Lunch is served, there's lots of playing and hanging out time and one Saturday a month they celebrate everyone who was born in that month. There are lots of presents, chocolate cake, laughing, games and so on...

So I brought the stickers to Papa's house... about 160 for all the kids and all the adults. It was a sticker frenzy! Not only a sticker frenzy, but each kid had colored all of the sticker label even though it had a sailboat or a power ranger on it. The paper the sticker had been stuck to was a valuable commodity too! Used sticker paper was flying everywhere!

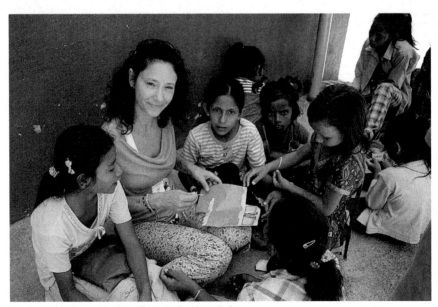

Marni and her famous stickers. Photo by Candace Koslen.

So now because everyone wanted a piece of paper I had to figure out how to cut and ration the paper so everyone got a piece! Needless to say everyone wanted to color a picture! I was so happy they liked this project but also a bit stressed because I wanted to make sure everyone got a piece on which to color. When we ran out of paper, they started tattooing my arm and we drew hearts on our hands... so fun! Even though I still cannot remember all of their precious names they are all in my heart!

_____*Marni Task*

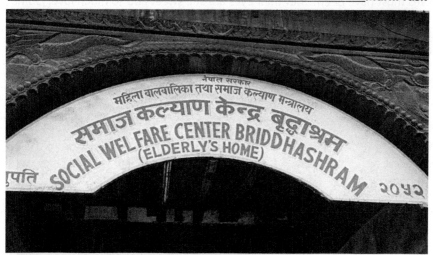

The sign outside the Elderly Ashram in Kathmandu. Photo by Tingting Peng.

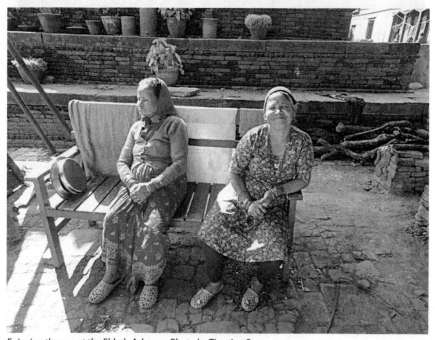

Enjoying the sun at the Elderly Ashram. Photo by Tingting Peng

Elderly Ashram

I watch the people…their daily activity. Lots of the women work in the fields and sweep the streets. You can tell by their old crippled figures what kind of work they endured. One woman's back bent nearly in half – she worked the fields. Another only half-bent swept the streets. Can't imagine how hard their lives must have been…but their eyes are still sweet and so much love. Some slept. Some stayed by themselves. Others smiled and wanted their picture taken. I am blessed to have laid eyes on them…they have touched my heart and left me forever changed.

Candy Koslen

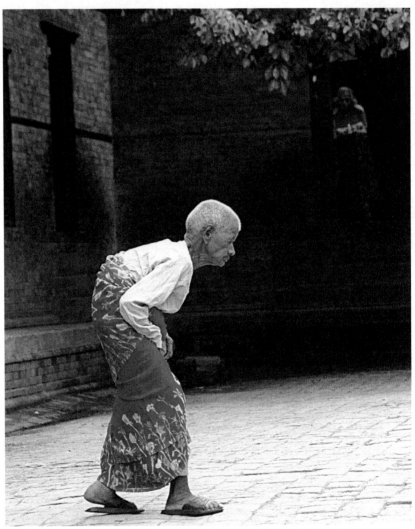

An old woman, bent but not broken, from years of hard work. Photo by Candace Koslen.

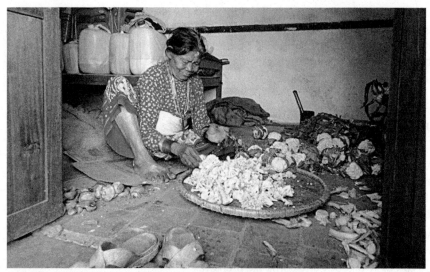

Preparing a meal at the Elderly Ashram. Photo by Tingting Peng.

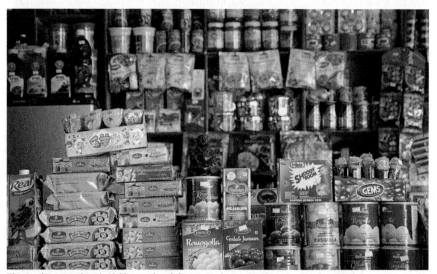

This is what munchies look like at a local shop in Kathmandu. Photo by Candace Koslen.

June 27, 2010

I definitely love the chili momos, and the veggie momos, [but] I am longing for some of my American creature comforts. I've been away a lot in my life, and I've traveled the world, and I never usually get homesick, and I find now that about, maybe 5 or so days into the trip, I am getting homesick. And I'm specifically homesick for simple things like my seltzer or bubbly water with lemon and lime, and I was so excited when we went to one of the more Americanized restaurants to see lemon soda on the menu. And lemon soda was, of course, club soda with a big whole lemon squeezed into the drink. Of course, they served it to me with salt in the drink, and I nearly yakked my head off, but, you know, 'swhatever'... "Swaha." That means "I give it up." I find that I am giving up, "swaha-ing," a lot in Nepal; I am letting go, surrendering to this culture, and really we have to do that, I guess, on a daily basis, wherever we are, but especially, here.

_____*Marni Task*

June 28, 2010 _____

Very powerful meditation – had a heavy heart in the beginning. Tingling in my skin – lots of energy held in my hands. JZ cried. Put my hands to her head. 108 prayers – mantras – *om mani padme hum* – may the wisdom in my heart be revealed.

We went back to the monastery at Boudhanath this morning. Yesterday it rained, so we did not see *prenam*. Today we walked, and as the people – so devoted – walked... and some did *prenam*.

The shops are beautiful. The *malas* and trinkets that are made here are amazing: rugs, sweaters, prayer flags, wheels, singing bowls, and deities.

We watched a woman feed a million pigeons! So many dogs everywhere, sleeping in the streets, eating garbage or whatever a passerby will offer.

Life is hard here for everyone, so very hard. You see it in their bodies, their faces, their eyes. But they are strong, hopeful, and loving.

_____ ***Candy Koslen***

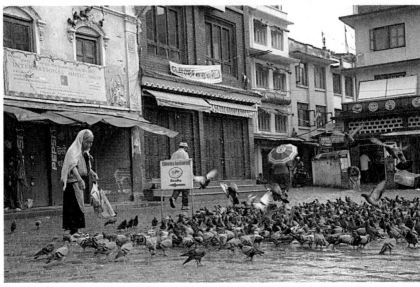

A woman feeds the pigeons in Boudhanath. Photo by Candace Koslen.

June 27, 2010 _____

The microbuses [here] are so old and broken down, but they work! I could drive a bus like this, it works! It goes. That was amazing to me. They really, literally use everything 'til it's done. They don't throw out something that's just half-new or lightly used. They use it 'til it's used up.

_____*Marni Task*

June 28, 2010 _____

Boudhanath in the AM with the monks :)

Cried for 3 straight hours... breakfast at Heavenly View restaurant and then to old city of Kathmandu. Gone all day there. Home for homework... dinner. Marni moves upstairs, 'cause the mattress on our bed doesn't fit the frame so we have been sleeping sorta upright for the last week.

_____ ***Jennette Zimmerman***

June 29, 2010 _____

Bakhtapur, the Old City

It took an hour or so to get here. Riding in buses is hard for me. I need to be by the window, because of all the people. I need air, but not sure which is the worse of two evils, because the air is so dirty. Some people wear masks all the time, mostly children, but some adults, too. There is a lot of dust, because the roads are dirt. When it rains, they turn to mud. There is garbage that lines the sides of the roads – it is everywhere! Some places more than others, but it's everywhere. Sometimes I can't believe what my eyes are seeing. I close them, then I think when I open them again, I'll be somewhere else. Or that this reality will somehow be different, but it's not. These people will never know fresh air, clean water or streets…

I think of their lives and my heart is so heavy. Children play and smile, just like mine do at home. This is what they know. The only life – the only way – I wish and hope one day they will have what I have. I wish I could do more than just witness their reality. If there was something more I could do…Nepal feels to me hopeless at times. But despite it all, there is beauty. Flowers and prayer flags find their way between the barbed wire fences. Under the masks are smiles from the children. They wave and say "Namaste" with much curiosity, as I snap my camera. The textures on the buildings against the sun are magnificent, and the colors so beautiful, despite the weathering of the wind. There is beauty everywhere, because that is life.

We lost Jennette and Marni in the old city, in its tiny little streets off the main square where the temple is. Shivoni (one of the volunteers) and I were going in

311

one direction and they the other. A couple of boys returned them to the group. They went up to them and said "You know your friends are over there looking for you." The people here are gentle and very kind. The animals are treated well... Cows are not eaten, because they provide milk to nourish our bodies. Cows roam the streets in Kathmandu. Cars stop and wait for them to pass. Nepal is full of the unexpected. You never know what your eyes will see next.

Candy Koslen

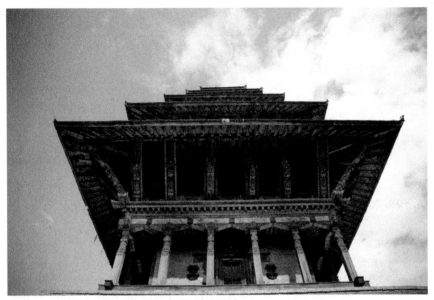

An ancient temple in Bakhtapur. Photo by Candace Koslen.

June 30, 2010

Yoga is not just on your mat... I think that was what I realized most about this trip—the yoga that happens off the mat. I noticed when I was in Kathmandu meeting all these new people, the people who I was drawn to and the people who really repelled me, and having to sit with all those feelings that are uncomfortable. "Why don't I like this person? Why don't I like everybody? I wanna love everybody." Just sitting with my discomfort....

I just thought, as much as the trip was so super hard, it was an opportunity for me, and I think everyone to really practice their yoga. I don't know if everyone got that, but I thought this trip was like a bed of nails, like the austere yogis in India who in the dead of winter sit outside in a loin cloth and have a bucket with cold water dripping down their head. They sit outside for three hours in the freezing cold. Crazy, austere stuff. This was an austere trip. And who were we going to show up as? Were we going to show up as calm, cool, and collected yogis so we could do the work that needed to be done? Or were we gonna flip out? And it was hard. It was very hard. I definitely struggled a lot on the inside, but I think in the end we all made it through. And I think we did a great—I don't know, I guess what I would call a great job, really finding our way.

_____***Marni Task***

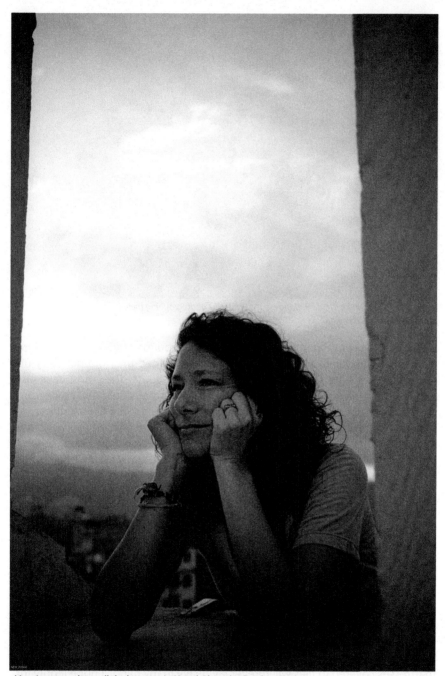

Marni contemplates all she has seen in Nepal. Photo by Candace Koslen.

Namo Buddha

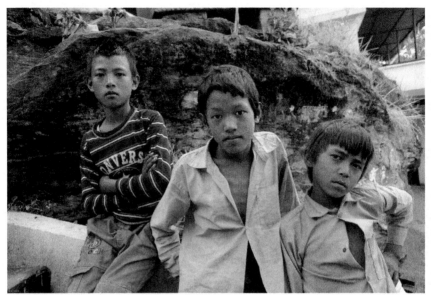

Three young boys living in Namo Buddha eye the Westerner photographing them with a mixture of curiosity and skepticism. Photo by Candace Koslen.

I have found a spot…perched on the hillside surrounded by prayer flags. Two boys gave me a silent tour of the monastery. I helped their mother carry up two buckets of water, and she let me see the baby goats. They must have just been born, safely tucked under a basket. I asked if they could drink milk from their mother, and she complied – such beautiful pictures. The boys showed me statues and caves, until one of my friends offered them chocolate. (I became less interesting…) We hear the gentle breeze and the sound of crickets (ahhh!) I can appreciate so much from coming to Kathmandu. I haven't inhaled this deeply in over a week.

Fresh air is just what I needed. I am grateful. I have seen more than I bargained for over the last two weeks. At times, I must admit feeling hopeless and despair. [Now] I sit in a place of acceptance… I have seen children dirty and rolling in the streets begging for rupees, one with no arms or legs. I have contemplated how this came to be, a birth defect or crippled to be used to gain attention of tourists. It does not matter – it just is and I accept it. I do wish there was more I could do. I have bathed, fed, and changed the diapers of many babies. I have looked into their eyes, held them, and gave my love for such a short time. It's not nearly enough, but it's all I have. I go to sleep thinking of them…if they are crying will there be someone to hold them? Will they have enough food to eat? What kind of future will they have? A room full of babies lying on pee soaked mattresses covered in flies will forever lay heavy in my mind. I hope if only for a few moments they felt my love. If I could have duck-taped [one child] to my belly, I would have, as she clung to me like a monkey the last time I put her down. As I walked away I could hear her cries. But her smile and her bright eyes will always be in my heart. I blessed them, each one, to be safe, healthy and happy. I pray to God, with eyes full of tears, to keep her eyes bright to watch over her – all of them.

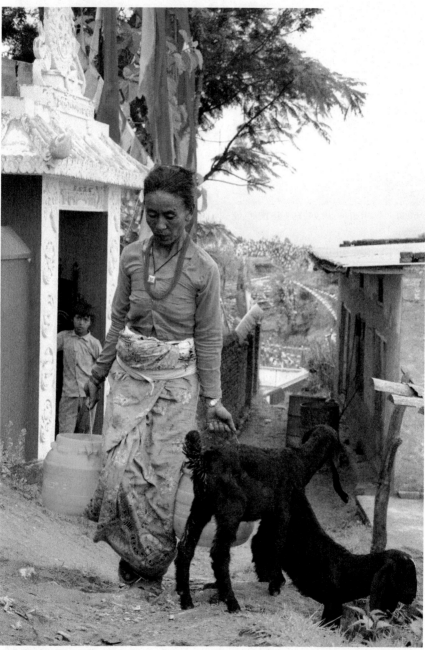

A mother hauls water for her family, and their goats, in Namo Buddha. Photo by Candace Koslen.

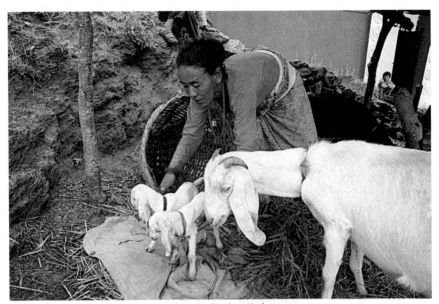

Feeding and caring for the baby goats. Photo by Candace Koslen.

Some people might question a God who could let this happen. I say if you question God, come to Nepal… you will go home a believer. Amongst the chaos there is space. Where there is space there is peace. Where there is peace there is God. You will find God in a microbus much faster than meditating on a hillside… (Trust me, I know.) You may ask, why so much suffering? God knows I have. There is no answer and there never will be, and that has to be enough. The beauty is the people, the faces, and the love seen in their eyes. I cannot save or change them, but maybe inspire and teach them a different way, one child at a time. For children will grow up and hopefully remember.

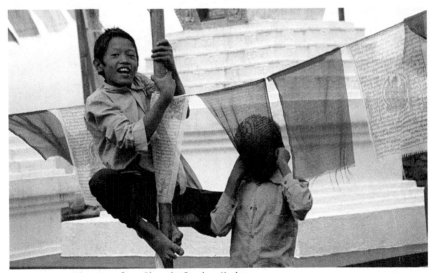

Playing among the prayer flags. Photo by Candace Koslen.

And so I wondered how all these prayer flags came to be…and a child climbed a tree. I cry not for sadness, although I am sad. I cry for happiness, because I am so happy. Especially in Nepal, I am happy.

"For all the darkness in the world cannot put out the light of one candle" ~unknown.

This gives me hope and with hope all things are possible. I am a fellow traveler in search of something more…I am grateful for Nepal. I miss my children. 3 more sleeps. HOME.

Candy Koslen

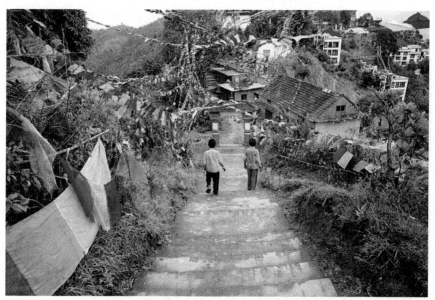

Candy's young guides take the steps back down to their home. Photo by Candace Koslen.

July 1, 2010 – Namo Buddha

I really wish the more enlightened me would just show up already and pull me thru this. My heart is so heavy. I haven't felt this helpless or truly sad in such a long time. I know this is how it must be, suffering, being part of the deal. I just had no idea that the suffering I was going to witness so closely in Nepal would be my own.

I got onto an airplane 13 days ago with a rather Pollyanna perspective of how I would be spending my time in one of the poorest countries on the planet, volunteering my time to girls who of all things, had been slaves… The unspeakable ongoing practice of kidnapping, selling, and raping children. Girls who have lived and breathed, and were swallowed up by the darkness of mankind in their tears and in their screams. Hopelessness…

I am a witness now, and the visions are burned into my memory as a reminder

317

not to make light of either the suffering, or the commands that you give the universe. I had made a game of the do-gooder role, and the house always wins.

All I wanted now was to be home in my bed, watching the trees and the moon. Sleeping babies downstairs tucked away together dreaming of ice cream, and waterfalls, and puppies. They themselves knowing very little of suffering, and I am grateful for that. More in this moment than ever before in my life.

Home feels like another lifetime. I've almost opened so much to the suffering that my life back home feels like a dream. Like a fairytale [one of the girls] and I wrote of a life that only exists in American T.V. and magazines. Somewhere a million miles away and the idea [of it]...feels as unrealistic as a day trip to Jupiter.

The children here are survivors. They expect neither sympathy nor coddling. "They live for the buck, they get for the family", (I love M.I.A.)

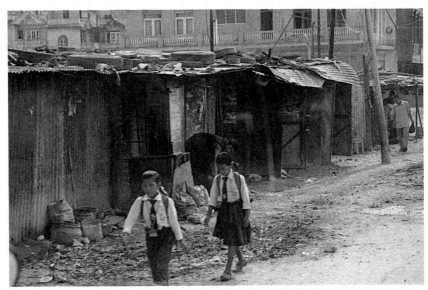

A young boy and girl walk to school in Kathmandu. Photo by Candace Koslen.

So as I sit here on a decidedly silent (sorta) day of reflection at Namo Buddha monastery high in the Himalayas overlooking some of the most gorgeous countryside in all of creation, I am feeling safe in this sacred space. I am ready to speak about what I have witnessed....

12 hours at a Buddhist monastery is exactly what the doctor ordered when you are on the brink of an all-inclusive breakdown. After only 12 hours here I am able to take deep breaths again. The choke hold around my heart has lifted a little and the painful knots in my stomach have started to ease their relentless grasp. Here I feel God. I feel compassion.... and mostly I feel safe to let it flow thru me in the shelter of the sky that the mountains provide.

...There is something decidedly different about friends made in Nepal. A five minute conversation with someone new at the VH, head out into the city, and you might as well be sisters, brothers, long lost friends...

Marni is my yoga teacher and I love her even more after this journey, which I would have thought an impossibility. She is a gift to all of humanity. Candy and I have a history that includes some of my most favorite memories and some of my darkest... (She is also a gift to us all, and I pretty much would lick her feet at this point in time).

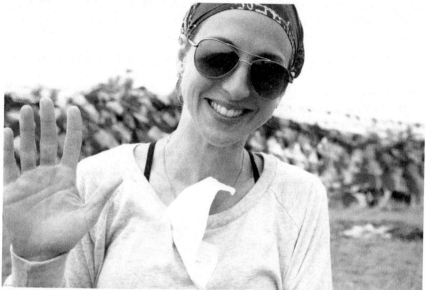

Photo of Candy taken with her camera by one of the young Nepali boys who accompanied her on the day of silence around Namo Buddha.

Truth be told, every single volunteer that I met in Kathmandu was amazing....

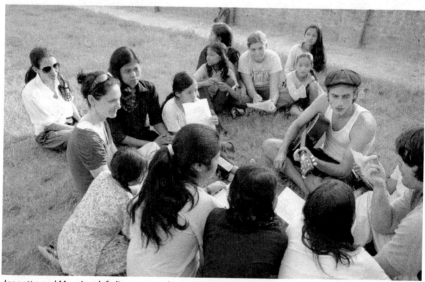

Jennette and Marni, at left, listen to a volunteer teach the NOH kids songs on the guitar. Photo by Candace Koslen.

… I see the faces of my children in every child here… All I can do is cry, wiping the snot and the tears on my (really nasty) sweatshirt, losing my breath, catching my breath, and I am lonely, and I am sad, and I am sorry. I am so sorry that there is no action to take other than tears. Tears are the holiest and purest form of support that I can give the people of Kathmandu. Tears of horror and fear. Tears of devotion and compassion. Tears of hopelessness and helplessness. Tears for not doing more, for not giving more, for not being more. Tears of confusion, of shock. Tears of gratitude for my life... and mostly tears of pure love.

I don't care who you are or what you've done. Your experience can a monster make, I have love for you too. Love for the ones who never had a chance. Love for the ones who had to harden to survive. The ones who were abused and the ones who ultimately become the abusers. Tears for the old who have seen lifetimes of suffering and the young who have yet to walk in the pain. I cry for the children that could never imagine it having been any different for them. I am not afraid of the pain anymore; I will sit here with you. I will never leave you.

Jennette Zimmerman

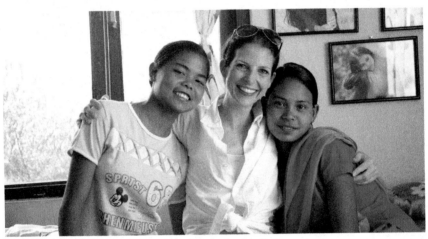

Jennette with two of the older girls of NOH. Photo by Candace Koslen.

Untitled Poem

Go to the edge.

don't let fear stand in

your way

for at the edge

there is no fear

only love.

And when you stand

in love you stand

in awe for

awe is all there is

and all that ever was.

Sometimes you have to lose

your mind to come

to your senses.

Candace Koslen

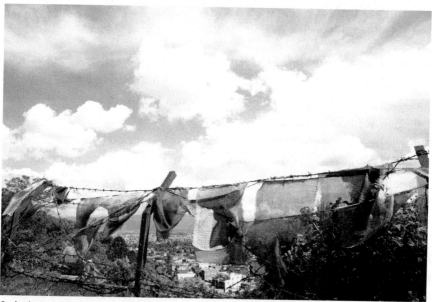

Barbed wire and prayer flags. Nepal is full of contradictions like this. Photo by Candace Koslen.

Day 12 of the Trip, continued...

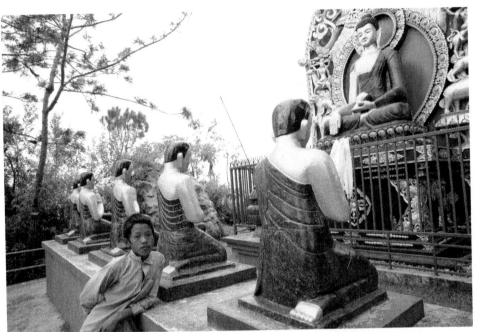

A boy rests on the statues of Buddha's disciples at Namo Buddha. Photo by Candace Koslen.

After hearing Candy, Marni and Jennette talk about what they had experienced these last 10 days in Nepal, we were all quiet for a while. Seeing Candy choke back tears as she talked about the babies at the government orphanage was sobering. Even though we had all been in Nepal at the same time, their experiences had quite clearly been different from ours, and we were just now realizing how different. Many in our group got fired up again, wanting to do something, anything to help make the situation better here. The talk returned to leaving Namo Buddha early to spend more time with the kids at NOH.

As Candy finished, and the group started venting their frustrations again, something in me clicked, and I spoke up. I said we were not being realistic here. We were being too hard on ourselves. We were only in Nepal for two weeks. In such a short time, there was little we could do to affect the situation here. It had developed over generations. It would take a generation at least to solve the problems of even a small third world country like Nepal. And they wouldn't be solved by us, Westerners, coming here and trying to fix Nepal. That, I said, was a very Western way to look at the world. The only people who could really solve the problems of Nepal were the people of Nepal. They had to make the change. This was their country. All we could do is support their efforts. Help them educate the children, like Michael Hess was doing at NOH. Advise them, point them in the right direction. Do what we could do. And trust that good, honest, educated, hardworking Nepalis like Basu and Subash could do the rest.

I watched Basu nod his head in agreement. Maybe I'm right I thought. I wasn't sure, but it felt right to say it. Subash then spoke. He said he and his fellow Nepalis were deeply grateful for us and people like us coming to Nepal and showing that we care. They were grateful for us donating money, and even more grateful for us going back home and telling the world about Nepal. But they all knew that if Nepal was going to get better, they were the ones who would have to make it happen. When he was through speaking, I had a huge lump in my throat. But somehow I also felt better. I think we all did.

July 1, 2010 _____

They [Candy, Marni, and Jennette] have seen so much and in comparison, we have seen so little. Their experience put things into perspective. NOH is a safe haven for so many children because it's a place where they can be nurtured and grow, whereas the children in the state run orphanage have no hope.

It's sad we can't do more to help, but really we are powerless to help. More than ever, I want to come back to Nepal and spend time at the orphanages and support their efforts. I will come back. I will.

_____ *Minling Chuang*

Then Deanna, Jaime and Rachel arrived. They had missed yoga and missed the stories from Jennette, Candy and Marni. They only caught the tail end of our discussion about Nepal. When Jesse reiterated the instructions for the day of silence, Rachel and Deanna spoke up. They were still upset about the previous night's bus ride and asked to leave early. Rachel said she had a responsibility to Jaime, that she had made a promise to her mother, to take care of her on this trip. Even in the daytime, she said, Jaime was still terrified to be up here. She wanted Jaime taken down the mountain today. Deanna and Rachel were also privately worried about David being alone in Kathmandu. The two women were friends with David, and they felt a certain responsibility to make sure he was okay, too. They wanted to go to Thamel, they said, spend some time with the kids at NOH, and meet up with us the next day. This did not go over well with the rest of the group at all, and another heated debate began.

The group is fracturing again. Can we ever be whole?

Minling Chuang

Finally, someone asked Jaime what she wanted to do. Did she want to go, or stay here? Jaime, to her credit, didn't hide behind the others. She spoke up, saying that while she thought the monastery here was beautiful, and that she wished she could do the day of silence; her fear of heights was overwhelming. She didn't think she could comfortably spend an entire day up here. She would really appreciate going down the mountain in daytime, and preferably today.

Jesse and Basu conferred briefly, and then obliged Jaime. Basu ordered up a jeep that would pick up Jaime in an hour or so, along with Rachel and Deanna, and take them down to the International Guest House where we were all going to be staying for the last days of our trip. Basu arranged for them to get rooms there a day early. Surprisingly, Marc chose not to join them, despite his own acrophobia.

Once that situation had been resolved, Jesse went on to explain what those who would be participating in the silent meditation would be asked to do. First, we had to take a vow of silence from right after breakfast at 9 a.m. until evening yoga practice at 5. That meant not uttering a single word to another human being for 8 hours.

Vows of silence are not uncommon in the Buddhist tradition, or among monks of most religions for that matter. Silent meditation can be a powerful, moving experience if you take it seriously. That is why monks take vows of silence that last weeks or months, sometimes even years. We were merely getting a small taste of it. But even a short day of silent meditation can put you in touch with your deepest feelings, let you tackle your most troubling thoughts or problems, and ultimately clear your mind and give you a great sense of inner peace. It is pretty challenging, though, keeping quiet when you're around other people. Human nature is all about communication. Your first instinct here in Nepal is always to greet someone you run into with a friendly "Hello" or a "Namaste". I knew I could probably go the day without uttering a word, because I've done it many times. I'm a writer, and it's a solitary craft, and you can easily go a day without saying a word when you're deep into a writing project. But actually remaining silent in this group? That was going to be pretty difficult for all of us, myself included. Nevertheless, I resolved to embrace the challenge. If silence was the plan for the day, then silent I would be.

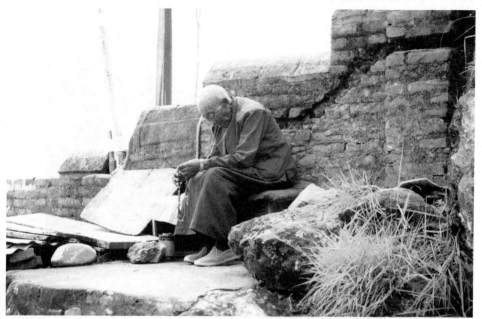

A solitary monk meditates with prayer beads at Namo Buddha. Photo by Candace Koslen.

While we ate our simple monastic breakfast, Jesse handed out safety pins and slips of paper with the words "Today I am silent" written in Nepali on them. He told us once we finished breakfast, to affix the slips of paper to our chests like name tags, to let everyone at the monastery know, especially those who didn't speak English, that we were practicing silent meditation. He then told us that after we finished eating we were free to wander the grounds for the rest of the day, to journal about our silent meditation, sleep, read, eat lunch, do whatever we wanted. We would meet up again as a group eight hours later, at 5 p.m., to take off the tags and then practice yoga again before dinner.

As soon as I finished my meal, I pinned my little 'Silent' tag on my chest. I was looking forward to the rest of the day, and the promise of peace and quiet. I think everyone was after all the sturm und drang of the last couple days. Following breakfast, each of us went off on our own to silently meditate in whatever way we saw fit.

Jaime, whose fear of heights had partially been the catalyst for this morning's big meltdown, steeled her nerves and made the decision to climb up to the uppermost temple of the monastery. Jesse and Minling went with her, and when they finally got there, Jaime looked around, breathed in the cool morning air, and took in the spectacular views of the valley below. She had faced one of her biggest fears, and for the moment she'd conquered it. It was not an easy climb though, physically or emotionally...

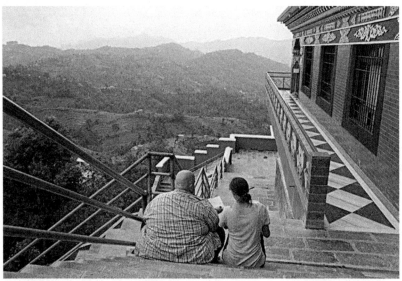

Jesse talks to Jaime about leaving Namo Buddha early. Photo by Minling Chuang.

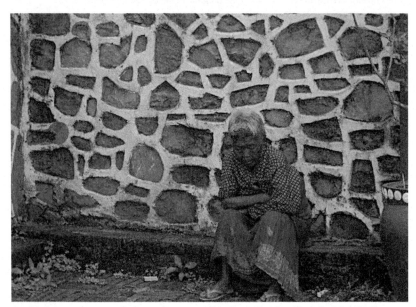

An elderly woman rests at the base of a stone wall at Namo Buddha. Photo by Jaime Furda.

I'm on the top of a mini-mountain by what I think is a shrine surrounded by hundreds of Tibetan prayer flags. On my way here, a very short and very old woman was walking toward me and she looked concerned. I wanted to say something, ask what was wrong, but I didn't know how. As I started to walk away, she tapped me on the left hip to get my attention. I turned to look, but all I saw was a troubled expression of concern/worry/confusion... I don't know what else. I am crying, and I don't know why.

Jaime Furda

Having done what she set out to do this morning, Jaime then headed back down to the parking lot to meet the jeep that Basu had arranged to take her down the mountain. I ran into her just as she was getting back. The smile on her face was enormous. Rachel and Deanna were with her, and they were giddy with excitement too. Rachel started talking a mile a minute about how Jaime had done it, faced her fears and climbed up to the temple for a look down.

"Can you believe it!?" she said.

I pointed to my "Silent" tag, simply smiled, and gave Jaime a big hug. They got into the jeep and disappeared down the mountain, yelling that they would meet us all in Thamel tomorrow. I waved goodbye, and then took off back up the road to explore the monastery grounds myself... in silence.

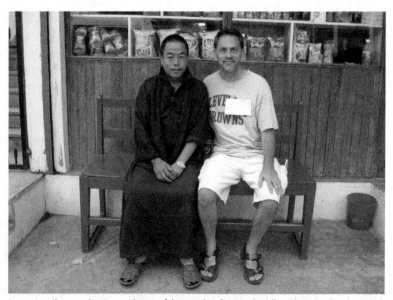

I practice silent meditation with one of the monks of Namo Buddha. Photo by Candace Koslen.

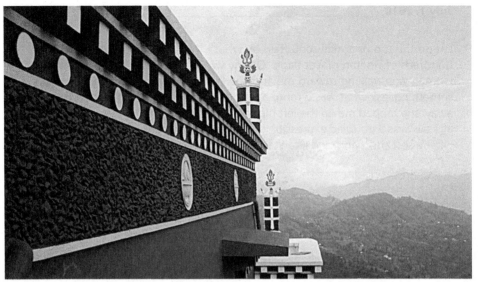

The architecture of Namo Buddha was as impressive as the landscaping. Photo by Kathy Hayes.

Many people brought their journals with them that morning, no doubt to take advantage of the solitude and get some thoughts down on paper. We'd been given a lot to think about in the last 24 hours, and people took to writing, using this time of meditation and journaling to try and come to some larger understanding of the world as seen through the prism of their own recent experiences...

July 1, 2010 _____

[This morning] Jennette, Candy and Marni shared their experiences in Kathmandu. On a daily basis they taught yoga to the children. While the kids were in school, they volunteered at a babies' orphanage. Their experience was in stark contrast to ours. We had a touristy vacation with brief encounters with orphaned children. They experienced true hardship...

_____ ***Christina Jankus***

July 1, 2010 _____

Our spirit and our love want to fix something that is not broken, want to protect something that does not have to be fixed. If everything was fixed, there would not be any more lessons and we would be back home (as one). That's the beauty, that's the miracle....

I have learned that conflict is duality, yet what can be done with conflict? Right now I am trying to write and the gentle, yet pleasant wind is blowing the pieces of the journal causing me conflict with my writing, yet I enjoy being here, I enjoy the breeze the wind is creating. What is my solution? My conflict is a physical one that can be handled with a simple solution of an adjust[ment] in mind and body. Why can't humans look for the simple solution? What happened to our group? Why does it have conflict? Who has the conflict? Should I let the conflict bother me? Am I selfish if I feel comfort within the conflict when others suffer? Buddha says life is suffrage yet we choose to suffer. But if I choose not to suffer do I lack compassion? So what is compassion? Does Michael Hess or Jesse Bach have more compassion for the children of Nepal than me? Just because of the work they do? I say no. I admire their spirit, but the same spirit makes me feel sad for the conditions they live in and the lives they lead. Kamlari is a way of life worldwide, it is here in Nepal, it is in the U.S. What can we do about it? Education? Open eyes with protests? Or going back to this morning, is everything perfect? I want to believe everything is perfect and what we see is our teacher. How we react and what we do may be not exactly the same but it is how it is supposed to be. The outcome will be the way it is supposed to be…

_____**Robb Blain**

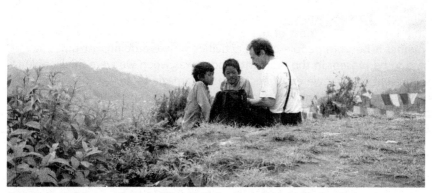

Robb sits like Buddha atop Namo Buddha with the local boys. Photo by Candace Koslen.

The serene surroundings of Namo Buddha had transported those of us who stayed into a more contemplative frame of mind. We all seemed to relish the gentle quiet, nourishing our spirits with it. This day was giving us time to breathe, to relax, to explore our thoughts and emotions, and come to grips with our feelings, in a way we hadn't been able to until now.

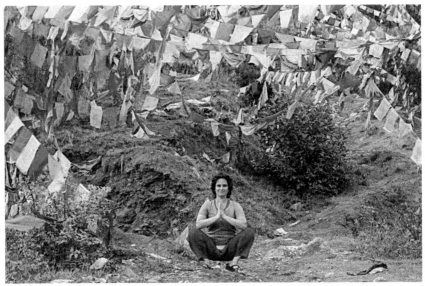

Gabby in Malasana (Garland) pose under the prayer flags of Namo Buddha. Photo by Minling Chuang.

July 1, 2010

The grounds of Namo Buddha were so beautiful and peaceful. I walked all over the place, but my favorite views were the ones from where the prayer flags stood in the distance — they overlooked the monastery and you could see the gorgeous views of the mountainside.

Being here is so different than the Korean monastery in Lumbini. I felt a peacefulness that resided within me. Even though I was scared at first, this is exactly what I needed. For most of the trip, there was always some sort of action, whether it be from people or the activities we were doing. At times, it was hard to be present in the moment. Today was when we were finally able to be present to what we experienced on this amazing journey and our beautiful surroundings. I think I formed closer bonds with people today than before because I couldn't rely on my voice to express my feelings. We had to search for other ways to communicate and I ended up feeling people's souls with a look in the eye or a hug. Today I felt people's love for each other and it was so intense. It's a connection we'll always feel and something that I will always cherish.

As I reflect on our journey, I'm overcome with emotion. Today is the first time I'm able to digest all that has happened and it's finally sinking in. The physical, emotional, and spiritual journey is nothing like I've experienced before.

These are the most amazing people that I've met and all have a heart of gold. We are making a difference and I didn't even realize it until today. Hearing Marni, Candy & Jennette's stories and experiences was so valuable. Even though we didn't see the conditions of the state run orphanages, I now realize what a difference NOH is making in Nepal. The kids at NOH will be the ones who impact Nepal and change it for the better. NOH is the future and we are here to help foster that, not pull them out of their situation. It's funny, as Americans we want to save people, but in reality, people can only save themselves. This is a shift in my perspective, as I thought I came here to save these kids. In reality, we are here to foster them and support. I think in the end, they have actually made a bigger impact on me.

_____ Minling Chuang

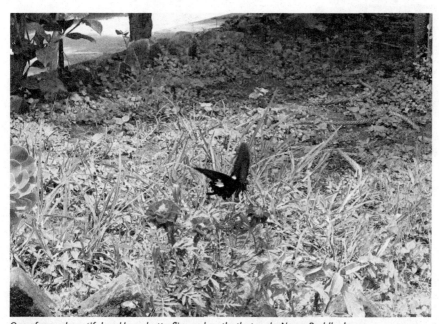

One of many beautiful and large butterflies and moths that make Namo Buddha home.

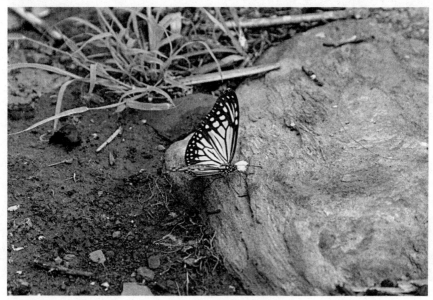

Nepal has over 650 species of butterflies. Photo by Candace Koslen.

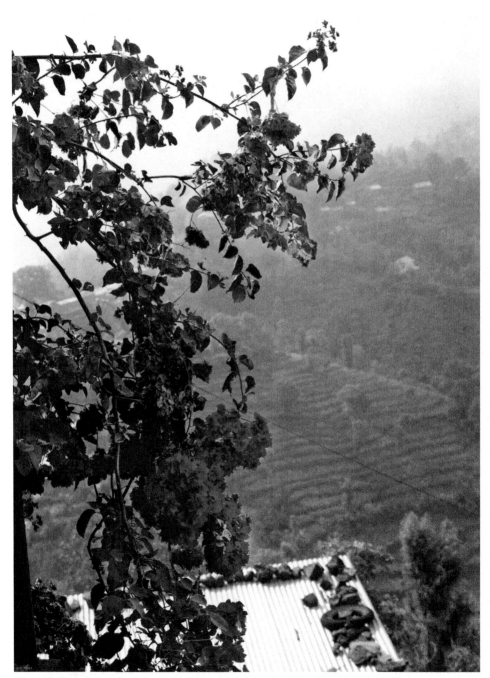

A beautiful flowering rose bush overlooking the surrounding valley below. Photo by Candace Koslen.

Reflection can not only bring peace, but it can also sometimes bring sadness. And that's not necessarily a bad thing. We have as much right to be sad as happy. We are corporeal creatures, living a finite existence in an infinite universe, and acknowledging that can be difficult. A place like this, and a day like this, allowed us to explore that side of ourselves as well.

July 1, 2010

Day of Silent Meditation

I am feeling sad. I am sad that the trip is ending, and yet I am so ready to go home. It is still a long journey to get home. I have been through so much on this trip. Everyone has. I love most of the people I was with: Terri (of course), David, Marc, John, Rachel, Ming, and Ting. The others I didn't really get to know that well. I will make an effort to keep in touch with all of them.

Am I glad I came here? Yes, absolutely. I think all Americans should go experience a third world country. Why? Because you will never complain again. After spending time in this country, I feel as though I never will [again]....

Real Knowledge is the Knowledge you can only get from experience. This is discussed in the yoga sutras… How does it feel to be in a third world country? What are the smells? Goats, exhaust, rotting decay.... Dirty water and trash piled up everywhere... Your feet are always dirty. Your hair and clothes are never clean.... Cows, goats, chickens, and dogs are running in the streets. Cars, busses, motorcycles are going in every direction – honking, no order, just complete chaos. I want to leave this place. I am feeling very alone.

Eve Ennis

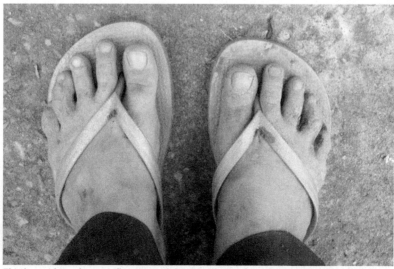

The downside to always walking in sandals in Nepal. Dirty feet. Photo by Christina Jankus.

It is the second to last day of YFF and it's finally our day of silent meditation. After a long morning... I found that the only way for me to resolve my frustrations about all the drama was simply to accept people for what they believe and how they feel, to truly let go of all judgment and expectations. The group as a whole can make collective decisions but at the same time, the group is made up of individuals who have the free will to make their own choices, and when the two are not aligned, there is and will be disharmony....

Candy, Jennette and Marni, three other volunteers who had spent the last week at Volunteer House, shared their experiences this morning. What they had seen and heard and felt moved them to tears even as they recounted their stories. There is so much suffering in Nepal, everywhere you look and it is hard to feel so helpless because there are so many people who need help....

This is the site where Buddha in his previous incarnation as a noble prince gave his own flesh and blood out of compassion for a starving tigress. What good is the body, what is the ultimate purpose of life if not to serve others? Yet how can we give someone something if we don't possess it ourselves? How can we bring peace and happiness to the kids of NOH tomorrow if we don't even have it within ourselves?

...I wish Rachel, Deanna and Jaime had stayed to witness how today unfolded, but their journeys are not up to me and theirs will be perfect however things turn out.

Tingting Peng

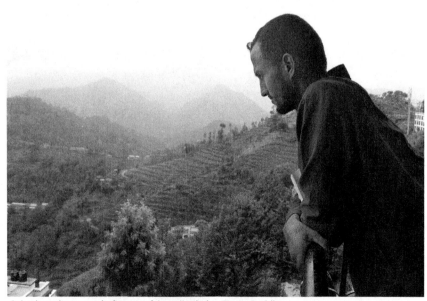

Subash meditates on the beauty of the valley below Namo Buddha.

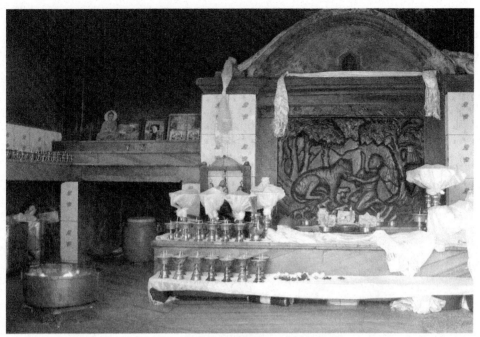

The shrine to the Buddha's sacrifice of himself to the starving Tigress with cubs.

For me personally, those eight silent hours at the mountain monastery in Namo Buddha were some of the very best hours I spent on the trip. I climbed up to the cave where, as Tingting described, the Buddha in his previous life had sacrificed himself to the tigress and her cubs.

At the shrine commemorating his sacrifice, candles were burning and offerings of money and other things had been laid out before the entrance. There was also a snack shop nearby, which made me laugh, silently, to myself. Commerce always seems to follow religion at holy sites the world over, and here it was no different.

I continued walking the grounds and came across a large sheet of burlap spread out on a wide concrete patio. On top of it hundreds and hundreds of chili peppers lay drying in the sun. A dog was curled up, asleep in the shade next to the harvested peppers. He barely stirred at my presence. I looked around, wondering where the farmer was, and where the garden that had grown all these peppers might be hiding. Everything around me was concrete and stone. Where did they grow all this food?

Looking down over the wall behind the drying peppers, I spotted a large field that looked like it had been worked recently. Question answered. As I stared down at the field, I could see a small grove of widely spaced trees right below me. Sunlight was streaming through the leaves of the trees, and flitting between them were dozens, maybe even a hundred, dragonflies. I'd never seen so many of these insects in one place. It was mesmerizing.

Above and behind me, I could see prayer flags adorning many of the trees all over the mountainside, as well. The grounds all around the monastery were well kept, and you could tell that a lot of thought had gone into the landscaping. As I walked and read from a guide book I had picked up at the monastery gift shop before breakfast, I learned that one of the missions of this monastery was to preserve the wildlife and the wild plants in the area as a tribute to nature and the sacrifice the Buddha had made.

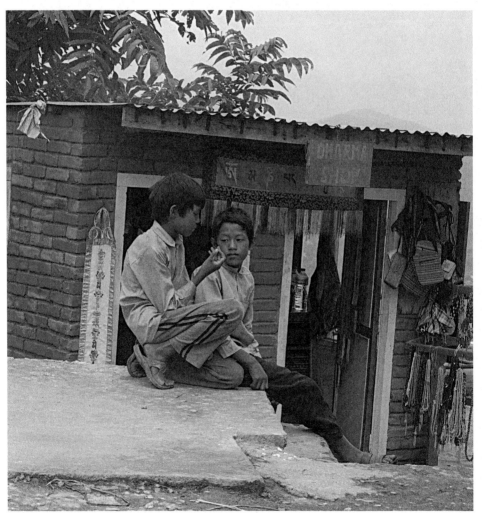

Local boys hanging out in front of the appropriately named gift shop atop Namo Buddha. Photo by Minling Chuang.

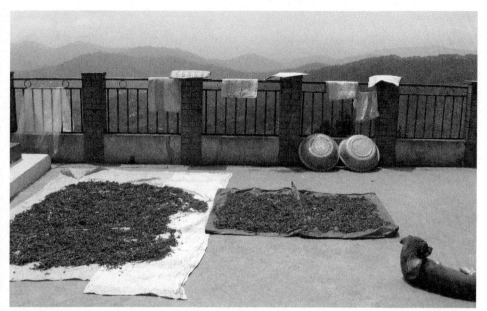
Chili peppers drying in the morning sun atop Namo Buddha.

I continued hiking up into the upper reaches of the monastery stopping to take in the view every few minutes. At one point, I found myself in what looked like someone's back yard. It must have been one of the caretakers' places. As I watched a couple of roosters strut around pecking seeds off the ground, a woman came out carrying a baby. She didn't realize I was out there, but she didn't seem the least bit startled by my presence when she saw me. In fact, she looked so peaceful and beautiful, holding her infant child in her arms that I quickly decided that I had to take a photo of her. But how could I do that and not break my vow of silence?

Instinctively, I pointed to my camera, and then to her, shrugging my shoulders and tilting my head in a questioning sort of way. Only afterwards did it occur to me that it would have done no more good to have spoken to her than using those simple gestures. I'm sure she wouldn't have understood a word of my English, nor I of her Nepali. In that moment, words didn't matter. She understood me quite clearly. Standing tall, holding her child in her arms, she waited for me to snap my photo. In that quiet moment, right before I snapped the picture, she looked to me like a Nepali Virgin Mary holding a little baby Nepali Jesus in her arms. It was the single most beautiful sight I saw on that whole trip. Now, I'm not one to see the Virgin Mary in a piece of toast, or on a weeping stone, or in the bark of gnarled tree. That's not my thing. It's not that I'm not religious, but that I'm more spiritual I guess than dogmatic. But what I felt there, seeing this woman standing and holding her child, was something I hadn't felt before in Nepal.

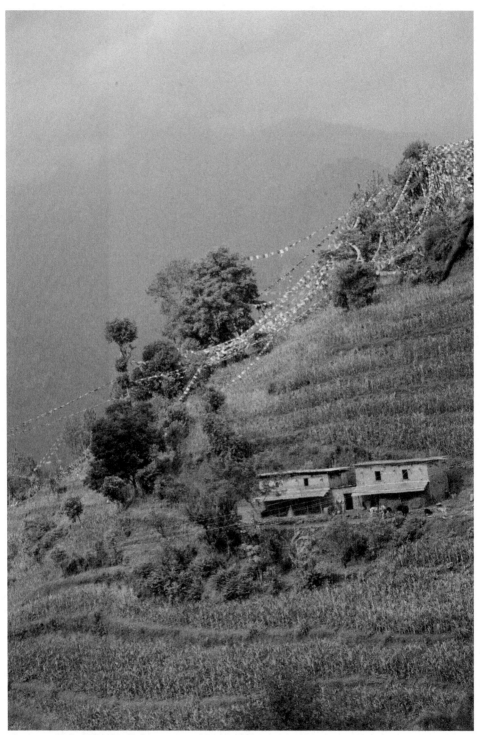

The terraced hillside farmland below Namo Buddha covered with corn. Photo by Candace Koslen.

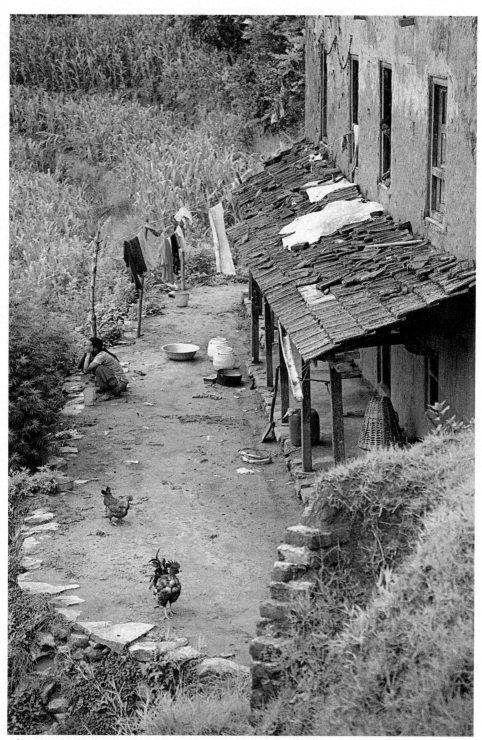

A farmer washes her face on the back patio of her home at Namo Buddha. Photo by Candace Koslen.

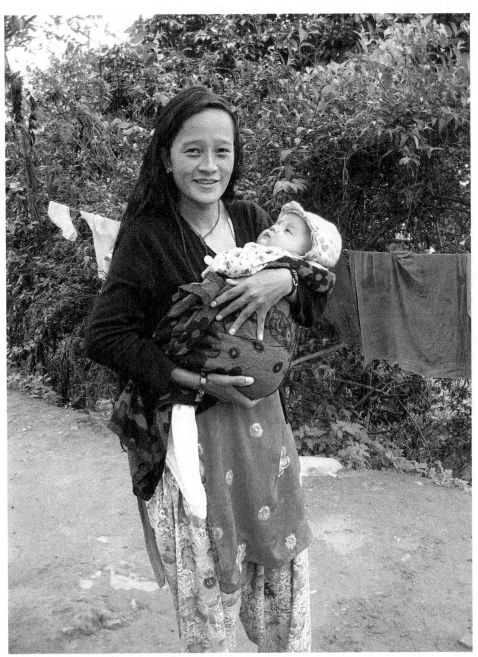

Mother and child. She holds the future of Nepal in her hands.

After spending time with hundreds of orphans at NOH and Narti, after watching Born into Brothels and reading Sold, after hearing about SWAN and their battle to eradicate the Kamlari system, after listening to Candy's and Marni's and Jennette's moving stories about the babies neglected at the government orphanage, I think I'd given up hope for Nepal. But here before me was a quietness, a strength, the gentle, unselfconscious naturalness of a woman holding a healthy, happy, chubby cheeked baby in her loving arms, just being there perfectly in the moment, that defied all that darkness. It was a truly beautiful sight, and it gave me more hope for the future of Nepal than anything I'd seen, heard or done in the nearly two weeks I had been here.

I left that young woman there behind her simple home, with her child, nodding my thanks to her for allowing me to photograph them, and spent the rest of the day snapping more pictures. Around noon, I stopped in the dining area for lunch and ate silently with several of the folks from the group. We conversed non-verbally, with smiles, nods, and finger pointing. At one point someone wrote out a question in their journal, and someone else wrote the answer. The rest of the afternoon I napped, read a bit, and wrote some in my journal. It was hard not to speak for eight straight hours, but I took my vow seriously and managed to make it to just before 5 o'clock without uttering a single, solitary word.

Then as I was walking up the hill towards the guest house and my room, to get changed and grab my yoga mat in preparation for the evening practice, my thoughts drifting around aimlessly in my head, daydreaming about who knows what, I ran right smack into Jennette. And I blurted out, "Hi!" in a loud, happy, friendly voice. The shock of hearing myself talk snapped me back to reality. I had to laugh then at my failure to go the full day in silence. Maybe it wasn't meant to be, or maybe it was just time to start talking again.

July 1, 2010 _____

After we broke silence some of us went to the temple to watch the monks pray. Some of the monks were startlingly young. The young monks were completely distracted by our presence. After their prayer, they exited, and we got a mini tour of the temple. There were offerings of orange Fanta and cakes and cookies to Buddha. At first we thought that was funny. We then realized these things were a luxury and very precious to those who offered them.

_____ *Christina Jankus*

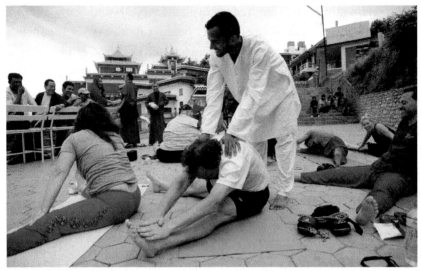

Subash helps Robb stretch out the hammies with Parsva Upavista Konasana (Side Seated Angle) pose as curious monks look on. Photo by Candace Koslen.

That evening, we practiced yoga again in front of the curious monks, and then had dinner once again in the upper dining room. Afterwards we watched some young monks play a game that was something like a cross between pool and checkers. You slid little white round pieces around a square table, trying to knock as many blue pieces into holes around the edges of the table as you could. A couple of the monks were really good at it, and one of them easily ran the table in short order. He would have made a great pool shark.

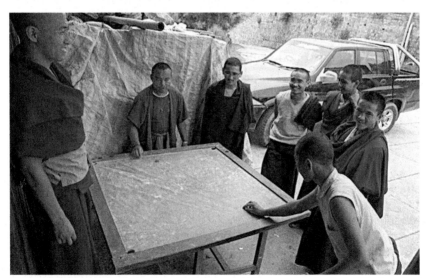

The Namo Buddha monks playing Carrom, a table game of Eastern origin similar to billiards and shuffleboard. Photo by Minling Chuang.

From our mountaintop retreat, we watched the sun set on another spectacular day, and then, with not much else to do at a monastery once the sun goes down, we all drifted back to our rooms to crash for the night. For the second evening in a row, we had perfect sleeping weather, and once again I slept amazingly well. Tomorrow we would head down the mountain, and as I drifted off to Never Never Land, I made a silent vow to do what I could to keep the ride down from being anything like the ride up the day before.

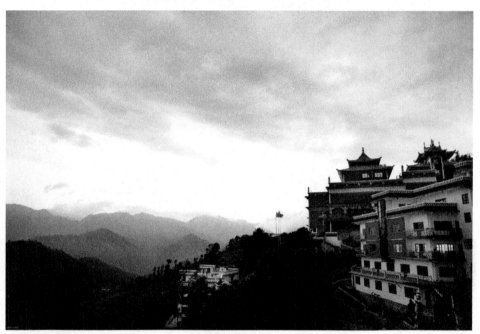

Evening approaches at Namo Buddha. Photo by Candace Koslen.

July 2, 2010

Day 13 of the Trip

Together but Apart

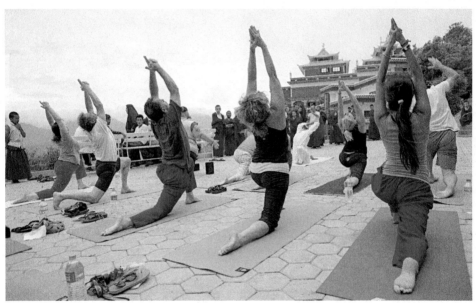

We move through Surya Namaskara at Namo Buddha. Also known as Sun Salutation A, this series of poses is often the initial vinyasa within a longer yoga series. There are 8 different asanas (or poses) in the sequence and 12 asana changes. Some poses are repeated twice in the cycle. This particular pose above is called Aekpaadprasarnaasana, also known as Third Eye pose. Sun Salutation is generally practiced in the morning before breakfast.[14] Photo by Candace Koslen.

We practiced yoga with Subash in front of the temple and the monks one last time early this morning, then ate a quick, simple breakfast. Afterwards we loaded the bus with our gear and ourselves for the ride down the mountain to Thamel. As we started down, this time in broad daylight, we hit the first bumpy patch of road,

[14] Source: http://en.wikipedia.org/wiki/Surya_Namaskara

and a few people quickly, instinctively uttered loud, frightened "ooh's" and "whoa's". I asked everyone to please make a pact to practice silent meditation on the trip down the mountain, just like we had yesterday around the monastery... we should do everything we could to make this ride as stress free as possible.

July 2, 2010 _____

Amazing what silence can do. It's making me think about if I need to say so much in general. Why do we talk so much? We really don't need to in order to enjoy the experience. Something I may want to try when I get back home... more silent meditation. I never thought I'd say that.

_____ *Minling Chuang*

As we wound down the mountain that we had driven up two nights before, we could see now in broad daylight that this was hardly a death defying, stomach turning, cliff hugging road that we had traveled. I wondered what those who'd left early felt on their trip down. What looked like a thousand foot drop into the abyss in the darkness was hardly more than a 10 or 20 foot hillside that you wouldn't be afraid to travel on with a bicycle, let alone a microbus, in the morning sun. Our minds had supplied most, if not all of the terror on the night ride up.

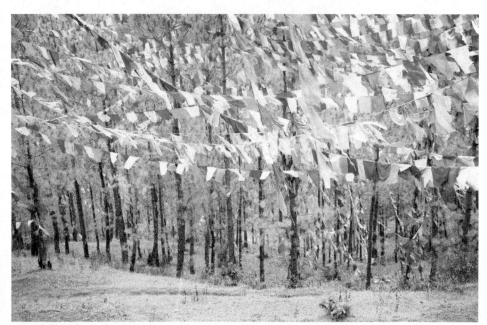

The view from the window of the bus on the way down the not-so-scary hillside at Namo Buddha. Photo by Candace Koslen.

It probably would've been funny, that recognition that the fear wasn't based on anything really dangerous, except for the fact that Marc was just as scared on the ride down as he had been on the ride up. As Buddha expertly navigated the bus, the rest of us managed to remain fairly calm and quiet the entire trip down, as much out of respect for Marc as perhaps out of shame for having been even remotely scared by what was clearly a wide safe road up the mountain.

July 2, 2010 _____

We / I made it down the mountain. I laid down in the back of the bus, put on some headphones, and prayed during the 45-minute trip. I made it. And the people that didn't leave drove in silence, so the air of fear left the group and the bus.

_____*Marc Nathanson*

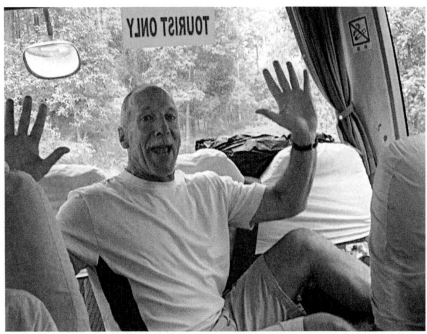

Marc makes it successfully down from Namo Buddha without panicking. Photo by Terri Bahr.

Safely down the mountain, our ride into town was smooth sailing. Kathmandu seemed to greet us with open arms, like an old friend back from a long trip. Our final destination on this two week journey was the International Guest House in Thamel, the center of the tourist industry in Kathmandu. Thamel sits between two of the original hotels in the area, the International Guesthouse and the Hotel Utse.

International travelers have flocked there for over forty years. Perhaps it's because its narrow streets are lined with small shops selling everything from food and provisions to clothes, hiking gear, CD's and DVD's (mostly pirated), and excellent native handicrafts. The area also boasts some very good restaurants. Although prices tend to be higher in Thamel than in the non-tourist areas of Kathmandu, the food is generally a lot better. Thamel also acts as a popular stop for mountaineers who flock to Nepal to climb the many nearby Himalayan peaks. You can find climbers from every continent here, picking up their climbing equipment at a wide range of mountaineering gear shops, changing money at the numerous foreign money exchange booths, and drinking and eating at the many pubs, clubs and local nightlife spots.

Thamel is also unfortunately the home of Kathmandu's red light district, and on the way into town, Jesse warned us that we might come across young girls here working the local brothels. The under-age girls were kept inside these places, and if you mistakenly went into one thinking you were going to a local bar or dance club, you might easily find yourself in the wrong place at the wrong time, and witness to the horrors of child sex trafficking. He urged us all, no matter where we went in Thamel, to stick together, as there was safety in numbers. None of us had any intention of exploring the dark side of this place.

As we entered Thamel, Jesse told us that he had arranged for us to spend the afternoon with the kids from NOH, first at a local swimming pool, then later on at NOH. This was exciting news. And Jesse said he thought that Michael Hess would be dropping in at NOH to give us a talk about the work they were doing there. We all badly wanted to meet this incredible man we'd heard so much about. We had so many questions we wanted to ask him, but both Jesse and Carola cautioned us that Michael was extremely modest, almost shy, and it was a rare thing for him to speak in front of large groups. However, Carola also said that Michael was so impressed that twenty of us had come all this way to Nepal to support and bring awareness to the orphans of NOH, that he was going to make an exception and meet with us. That got everyone pretty psyched.

As we approached the International Guesthouse, winding our way through ever narrow city streets, our bus was forced to stop short of the hotel, unable to make the last turn onto the road where the entrance was located. So Buddha parked at the corner, and we hoofed it the last block to the International Guest House. The hotel itself looked very nice, especially the lobby with its dark wood, marble floors and staircases, soft couches, and loads of local Nepali artifacts.

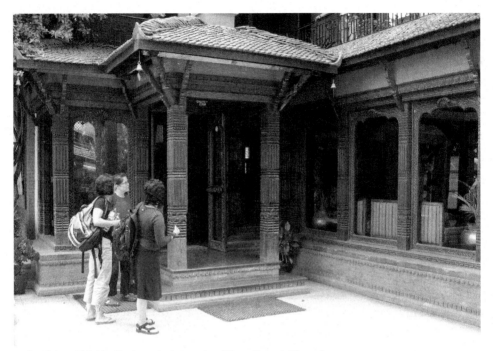

Kathy, Chris, and Gabby check out the International Guest House in Thamel.

Inside we saw all kinds of people from different countries sitting talking in various languages, German, Italian, French, English; sipping Coke or Sprite or Nepali coffee, checking in and checking out. David, Rachel, Jaime and Deanna soon showed up, and though they seemed in high spirits, it felt now like our group had been divided. My roomie David seemed happy to see me, and I was certainly happy to see him, alive and well. He had already been in Thamel several days now, and had arranged for a double room that I would be sharing with him this last night in Kathmandu. Everyone else got quickly situated in their own rooms, and then we all rushed back down to the bus for the ride to the swimming pool.

July 2, 2010 _____

Quickly dropping off our things, we changed for the kids' pool party at the Nature Club nearby. By the time we got there (in Nepal time, of course, 20 minutes late), the party was in full swing.

_____ ***Tingting Peng***

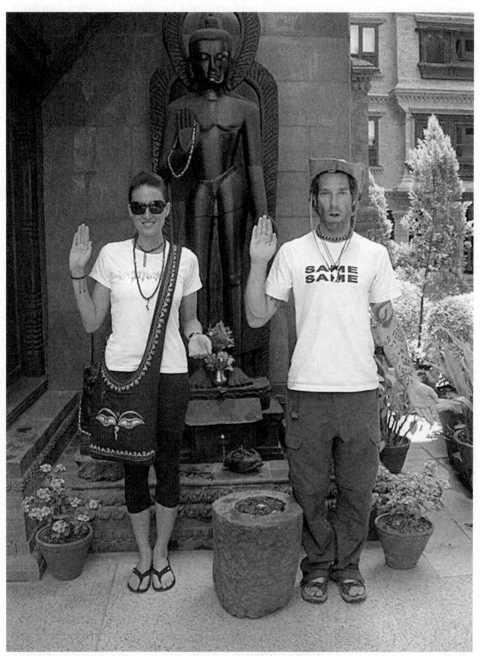

David and Deanna stand before a statue of the Buddha, all in Tadasana (Mountain) pose with Abhayamudra, the gesture of reassurance and safety (the open hand), which dispels fear and accords divine protection and bliss to the devotee (Source: http://en.wikipedia.org/wiki/Abhayamudra). Same Same But Different, as the Nepalis like to say. Photo by John Vourlis, courtesy of Deanna Lee.

The pool was located at the local Nature Club in the heart of the city. Once every month or so in the summer, Michael arranged for the kids to spend an hour swimming there. The pool, one of the very few public ones in all of Kathmandu, is rented by the hour. One of the volunteers was getting married soon, and as a gift to the kids of Nepal Orphans Home, she bought them an hour of swim time on this day. Like kids anywhere on a really hot summer day, the kids of NOH were over the moon excited to be playing in the pool. And, surprise, surprise, right smack in the middle of the fun was Michael Hess himself, wearing his favorite Cleveland Indians baseball cap in our honor.

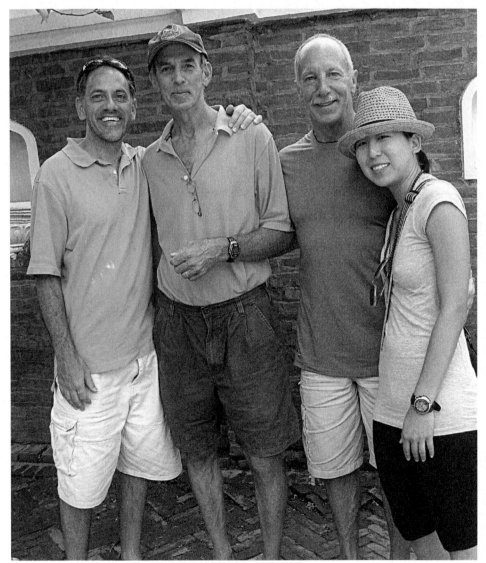

Michael wearing his famous Cleveland Indians baseball cap on Swim Day.

Michael didn't look at all shy here. In fact he looked completely at home. Several of us took the opportunity to introduce ourselves, and he thanked us for coming to Nepal and for everything we were doing for the kids. I found myself liking this guy instantly. First of all, there was that Indians' hat, which sat comfortably worn and faded on his head above a pair of clear, bright eyes and a gentle smile. Michael was warm, friendly, intelligent, and one-on-one, quite talkative. It was apparent almost instantly why the kids adored him, and why the volunteers revered and respected him so much. He was quite simply, a great guy, the kind of guy you'd happily hang out with anywhere, any time. We took pictures with Michael, and with the kids in and out of the pool, and we all had a fantastic time. My only regret, personally, was not bringing my swim trunks with me so I could have enjoyed the pool too. But that oversight didn't stop some of the others. Tingting, Marni, and several of the volunteers jumped right into the water, in their street clothes, and splashed around with the kids.

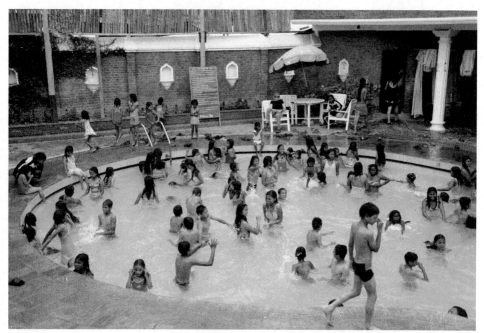

The NOH kids having a ball on Swim Day at the Nature Park. Photo by Candace Koslen.

July 2, 2010 _____

The YFF group, reunited with David, Rachel, Deanna, and Jaime, jumped right in to play with the kids – some of us got wet swimming and teaching the kids how to swim in the pool while the rest also got a little wet sitting by the pool's edge from the crazy splashing ... There was so much joyous laughter, screaming and shouting. As soon as I got into the pool, it seemed like a hundred little arms all grabbed for me at the same time, "Sister! Sister!" the kids kept shouting...

_____ ***Tingting Peng***

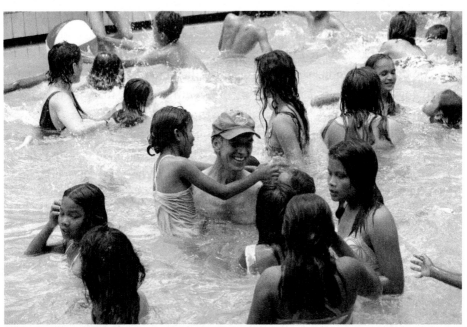

Michael happily joins the kids in the pool. Photo by Candace Koslen.

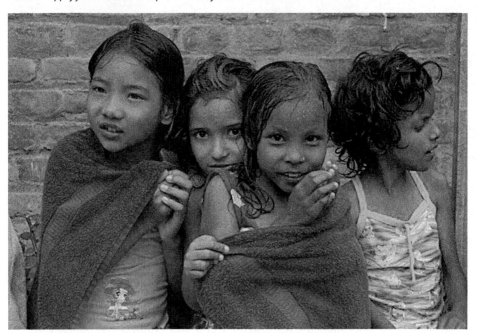

The NOH girls snuggling to stay warm while out of the pool. Photo by Minling Chuang.

After the hour of pool time was up, all of us, grown-ups and kids went outside the pool area to a large grassy courtyard to have lunch. The kids had all donned black and yellow warm-up suits that looked like they'd been created by a Pittsburgh Steelers fan. They looked like little Olympic athletes as they marched out of the pool area into the yard with huge smiles on their faces.

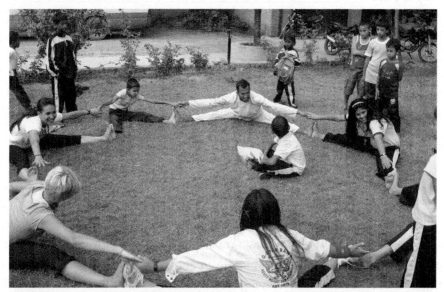

After swimming, fun with yoga. Will the circle be unbroken?

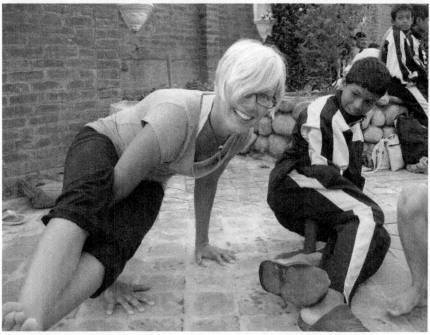

Rachel teaches one of the NOH boys the very challenging Astavakrasana (Eight-Angle) pose.

As the Nature Club staff prepared our meal, some of the yoga teachers, including Rachel and Deanna, began teaching the kids yoga. The kids dove right in. It was hilarious watching them try all the poses, fearless and just having fun.

July 2, 2010 _____

The kids were imitating all sorts of yoga poses and were completely unafraid to do silly and crazy things. Wheel! Ok! And landing back on their heads. Or, handstand! Ok! And flip flopping over, also on their heads. They were carefree, open and eager – like sponges, soaking up everything they see and hear, everything they experienced. It was an awesome time, exhausting at the same time, trying to keep up with their level of energy.

_____ *Tingting Peng*

When the lunch bell rang, we all sat down in a giant circle around the courtyard to eat. Several of the girls, along with staff from the Club, served everyone fresh hot buckwheat noodles cooked with vegetables, and washed down with Orange Fanta or bottled water. It was now past noon, and quite hot, but we were all hungry, especially the kids, who had built up quite an appetite playing in the pool, and in no time we had wolfed down heaping plates of food. When we had satisfied our bellies, the kids cleaned up the plates, utensils, and empty cans and cups. There was no moaning and groaning about having to do these chores; they all pitched in and got the job done enthusiastically.

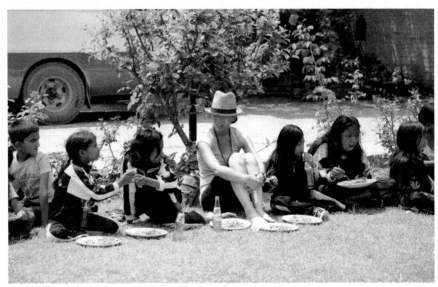

Minling lunching with the little ladies of NOH. Photo by Candace Koslen.

After all the garbage had been picked up, it was time to head down to NOH, to Imagine House and Papa's House, to see what things were like for the kids at school. Apparently the four prodigal members of our group had been up late partying the night before, and were now exhausted. They hopped a cab back to the hotel, telling us they would catch up with us at Papa's House later with the yoga mats we had brought for the kids, and then went back to their rooms to get some sleep. There was little outward reaction from the rest of the group. We simply made the short trip down to Imagine House, where we'd first met the NOH kids. We only stayed briefly at the first stop, just long enough to say hello to some of the kids we'd met earlier, the ones who hadn't made it to the pool. Even though we had only met them once, and for just a short time, the kids greeted us all like long lost cousins.

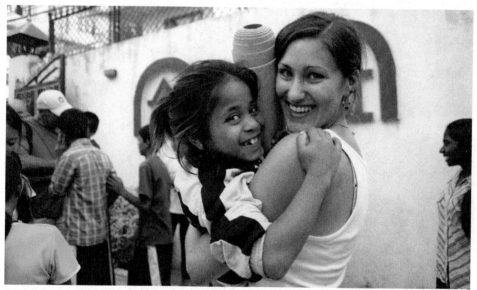

Jaime delivers a Kulae yoga mat to the delight of one little girl. Kulae donated 20 mats for the trip which we gave to NOH on our last day there. Photo by Candace Koslen.

July 2, 2010

On the first day we arrived at the orphanages, after greeting the children, Jesse pointed out Kancham. This is a girl he had told me about. Even though she had never met me before, we embraced. Just the stories that Jesse told me prior to the trip about her, made me want to hold her forever. In the midst of all the exchanges of excitement, I took off my Namaste necklace and put it around her neck. She was surprised, but shining with pride. She is one of the older ones, and I know she has had it really tough. She is very shy, but really expressed so much beauty from her heart when she received this gift.

When we returned [today], she was looking for me, sweaty with anticipation to give me a gift. It was rumpled and wrapped in newspaper, but given to me with so much pride. It was a bright blue scarf she knitted for me. The thought still brings tears flooding down my face. It's so hard not to want to bring these children back to the U.S. with us.

Terri Bahr

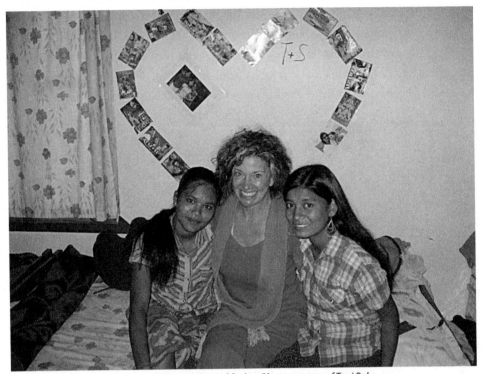

Terri showing off the scarf that one of the girls knitted for her. Photo courtesy of Terri Bahr.

Following the short, emotional stop at Imagine House, Carola asked us all to walk up the hill to Papa's House with her. She wanted us to drop in on the kids during school time so that we could see what it is like for them in their classrooms. We had to hustle before their study period was finished if we wanted to see the kids at work, so up the street we all marched, single file, the kids looking like little black and yellow ducklings following momma duck Carola back to the nest. As we made our way up the hill, one of the older girls began questioning us about our soccer allegiances. Who did we like to win the World Cup, she wanted to know? She was all for Argentina to win it, she said, and not because she thought they were the best team, but because she thought the great Argentine striker Lionel Messi was the cutest of all the players. Another girl wanted to know who our favorite singer was. Hers, she told us without a trace of irony, was Brittany Spears.

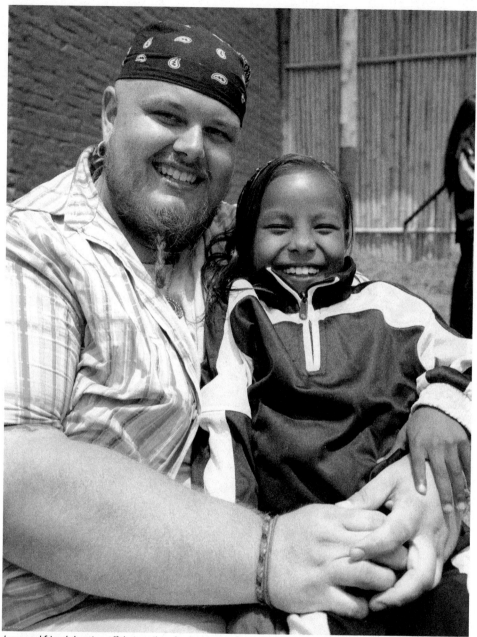

Jesse and friend showing off their smiles after Swim Day. Photo by Candace Koslen.

July 2, 2010 _____

One of the girls was particularly fond of me. She kept asking me if I knew Justin Bieber and sang his hit song "Baby" repeatedly. She even showed me to her room, which was small, with 3 beds crammed inside, and played the song on her cassette player (I have not seen one of those since I was in middle school). As she proudly showed me her schoolwork and certificates of achievement, I felt so proud of her for working so hard, for really appreciating the life and opportunity that she has been given. Some people... don't even realize the kind of privileges that they have...

_____ ***Tingting Peng***

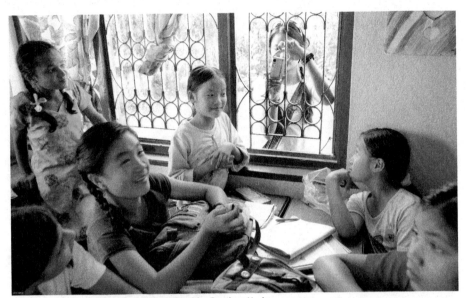

Tingting peeks in on the girls studying. Photo by Candace Koslen.

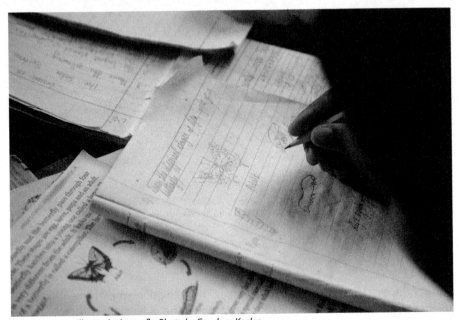

From the caterpillar to the butterfly. Photo by Candace Koslen.

At Papa's House, we found a small group of kids studying in the large classroom. Several volunteers were working one on one with the children on various subjects like math and English. One of these volunteers, Jake Hickey, was a tall, young Aussie who had been at the pool, and in the pool, and was planning on spending quite a while, three months perhaps, volunteering at NOH. The girls in our group, especially the ones who had worked with him as volunteers, all adored Jake. In fact, we all liked Jake. He had an easy-going, friendly manner, and he clearly loved the kids and they him. He hung out with Jordan Boehler a lot, a volunteer from New York, and the two of them were keen on joining us later that night when we all planned to go out on the town in Thamel.

Once the kids had finished their studying, we all went outside for a bit of fun. A few of the boys played basketball; the others played a little volleyball. The girls asked us to teach them some American songs and dances, and after watching Minling and Marc do quite well at it, I was coaxed into teaching them a little Greek dancing. Everyone seemed to get a kick out of my version of Zorba, and I was once again sweating up a storm when it was all over.

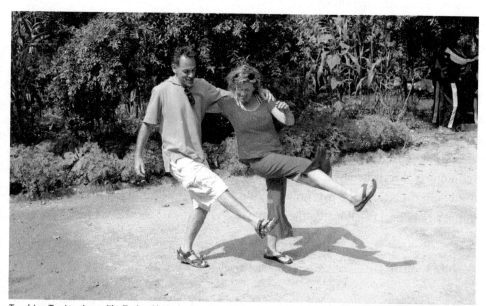

Teaching Terri to dance like Zorba. Photo by Candace Koslen.

Then Carola ushered us back inside to give a talk about NOH. She stood before us all and said she wasn't sure if Michael would come, but if he did, now had been the time that he had scheduled to meet with us. She told us all not to take it personally if he didn't show. The other volunteers said the same thing, they all loved Michael and being very protective of him, they were probably more surprised than we were that just as Carola was about to launch into the talk without him, he popped his head into the classroom. Without fanfare, he joined the discussion, and soon we were learning all we wanted to know about the kids and NOH.

July 2, 2010 _____

We did have a chance to talk with Papa Michael Hess. He is a lovely man. He kisses each child goodbye when they leave for school in the morning and kisses them when they return from school.

Michael gave us his background and what his plans for the future are. Although in Nepal, plans can easily change. He told us a story of how he started another school only to have the government take it away from him. Michael also explained that sometimes he may have money tagged for certain needed items only to have the need change.

Someone asked Michael if he provided counseling for the children. He said it was an unnecessary expense as the children are happy and well-adjusted and very rarely does a counselor need to be called in... Michael is a beautiful person. He radiates goodness.

_____ **Christina Jankus**

The talk about counseling for the kids was a real eye-opener. It seems early on, Michael had felt the way most of us did, that these kids must be badly scarred from their experiences as orphans and child slaves. So he brought in a psychologist to evaluate them. And the psychologist came to the conclusion that these kids showed virtually no psychological damage from their experiences. They were remarkably well-adjusted, well-behaved, hard-working kids. They loved each other, and they loved being at NOH. The psychologist told Michael the kids didn't need any counseling, so Michael re-allocated the money... to healthcare for the kids.

July 2, 2010 _____

The afternoon at Papa's House was incredible. We sang, we danced, we did yoga, we laughed and smiled, held hands and talked. We also got to meet Papa, Michael Hess, and learned about his incredible story in creating NOH six years ago and how he built it to what it is today. His compassion, selflessness, and dedication and love for these kids is simply inspirational. He told us what he hopes to create in the next few years – a campus where they would have their own school and technical school with enough space to support at least 200 kids. With NOH at capacity, and some of the older kids soon to be nearing college age, Michael hopes to be able to find a way to transition into something bigger that can see the kids to a solid and bright adulthood.

Tingting Peng

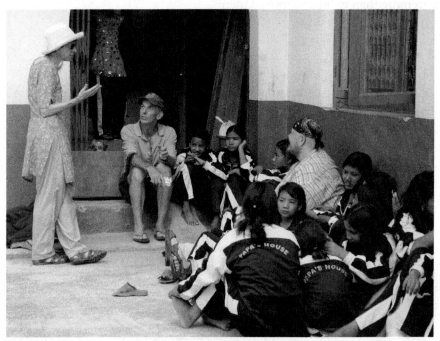

Carola gives Michael the lowdown on YFF. Photo by Candace Koslen.

Michael was very informative, answering every question with patience. We all came away from that meeting deeply impressed with him and the work he was doing in Nepal. You don't often meet people like Michael, people who devote their entire lives to the service of others, and who do it without ego, without fanfare, and with no regrets. I considered myself lucky to have had the opportunity to spend a little time with such a great human being. It was inspiring and very humbling, to say the least.

After the discussion with Michael and Carola, it was time to pass out some gifts that we had brought with us from home for all the girls and boys, so we gathered up the kids outside the house, just like we'd done with the girls at Narti, and presented them with earrings, bracelets, picture books on yoga, Frisbees, and all sorts of fun stuff. The kids were overjoyed. It was like Christmas in July for them, and we all got to play Santa Claus.

We spent an hour or two playing with the kids out on the playground, and everyone had a blast. They opened the yoga books they had received as presents, and started mimicking the poses. It was so much fun watching these kids playing, laughing, and enjoying their free time. And once again, the kids managed to surprise us more than we had surprised them...

7-2-10 _____

One girl gave me a pair of earrings that we had brought for them because she thought [they] looked nice on me; another girl, responding to my question "Who is your best friend?" answered "everyone here". They are a true unbreakable family... [One girl] wrote me a postcard as I was leaving. On it, she had written, "Always be happy. Never be sad." What a brilliant little girl! It took me about 25 years to learn that and finally be able to live it.

_____ *Tingting Peng*

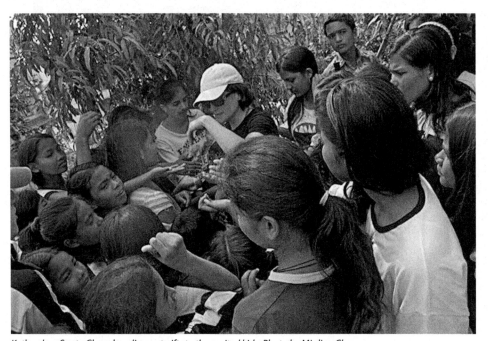

Kathy plays Santa Claus, handing out gifts to the excited kids. Photo by Minling Chuang.

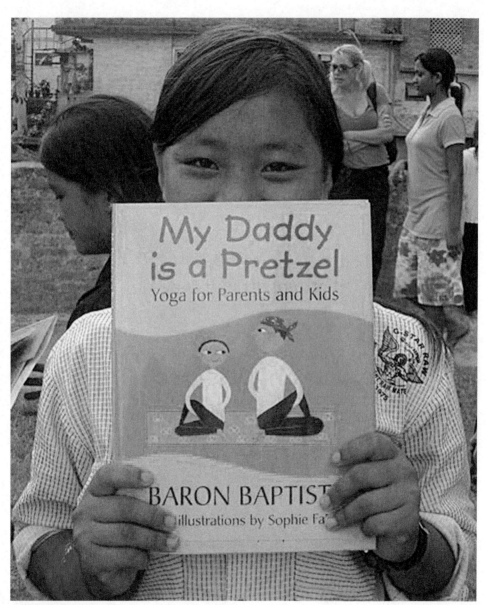

A gift for the kids on our last day with them. Photo by Tingting Peng.

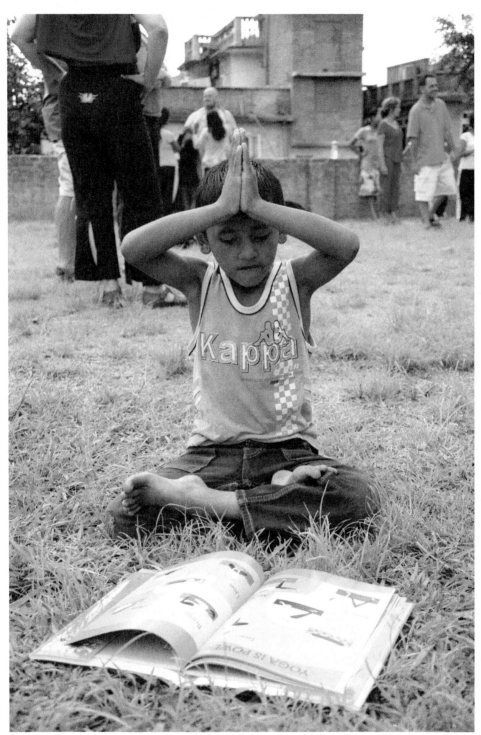

Wasting no time at all, this little guy starts practicing Padmasana (Lotus) pose with Anjali Mudra (hands above the head in a gesture of reverence). Photo by Candace Koslen.

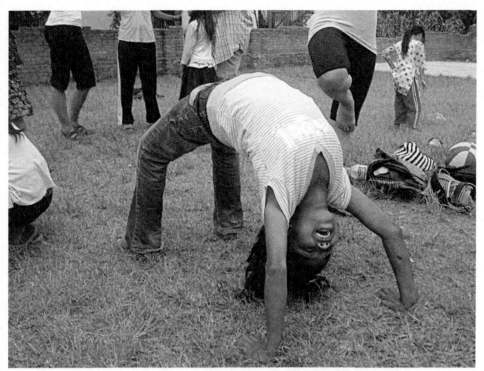

And this young girl tries Urdhva Dhanurasana, the Wheel pose, and nails it. Photo by Tingting Peng.

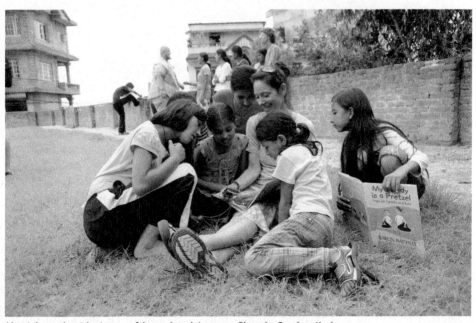

Marni shows the girls pictures of themselves doing yoga. Photo by Candace Koslen.

July 2, 2010

Day 13 of the Trip, cont'd

A Last Night In Thamel

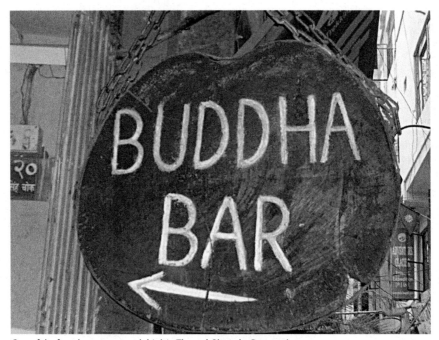

One of the fun places to eat and drink in Thamel. Photo by Deanna Lee.

We left Papa's House around 5 p.m. Back at the hotel, we had a light yoga practice in the courtyard, and then showered and rested up before heading out for dinner. The volunteers, Candy, Marni, Jennette, decided to wear the Nepali outfits they'd bought earlier to celebrate the night's fun, since we were going to a pretty upscale restaurant that Jesse highly recommended, and which even Basu and the other Nepali's were excited about. It was called OR2K. This popular Israeli-run vegetarian restaurant is a favorite among tourists, mountain climbers and other travelers. The menu included crêpes, soups, zucchini pie, coconut tofu, ziva (pastry fingers filled with cheese), and all manner of Nepali dishes. They also served pizza. The goat cheese variety was Jesse's favorite, he told us. They also served alcohol, and most of us planned on partaking, since we had all been planning on a major blowout for our last night in Nepal.

The mood inside the restaurant was cozy and warm, with excellent pop music playing over soft lighting, and low tables surrounded by cushions on the floor for seating. Jesse told us we had to take our shoes off in the restaurant, so we might want to make sure we were wearing clean socks if we didn't want to go barefoot. Jesse then informed us that dinner was on NOH, as a thank you to the YFF group for coming to Nepal. Since many of us had burned through most of our rupees during the two weeks of the trip, this was a much appreciated gesture on NOH's part.

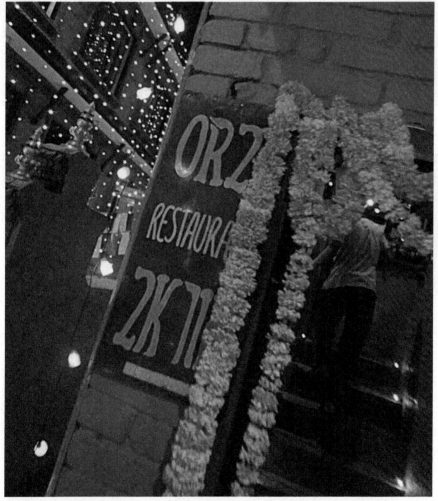

Our last supper in Nepal at OR2K, one of the best restaurants in Thamel. Photo by Tingting Peng.

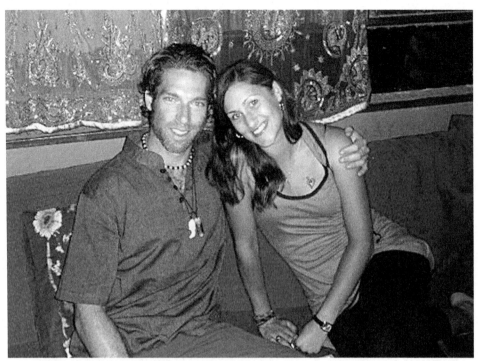

David and Jaime chilling out at OR2K. Photo courtesy of Jaime Furda.

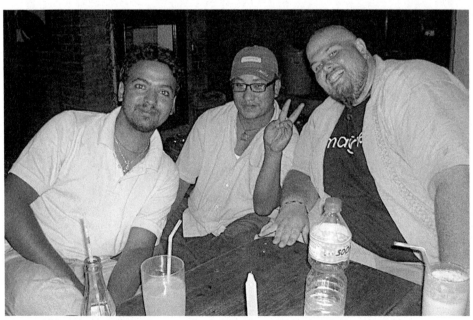

Basu, Buddha, and Jesse. The three amigos enjoying themselves at OR2K. Photo by Deanna Lee.

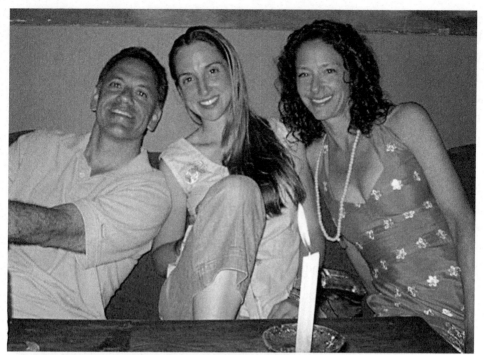

Me and the lovely Candy and Marni, all blissed out at OR2K. Photo by Terri Bahr.

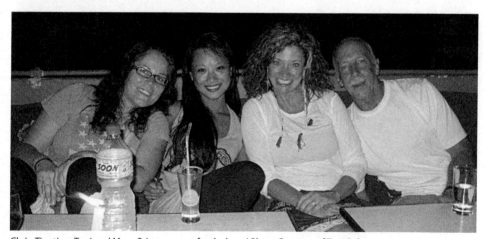

Chris, Tingting, Terri and Marc. Bring us some food, please! Photo Courtesy of Terri Bahr.

OR2K turned out to be a blast. The women all looked terrific in their finery, and everyone looked fit and tanned from nearly two solid weeks of yoga and sun. We ordered up everything on the menu that sounded even remotely interesting, and shared the feast amongst ourselves (those of us who wanted to drink alcohol dipped into our own pockets, so as not to roll up the bill that NOH had agreed to pay). Rachel, Deanna, David and Jaime showed up just after the main group had been seated. Even Buddha our bus driver joined us. He was decked out in his finest, wearing a pair of very cool shades, and looked every bit at home here. We gave him a huge round of applause when he sat down, and toasted him for his excellent bus driving skills, with Basu doing the translating from English to Nepali. You could tell Buddha appreciated our heartfelt words of thanks, and he toasted us all back just as heartily.

Jesse was a little subdued this evening, but once everyone was there, and we all had our first drinks in hand, he made a warm toast to the whole group, thanking us all for coming on this amazing journey with him. He would be spending the next few weeks trekking on his own in Nepal, and doing volunteer work at NOH. I raised my mojito, green with fresh ground mint, and toasted Jesse. He then loudly proclaimed to us all, "You made it! Have fun tonight, it's your last night in Nepal!"

And we took him to heart on that. We ate until we were stuffed. The food was delicious, from the appetizers, to the main courses, to dessert. We all had a few drinks, took loads of pictures, and shared stories and laughs.

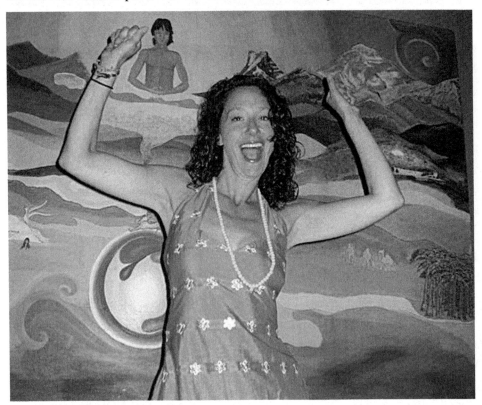

Marni rockin' it at OR2K. Photo by Terri Bahr.

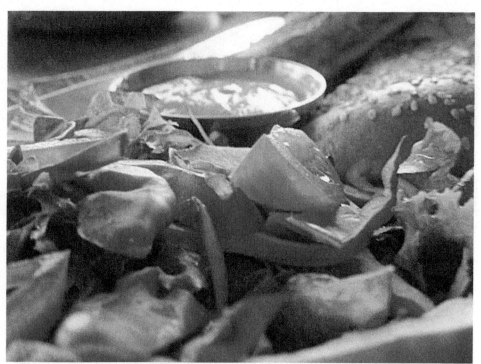

Mmmmmmmm…. Fresh and delicious food at OR2K. Photo by Jaime Furda.

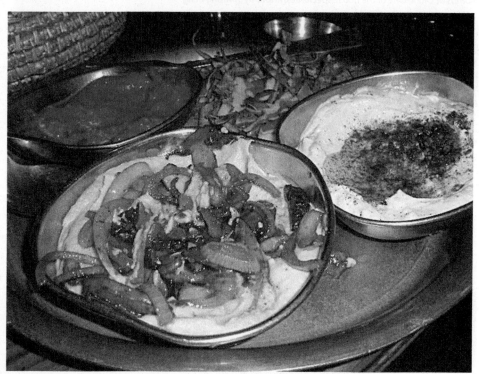

More OR2K yummies. Hummus topped with grilled onions, front and center. Photo by Jaime Furda.

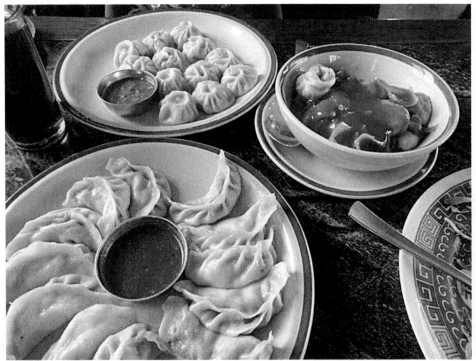

Momos at OR2K. One of the house specialties. Photo by Tingting Peng.

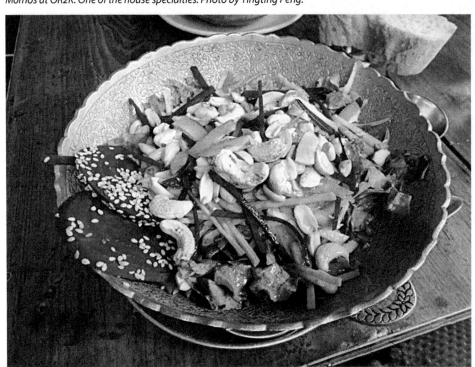

Beet and cashew salad sprinkled with sesame. Photo by Tingting Peng.

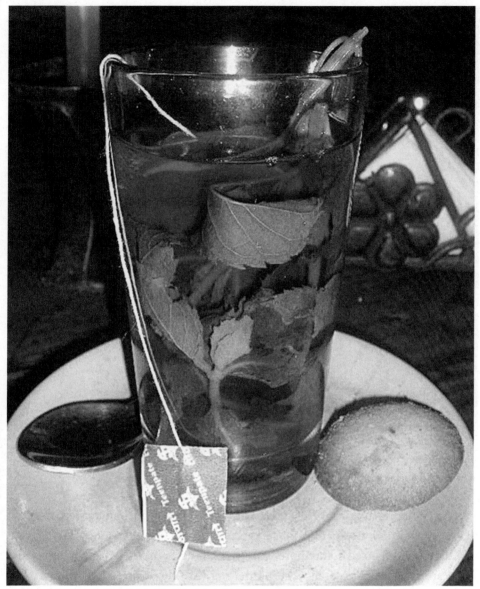

Mint tea and crumpets, Nepali style. Photo by Jaime Furda.

After a couple hours of merriment, we all decided to go find a bar to finish out the rest of the evening. We wandered Thamel, Jake and Jordan and our own volunteers leading the way.

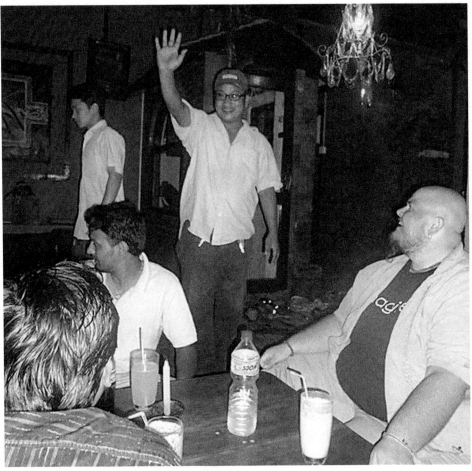

Buddha calls it a night. Photo by Eve Ennis.

We ended up at a local "Mexican" bar where the Nepali waiters were dressed like mariachis and the Spanish music mixed with modern pop songs. We danced and drank and danced some more, sweating our asses off, and just having a ball. I had a blast letting loose and cutting the rug with the ladies, all of whom were excellent dancers. We then moved to a second bar, just for variety, and continued the fun well past midnight.

July 2, 2010 _____

The rest of the evening was spent in a feeding, drinking and dancing frenzy as we lit up the final night in Thamel… I moved onto the next place (a Mexican bar) with the remainder of the crew to dance and take down some margaritas….

_____ ***Tingting Peng***

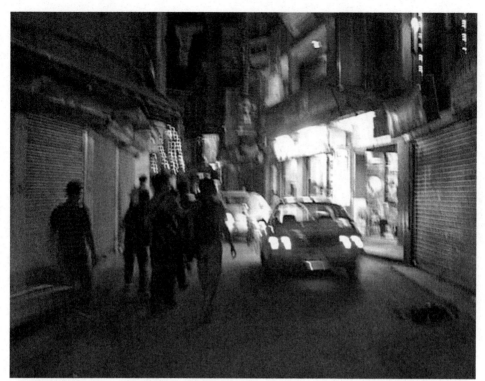

Street life, at night, in Thamel. Photo by Christina Jankus.

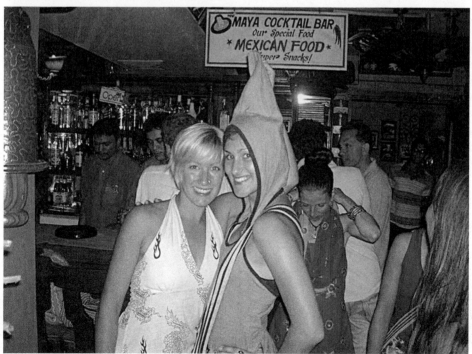

Rachel and Jaime, ready to party Nepali style. Photo by Deanna Lee.

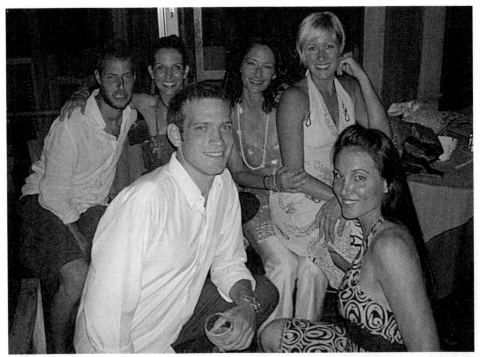

Jake and Jordan, NOH volunteers, hanging with our YFF ladies. Photo courtesy of Deanna Lee.

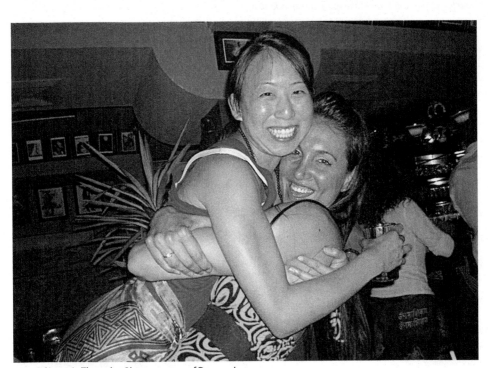

Huggin' it out in Thamel… Photo courtesy of Deanna Lee.

At some point, we decided to retire to the rooftop patio back at the International Guest House. It was very late, perhaps 2 or 3 a.m. when we stopped to pick up some refreshments on the way back. Once there, I went up to my room to get some cash to help pay for the drinks. I lay down on my bed for a second, to relax and rest my feet, and the next thing I knew, it was morning...

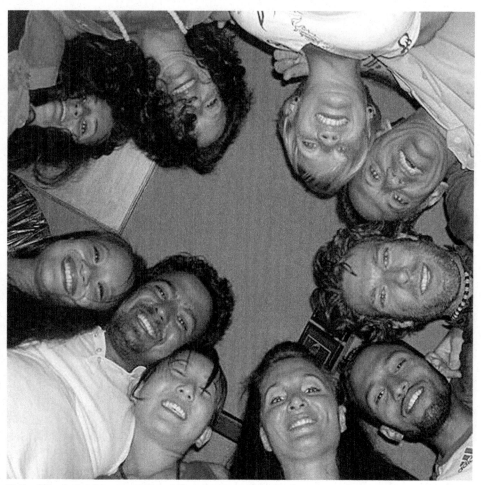

Circle of friends. Good times, good times! Photo courtesy of Basu Panday.

July 3, 2010

Day 14 of the Trip

Departure

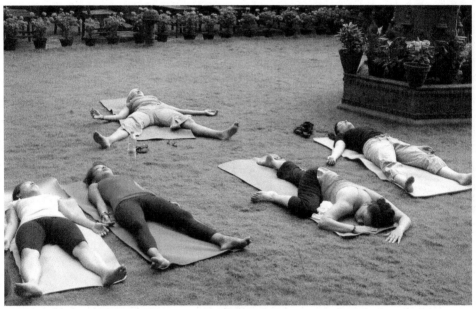

Our last morning in Nepal. Completely wiped out from the night before, savasana sounded like a good idea.

I'd fallen asleep on top of the wool blanket on the bed in my hotel room. Luckily we had a small fan in the room, and the windows were open, or I probably would have awakened soaked in sweat. When I did get up, a bit woozy and a little hung over, David was fast asleep in the other bed. I showered and went downstairs for breakfast. Outside the lobby, on the back patio, I saw some of our group, Minling, Tingting, Kathy, Gabby and Rachel all practicing some light yoga on the grass in the courtyard. Actually they were lying in savasana, which to me seemed like a great idea. Their powers of recovery were more impressive than mine, though. I couldn't muster the energy to join them. Jaime, Joyce and Chris were up too, and had already showered and eaten breakfast. I waved hello to the yogis, then went off to get some food. Aspirin and OJ would be a good start to this day, I thought. As I sipped hot tea and ate my toast and eggs, I felt a kind of melancholy rising in me, knowing the trip was over, and knowing it would be a long while, if ever, before I saw some of these people again.

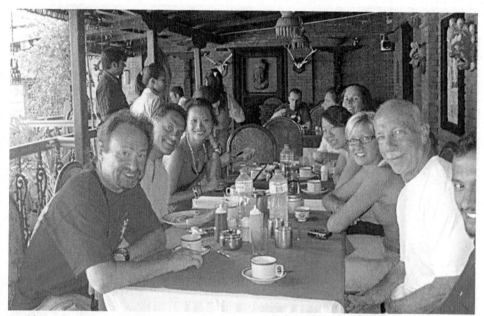

Breakfast at the International Guest House. Our last meal together. Photo by Kathy Hayes.

Basu and Jesse stopped by to organize the morning departures. I was leaving in the afternoon. David came down for breakfast, and he, I, Eve, Jaime, Minling and Tingting decided to do some last minute shopping in Thamel. Basu asked us to drop by his office as well, so he could show us where he worked. I went back to my room and finished packing up my things, leaving one bag open for any last minute souvenirs I might purchase.

While I was packing, Subash knocked on my door. He had stopped by with a gift, some CD's of Hindi music, which he'd thoughtfully labeled 'Gayatri Mantra in English and Hindi'. Subash told me this was very special music, very good for meditation and yoga practice. I came to find out that the Gayatri Mantra is highly revered amongst yogis. It's based on a Sanskrit hymn cited very widely in Vedic literature, including the Bhagavad Gita. Subash also gave me some special ointment he said would cure any aches and pains I might get. I told him it sounded perfect for my mom's arthritis.

I was really touched by Subash's gifts, and inspired to give him something in return. I remembered his interest in my Isherwood translation of the Gita, and quickly retrieved the book. I told him I would love for him to have it, as thanks for all that he had taught us about not only yoga, but about Nepal. I wrote the following inscription on the cover page inside the book: "To Subash Adhikari, My teacher, My brother, My friend. Namaste, John Vourlis," and then gave him the book.

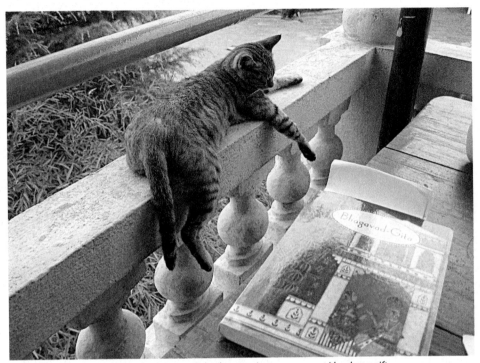

The copy of the Bhagavad Gita that I gave to Subash as a going away present/thank you gift.

Subash seemed very pleased with the gift, and asked me if I'd like to stop by his studio before I left. I said, absolutely, and told him to meet me down in the lobby in ten minutes with the others who were going shopping. I said I was sure some of them would love to see where he worked as well.

I re-connected with the others in the lobby and told them about Subash's offer to visit his studio. Several people jumped at the idea, eager to do some last minute exploration of Thamel, but there were a couple of us who couldn't come along even though they wanted to because they had to catch their flights. Joyce was the first one leaving, and we all hugged her warmly goodbye, and made promises to meet up again back in Cleveland. It was an emotional moment watching her wave goodbye to the rest of us as she got into Basu's car for the ride to the airport — the first real indication that this trip was officially ending. I tried not to think about the fact that I'd be leaving in just a few short hours myself.

When Joyce was gone, Subash led our merry little band off to wander the streets of Thamel one last time. We passed all kinds of markets, including an open air fish market, where I took a picture of Eve and a cart full of dead fish that still makes me laugh when I see it today.

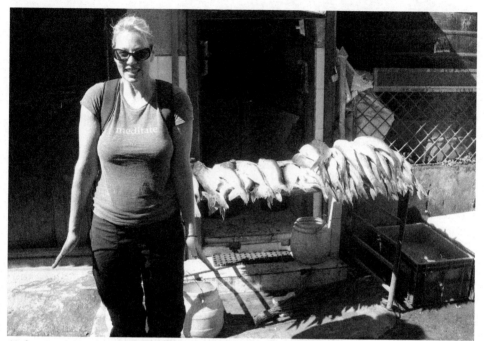

My favorite picture of Eve, freaked out by the fish at a local market in Thamel.

We also stopped by a studio where artists were painting mandalas, and I bought some beautiful hand-painted ones. Mandala is a Sanskrit word that means "circle". The basic form of most mandalas is a square with four gates surrounding a circle with a center point. Each gate is in the shape of a T. These mandalas have spiritual and ritual significance in both Buddhism and Hinduism, their sacred art often taking the form of a mandala. They are also often used as meditation aids. According to the psychologist David Fontana, their symbolic nature can help one "to access progressively deeper levels of the unconscious, ultimately assisting the meditator to experience a mystical sense of oneness with the ultimate unity from which the cosmos in all its manifold forms arises."[15] I just thought they looked beautiful.

---

[15] http://en.wikipedia.org/wiki/Mandala

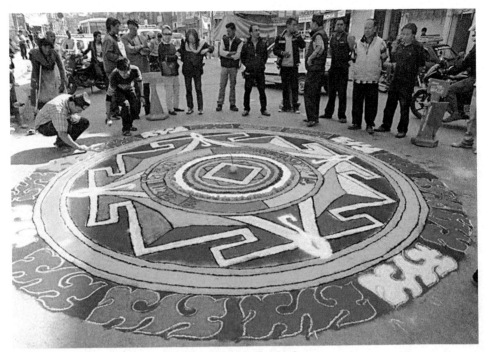

An exquisite chalk mandala. Street art in Thamel. Photo by Tingting Peng.

I also bought a small prayer wheel and a hand-painted red and black lamp shade at some other small shops. The women bought more clothes and scarves and some small handmade purses and shoulder bags. David helped Jaime once again bargain for a very good price on a handmade sun dress. After satisfying our last minute shopping urge, we stopped at Basu's office. He was already back from his quick jaunt to the airport. Subash left us there to attend to some business, and told us he'd meet us back here shortly. Basu's workplace was in the heart of Thamel, located right next to a "Hooters Dance Bar". We teased Basu about this, and he turned a bit red, shaking his head and saying no, no, no, when we asked him if the reason he had his office here was because of the "dance" club.

Basu then took us inside and showed us around the place. He and his good friend Ram Barakoti, a fellow Nepali, own and operate their own travel business here, which they call Nepal Social Treks. The two men arrange trips like ours, as well as treks to the Himalayas and other resorts and national parks in Nepal. I'm not sure what I was expecting to see, but what I found was a pretty modern office. There were several new computers, a couple desks with comfortable office chairs, and bookshelves lining the main greeting room.

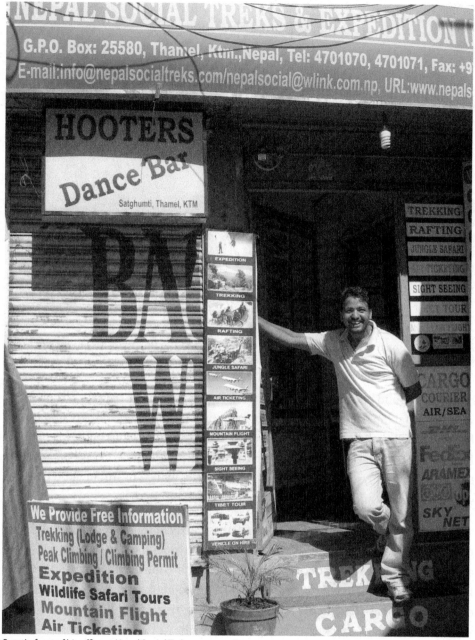

Basu in front of his office at Nepal Social Treks.

Basu led us back to his office, where he had a large desk covered with a map of Nepal and a map of the world. From a desk drawer, he took out a photo album and showed us his Everest pictures. I was blown away. Basu had climbed all the way up to 20,000 feet on Everest (about 2/3 of the way to the top), and he had photos of

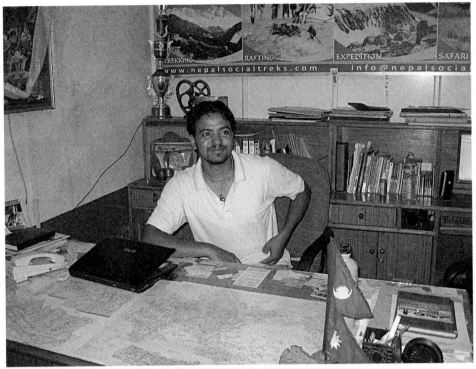

Basu in his office at Nepal Social Treks, www.nepalsocialtreks.com.

himself there and on some of the other great Himalayan peaks as well. The pictures were breathtaking. He told us he was organizing a trek to Everest base camp in the fall, and we all took down the information. As we took turns looking at his photos, Basu served us some Nepali tea, and we chatted a bit about his work. As I sipped the tea, I thought to myself, somewhere down the road, while I'm still in good enough shape to do it, I want to take that climb up Everest with Basu.

As we were finishing up our drinks, Subash arrived on his motorcycle to give us a tour of his place of business. We followed him through the winding streets and alleys of Thamel, stopping occasionally for some more quick shopping and picture taking. Our time in Nepal was running out fast. At a bookstore, I picked up a tome on yoga that Subash had highly recommended. Tingting, Jaime, Minling and I then went with Subash to check out his yoga studio.

Though Subash and Basu are both pretty humble guys, it was clear that they were also proud of what they were doing in Nepal. And they should be. Young, educated, hardworking people like these two are the future of the country, and luckily for Nepal, they are both capable and committed to their vocations. It's folks like Basu and Subash, in my opinion, who will pull Nepal up from its boot straps and into better times in the future. I am honored to have met them, and, even more than that, privileged to call them both my friends. In the words of Mr. Spock from Star Trek, "Live long and prosper, gentlemen."

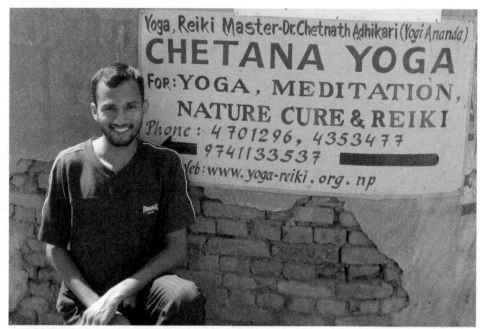

Subash in front of the sign leading to his yoga studio in Thamel.

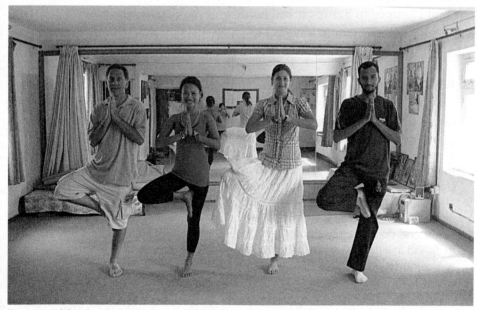

Tree pose with hands to heart, also known as Vrksasana with Anjali Mudra, in Subash's studio. Photo by Minling Chuang.

It was getting close to noon, and several of us had to get back to the hotel to finish packing to leave. I was one of them, and I can assure you I was pretty sad about having to go. We all were…

July 3, 2010 _____

The last day and I don't want to leave. We spent the day shopping in Thamel. Subash showed us the yoga book he used. I bought a copy so I could continue to practice when I get home.

_____ *Minling Chuang*

I went to my room and grabbed my luggage. David graciously said he'd do the check-out, for which I thanked him profusely. David had been a great roommate, and despite his own idiosyncrasies, or maybe more accurately because of them, I knew I would miss hanging out with him. He really was a good guy, and I'd been glad to get to know him. We gave each other a quick, manly hug, the kind where you shake hands homeboy style, chest bump, and slap each others' backs loudly and forcefully, and we promised to stay in touch back in Ohio. Down in the lobby, I gave everyone else a warm hug, and Rachel reminded me, as we embraced, that I still owed Jake money for the drinks last night. Grateful for the memory jolt, I fished out my last few hundred rupees and asked her to pass them on to Jake. Then Basu and Jesse and I jumped in Basu's car and headed for the airport. The others were soon to follow, just as reluctant to leave as I was, later that afternoon.

July 3, 2010 _____

Before we knew it, we were headed to the airport and on our way home. As a parting gift, we were given mala beads with an "om" symbol to remind us of our time in Nepal. We hugged Jesse and Basu goodbye and walked through the gates of the airport. It was weird being in the airport again. I feel like I've changed so much and gained a new understanding of myself. In the airport I felt like I was caught between two lives. What lies ahead of me is my old life and what's behind me is a new life I want to live. I want to travel and see the world and do something positive in the world. I don't want to be stuck at a desk and in a job. How I shift that is beyond me. I just want to cry and hold on to the journey.

_____ *Minling Chuang*

I had lunch, then Eve, Terri, David and I went to the airport. We reminisced about our adventure. I recalled my favorite line from David. In Narti he said, "Did I pee myself, or am I sweating that much?"

This was my horoscope today:

Scorpio

October 23 - November 21

You're much closer to someone today -- or maybe to a group of people! It's a good time to work together on big projects, or to make plans that assume this same kind of bond in the future.

My horoscope cracks me up!

_____ *Christina Jankus*

On the way to the airport Jesse and Basu asked me what I thought of the trip. "It was fantastic!" I said. "Do you think you will come back some day?" Basu asked. "Absolutely!" I replied. I believed it when I said it then, and I believe it now. I will go back someday, to make that trek up to Everest base camp with Basu, and to drop in on Michael and the kids at Nepal Orphans Home.

It was a short ride from the hotel to the airport, and in no time Jesse and Basu were dropping me off outside the terminal. As I got out of the car, I had a lump in my throat. Basu gave me a prayer shawl, and put some mala beads and the shawl around my neck. "Safe journey," he said. I shook his hand and gave him and Jesse both a big homeboy hug. "Thank you for everything," I said. "Namaste." "Namaste," they replied. I couldn't say any more, as the lump in my throat was now the size of an apple. I shouldered my backpack, and picked up my duffel bag and souvenir bag, nodded goodbye and headed into the airport. The others would soon be following, but for now I'd be on my own again until Delhi.

Tingting was the last of our group to leave Kathmandu that day. While we all traveled west, she was going to be heading east, back to Hong Kong.

30 minutes to check-out but still have at least 8 more hours before I head to the

airport. The last day was totally and utterly amazing. I am sad to say good-bye to everyone... already heading back to their respective homes and yet I'm so anxious and excited to begin work on helping Imagine and NOH continue their amazing work...

As people started to depart—Joyce was the first one to go—I suddenly realized that the trip was finally coming to an end. The few people with later flights took to the streets to do some last minute shopping. We stopped in Basu's office (Nepal Social Treks) to check out his digs and pictures from his past tours. Also had some amazing Nepali tea. There, looking at his pictures of Everest Base Camp, I decided that I am definitely coming back to trek to Base Camp.

In the afternoon, I waited for a ride to NOH... Basu helped me to carry everything (including some clothes and supplies for the volunteers) to a cab, and then we met up with Jake, an Aussie volunteer, to walk the stuff to the Houses. Seeing the kids again made my heart smile. I also wanted to thank the girl who had written me a lovely letter earlier in the morning, and passed it to Marni to give to me. I went from house to house looking for her and finally found her at Sanctuary House, the most remote house further down the village path. She was so shy when I hugged her good-bye, but as I was walking back on the footpath, Jake told me to turn around and there she was... on the 2nd floor balcony waving me farewell.

_____ ***Tingting Peng***

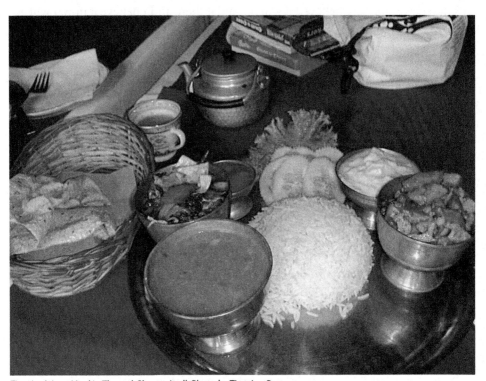

Tingting's Last Meal in Thamel. She ate it all. Photo by Tingting Peng.

At the airport in Kathmandu, I had a small lunch. It was early afternoon, and the airport was pretty quiet. I killed time watching episodes of some American Idol type show on the TV outside the gate. As the time for my departure neared, the airport began to fill with people, and soon we were boarding the Jet Air flight to India. I stared quietly out the window as we lifted off, watching the city of Kathmandu, and then Nepal, disappear below me. Namaste, Nepal. Thank you for an amazing two weeks.

The flight to Delhi was short. When I got there, the gate at the international terminal for my connection to New York wasn't open yet as it was more than three hours before boarding time. I had to go back to the main terminal and wait in the general waiting area. It was hot, crowded, and noisy. There was little to do, and I was feeling pretty tired by now. I hadn't slept more than 4 hours the night before, with all the partying we'd done in Thamel. I chatted with a young American woman, just out of college, who was returning home from a stay in India. Then I went to the food court and had some fairly decent Indian food for dinner. I still had several hours to kill before my next flight, so as soon as I could I entered the international terminal and wandered around until I found a TV. There was a World Cup game coming on, Germany vs. Argentina, and I parked myself in a chair, thankful that I had something to keep my mind occupied during the long wait. There were a couple dozen German travelers seated around me, and the game was an excellent one, from the German's perspective, as they crushed Argentina 4-0 with surprising ease. It was fun listening to their fans shouting excitedly in German as each goal was scored.

About an hour and a half before the New York flight was scheduled to leave, the YFF gang who were traveling on the same flight arrived. Minling, Kathy, Gabby, Deanna, Marc, Robb, Candy, Marni and Jennette were all sharing the flight with me. I was very happy for the company, and especially happy to see all of them again so soon. After one late gate change, we all boarded the 747 bound for New York. It was around 9 or 10 at night, and we had an 11 ½ hour flight ahead of us. We were scattered around the plane, with Kathy and Minling, lucky bums, seated comfortably up in business class. I checked out their digs. Nice big seats that folded back into little sleeping beds. They had upgraded with frequent flyer miles, sharp corporate ladies that they were. I wasn't a fan of sleeping on planes, I don't sleep well sitting upright, and I'm not ashamed to say that I was jealous of their accommodations. Resigned to a long flight, I settled in to watch a movie, but it wasn't more than an hour into the flight that I fell asleep.

From the tarmac in Qatar, on the way back to the good old U.S.A. Photo by Jaime Furda.

I awoke sometime in the middle of the night to go to the bathroom. I wandered around and found Robb and Marc. Marc was zonked, but Robb was up. We talked a bit, and he told me he was going to Florida from New York to see his girlfriend. We both had a good laugh wondering if it was going to be as hot in Florida as it was in Nepal. I headed back to my seat after a bit and did some stretching, then settled in for the remainder of the flight. I never even bothered to watch any TV. Just drifted off, my thoughts more about Nepal, and all that we'd done and seen, than on my return to Cleveland. The others, especially those with kids, had their thoughts focused elsewhere...

July 3, 2010 _____

The Flight Home

Can't figure out if I am
awake or asleep...
feels like a dream,
Kathmandu or
returning home.

When I was in Nepal,
I would close my

eyes and wish when
I opened them, I
could be home.

Now, that is almost a
reality.
I can't wait to look at
my children...
they don't seem real.

My life doesn't seem
like reality.

Neither does Nepal.

I am in transit...
processing all that
I have seen through
all that I have seen.
It feels like a dream.

I have not really cried
yet. Only shed a tear
here and there.
I know when I see my
family... I will finally
be able to let go.

I have been away for
two weeks.

My eyes have seen the
extreme poverty of
Nepal.

I traveled to the other
side of the world,
and return forever
changed and renewed.

I have so much to
give, and so much to do.
Nepal opened the door and
I walked through.

I am no longer afraid
of the space.
Where there is space,
there is peace.
I have so much space,
so much peace.

Where there is peace,
there is God.
I am grateful,
eternally grateful.

Candy Koslen

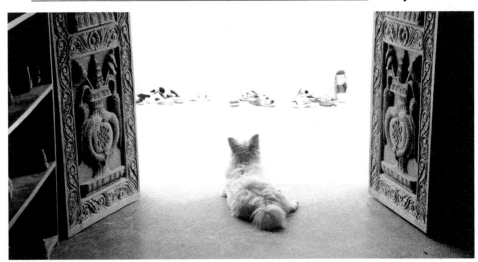

Snowball waiting for the NOH kids to return. Photo by Candace Koslen.

July 4, 2010

Day 15, the last day of the trip

Return of the Natives

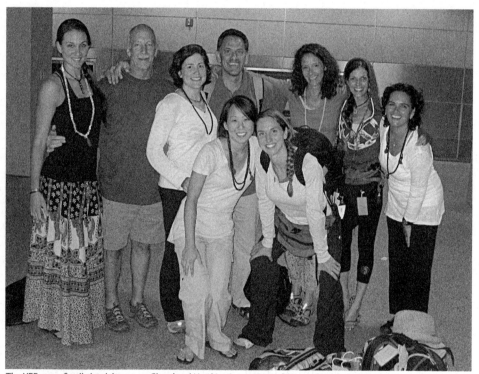

The YFF crew, finally back home, at Cleveland Hopkins International Airport baggage claim.

We arrived in New York just before dawn on the 4th of July. We regrouped at the gate, and then made our way first to baggage claim, then through customs and security, and finally to the domestic terminal at JFK, where we rechecked our luggage. A few people were hungry and grabbed a bit of breakfast. I think I had a cup of tea and a bagel. I didn't have much of an appetite. My mind wasn't really on food. Nobody's was, really... Our amazing Nepali adventure was over.

July 4, 2010 _____

Independence Day. I didn't feel very patriotic or a lot of freedom today. Being back for a few short hours, I already had a list of things I needed to do and take care of. All the stresses of life came back in an instant and I didn't want it to come back at all. I didn't feel free anymore. Why must life feel dreadful with all the responsibilities? Why can't each day be carefree? Maybe it's just me. I know I want to escape my current life and live a life that is more simple and free. But how?

_____ *Minling Chuang*

July 4, 2010 _____

Watched fireworks from the plane's descent into Cleveland with thoughts of freedom and what it means to me.

To me freedom means independence, hope, happiness, opportunity, safety, security, no fear, confidence, to vote and elect our officials, and having rights and privileges yet acting responsibly.

_____ *Christina Jankus*

Tingting also arrived home, to Hong Kong, on the Fourth of July. The irony and poignancy of returning on that particular day didn't escape her either.

July 4, 2010 _____

When I flew into Hong Kong it was morning and the skies were unusually clear. I saw the skyline of HK through new eyes that morning – 4th of July, America's Day of Independence. This is a city of abundance and of lack. It felt unreal to re-enter what most people would call normal society. I sat on my bed for a good while after I got home, just thinking. There's a lot I need to digest, even still.

_____ *Tingting Peng*

Back in New York, Robb was leaving us now for Florida, so we all said our goodbyes, promising to swap photos on Facebook and get together when he got back to Cleveland in a few weeks. It seemed like no time at all before we were back on board a plane again, this time for the final stop of our return trip — Cleveland, Ohio. That last flight was short and uneventful. Around 9 a.m., we finally landed. It was morning now, and our long overnight journey was finally over. After a short bathroom break, we made our way to baggage claim. As soon as we had our bags, we gathered for one last group photo before scattering off to our various homes.

Marni's, Candy's and Jennette's husbands were all waiting outside for them. Marc's son picked him up. Everyone was happy to be reunited with family. My aunt Nettie picked me up, since our extended family was coming to her side of town, near the airport, for a Fourth of July cookout. I was happy to see her, and must've talked a mile a minute until we got back to her place. I dropped my luggage in her spare bedroom, took a shower, and then lay down on the bed and went to sleep. It was a bright and sunny morning, but my body was telling me it was almost midnight and I needed rest. I tossed and turned, and managed to sleep a short while. My family arrived mid-afternoon, mom, dad, and sister, and I got up out of bed, sluggish and not very well rested, but really happy to see them. I spent the rest of the day enjoying our annual Independence Day gathering, eating, drinking, and watching a little baseball and soccer on TV. It felt good to be home with family. I couldn't put my finger on it exactly, but I somehow felt better, more appreciative of home and family than I'd felt in a long time. I wasn't sure why, but that didn't seem to matter. I just knew I felt better. Somehow different. Changed.

While the rest of us were now home and safe, Jesse remained in Nepal, doing his own work to process the last couple weeks...

July 4, 2010 _____

I hope everyone looks back at this activity with understanding. The understanding that for two weeks we lived our lives for others, our actions, our words for others.

Everyone showed their true colors, some were beautiful and some were horrific.

I know that I lost friends on this trip, but I also made some. I'm ok with that.

Now that everyone is gone, I can do what I need to do.

_____ *Jesse Bach*

It would be some time before he got back, and before we all would see each other again. That was probably a good thing. We all had a lot of thinking and processing to do before we could come to terms with what we'd experienced on our trip. We needed to be away from each other, and away from Nepal, to really understand and appreciate the journey we had taken, both as individuals and as a group. And now that we were home, we'd have the time and distance necessary to gain some perspective. I wondered, as I finally got home that night, after the cookout, what would happen to us, not so much as individuals, but as a group. Would we be able to hang together, to stay close, to keep in touch, or would we drift apart once we no longer had the trip to bind us together?

Part 3
Home

Believe nothing merely because you have been told it.
Do not believe what your teacher tells you merely out of
respect for the teacher. But whatsoever, after due examination
and analysis, you find to be kind, conducive to the good,
the benefit, the welfare of all beings – that doctrine believe
and cling to, and take it as your guide.

~ Buddha

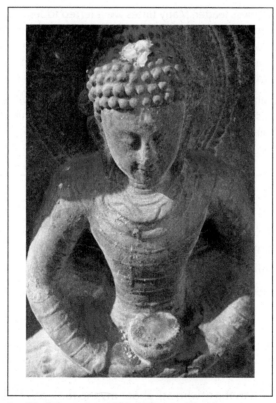

Small Buddha carving with bindi blessings. Photo by
Candace Koslen.

Summer 2010

Trying to Make Sense of it All

The attempts to make sense of the whole trip, to put it in some kind of perspective, began almost immediately once we were back. That's not really surprising; it's human nature. When you go through something as eventful and intense as our two weeks in Nepal had been, it's only natural to try to draw some meaning from it all. Many people were still focused on what happened in Narti, and on Jesse, still trying to make heads or tails of the events of that day, now over a week old…

July 5, 2010 _____

Jesse Bach, our fearless leader. Many times we referred to Jesse as our "fearless leader." It is indisputable that he took on an amazing task to bring us – a group of yogis, a group of veritable strangers – to an unknown terrain. All in the earnest attempt to raise awareness in our community back home. That was the mission. Well… mission accomplished.

I came home realizing that he was right. We were there to witness. We were there to witness, so that we could come home and spread the word. So that those beautiful girls can continue to lead the lives that Michael Hess is providing…

_____ ***Eve Ennis***

What Eve said was true, we were all still hanging on to Nepal, and we were also trying to come to grips with our feelings about the kids at NOH that we'd met… those incredible, resilient, wonderful kids. Friends and family were asking us about the trip, and that was forcing us to try and articulate what the journey had been like.

July 5, 2010 _____

My elevator speech to those who ask about my trip to Nepal is this:

Those children harbor no anger or bitterness toward their parents for having sold them, nor to their owners for having worked them hard and abused them.

They now only know happiness. They are present in their happiness. They don't lament the past or fear the future. They have nothing to hide, nothing to prove and nothing to lose. This is their truth!

I went to Nepal to help children and they helped me.

_____ *Christina Jankus*

We were all grateful to be home, safe and sound, with our families. We had been tested by this trip, just like Jesse had predicted we would be, and we had all learned a lot about ourselves…

July 5, 2010 _____

I am home. I am grateful to be home, and grateful for every minute spent in Nepal.

The group broke down the last couple days of the trip. It was not good, but the people that remained stayed strong and focused. It ended up seeming like a reality show, with people's limits and strengths being tested. Some great lessons were learned by all of us.

I asked one of the girls [at NOH] if she had a best friend. She said all the kids (150) were her best friends. What a great response, and what a testament to the program, the kids, and to Michael. I wish we could bottle up their family dynamics and bring it home with us. What a gift that would be.

_____*Marc Nathanson*

Now it was time to get back to our lives. Back to work, back to school, to the daily routine of our normal existence. That would prove to be more challenging than many of us thought. We'd seen too much to not look at the world back home now in a very different way…

July 2010 _____

After being back for awhile, I had some time to think. And I had time to process this experience.

What I know: At random times I find myself overcome with emotion, wishing I were back in Nepal. I'm missing it, and missing the closeness of being there with some of the people. Many I feel as close as family. Part of that is because some of what we went through together is indescribable to anyone who didn't experience it. My heart longs to spend more time with these children…

I have definitely returned, forever changed in some ways. The children, in their ability to survive, forgive, finding hope and happiness in their lives, is a constant reminder to me in my daily existence of just how good we have it here.

_____ *Terri Bahr*

July 6, 2010 _____

First day back at work. I didn't feel like my old self at all. I didn't want to be there. The chaos of work got to me, especially since my heart longed to go back to Nepal and be there. Luckily, Kathy was at work and could relate. It was surreal being back to something that was once so familiar. All the timelines and new products I have to keep track of. Does it really matter? Does this world really need a new product to make people money? I benefit from it because I get paid, but does anyone really need more stuff? I don't think so. There's so much product proliferation and waste in this world. Why? Corporate greed. But I am stuck. I'm stuck in that world of being in a corporation and I'm scared to get out even though that's what I long for. I'm scared to make that leap and move on.

_____ *Minling Chuang*

July 2010 _____

I got home, and I was so happy to be in the USA, but quickly found myself feeling really angry. I don't know what that was about, I don't know if it was because I wanted to be back there and wanted to serve and wanted to somehow make a difference. Or so happy to be in my clean house, and yet there's something so utterly, perfectly, Stepford Wife perfectly perfect-ish about the USA. And it's kind of, I don't know, fake and fabricated. And we always put a band-aid on it so it feels a little [better]. I don't know—there's something very real about living in the grit of life. I used to live in New York, and so I feel like there's something very real about New York. And I think, as Americans, we tend to pretend everything is super perfect. And there's something about sitting in stuff, just letting it all hang out.

_____*Marni Task*

July 5, 2010 and later_____

Back in the US things seem surreal—there is so much room on the streets and things are so orderly they appear hypnotized. The frantic buzz of Kathmandu is far behind and the quiet of the Cleveland suburb feels so tranquil that there is almost no pulse. My body is home; my mind is still journeying in Nepal, and my spirit? I feel like seeds of it are there—bits of it that don't take away from the whole, but like seedlings have fallen there hoping to grow. The faces of the children I see are those who are rescued and saved. I'm not yet haunted by the thousands who are yet to be set free. Perhaps that is because I saw the "lucky" ones—the ones who were safe, well cared for and loved; not those without enough to eat, no safe place to sleep and little rest when sleep finally comes…

I go to Vicarro's for dinner and feel a bit silly signing a $50 check for just one meal—now my currency valuation is always "how many days could a child at NOH live with this money" —so it's about 2 weeks! One meal of mine—2 weeks of shelter, food, school, clothing, medical. Seems so strange that this equation is even possible. But it is and here I am and there they remain.

How do we remember the trip? The actual trip was just 2 weeks—the anticipation was 6 months and the memory indefinite.

Kathy Hayes

Back in Nepal, Jesse was, strangely enough, struggling with the same perspective shift that we were wrestling with at home.

July 9, 2010

In Nepal, working with these children there are moments of pure surrealism. I had a conversation with a young rescued girl who was beating herself up over being "stupid" and "lazy" and an "idiot" and every other nasty thing…. She told me that she tries as hard as she can but still has difficulty. I knew exactly how she felt.

In that moment I got to tell her everything I wished someone had told me when I felt the same way, so many years ago.

I told her that she could do it, that she can do anything. She was smart and special and she was doing a good job. All that mattered was she tried as best as she could at everything. I let her know that sometimes an A isn't 100%, sometimes it's a C- and that's ok. I let her know that she has something special inside of her and no one can change that.

I told her how in school kids made fun of me, and teachers yelled at me. I told her about summer school and failing subject after subject. I told her how it took me 7 years to graduate from college and I almost failed out on multiple occasions. I told her how people still laugh when I tell them I'm a Yoga teacher and how people still make fun of me. I let her know that even though I'm not scared of anything I can still get my feelings hurt and I will cry, that the strongest people allow themselves to cry.

Her face changed slightly and I could tell that this was the first time an adult had talked to her like this. I could see that she truly heard what I was saying.

I told her that anything is possible if she just tries. A little confused, she asked if I was sure. And I told her to trust me, that anything is possible.

When I said that, I finally understood my own life. I understood what I was saying and for the first time I was thankful for it.

I'm thankful for everyone who's ever been mean to me, who's made fun of me and told me I couldn't' do it. I'm thankful for being called stupid and dumb. I'm thankful for failing. I'm thankful for my own pain and suffering. I'm thankful for special classes, testing and summer school. I am truly thankful for every negative experience that has ever happened to me. I am thankful for everyone who has ever let me down. I am thankful for everyone who has yelled at me and made me feel bad for just being myself. I am thankful for being called names and pointed at. I am thankful for detentions and abusive teachers. I am thankful for looking up to people and then finding out they are horrible human beings. I am thankful.

I'm thankful for them, because I understand where she was coming from. If I never had these awful experiences I would have never been able to empathize, I wouldn't have understood.

I get it now. I understand that I am a student, always, and life is my teacher. The only lesson I have to pass on is my own life and how I live it. I will pass on the best lesson I can.

I'll never be rich or famous. I'll never win a marathon or jump the Grand Canyon on a motorcycle. I'll never walk a red carpet or make a dramatic speech at the Lincoln Memorial. I will never be beautiful or handsome or having rippling abs. I will never have paparazzi fawning over me, or be on CNN with Anderson Cooper but I don't have to.

It's because I can. I can inspire people to act. I can hug. I can dance. I can sing and I can listen. I can cry and I can watch movies with you. I can have up to three children on my lap at any one time. I can understand and I can try and try and try and fail and fail and fail but keep trying. I can fall and get back up. I can encourage and I can help. I can let you know that everything is going to be all right and I can get yelled at and smile. I can get made fun of and pointed at and not care anymore. I can know that my days here are limited and I can't waste a single one of them worrying about the I can't's. I can see you and know you and love you and I don't need anything else, because I can.

Thank you for that.

_____ *Jesse Bach*

While the trip had stirred up a lot of complicated feelings in all of us, some of us also came back with a greater sense of calm, perhaps even a greater sense of purpose…

…back in the States.

In NYC… sitting at a sushi restaurant. Been here for 1 ½ days. It is the polar opposite of Nepal. CRAZY.

I must say my energy, demeanor, mood have been calm, reflective, appreciation for simple pleasures, appreciation, positivity. I'm so grateful for the people I traveled with and those I met on the journey, Americans and Nepali, that have all become family…

I walked around the city, ironically stumbled into a Nepali/Indian store (that sold the same items I saw every day in Nepal for soooo much more $).

_____ *Rachel Vincent*

July 8, 2010 _____

As I headed up the escalators, I walked by an old elderly homeless woman sitting on the side, almost crumbled over, begging for money. I took a 20-dollar bill out of my wallet and placed it in her basket, which only had two coins in it. When I walked away, I felt a sudden surge of sadness, and I thought back to the kids of NOH and felt even sadder.

There was a heavy feeling of universal suffering that bore down on me as I continued walking. I kept passing by well-dressed people who probably have no concern for the poor; they just walk by and go about their own lives. I began to feel angry and wondered if anyone else could see the suffering that happens right in their own city. Then I remembered what Candy had said at Namo Buddha, "We all do the best we can but we can't help everybody…" And I wonder how I might be able to do more. Pondering this, my eyes swelled up with tears. My life became trivial again. I could see that the higher purpose of my life (as an individual) was and is to do great things for the less fortunate.

Two years ago, being able to buy the latest Jimmy Choo shoes was my priority. Last year, it was about being free and happy to pursue my passion of yoga. This year, it is about impacting and empowering others, through all the tools that I have learned. Thinking about scaling back even more my consumption, and being more conscious about reaching out a helping hand wherever and whenever I can. I cannot wait to go back to Nepal. For now, I am taking a stand for the goodness that can be found in everyone.

_____ *Tingting Peng*

It has been almost a week being back in Cleveland. Slowly but surely, the physical part of me is getting back to normal. How am I? I find myself much more patient and getting less excited and worrisome over the mundane.

I am not worried or uptight about the first day on the job. Everything will be okay. I guess, after taking on the kids and their love, most everything else seems less important. Even my family which usually causes me to worry, or try to fix, has taken on less important significance. It's all good.

*_Marc Nathanson_*

Maybe it wasn't just being in Nepal that had altered our worldview. Maybe it had been those two weeks our group had spent together in Nepal that had changed all our perspectives on the world… maybe it was that attempt to make the trip from me to we that had most affected us all.

Jesse had things to do in Nepal, and he had his Imagine Foundation on which to focus his energies when he returned. The question for the rest of us was what were we going to do with our new perspective on the world? Ignore it? Internalize it, compartmentalize it, and then just move on? Or were we going to take it and do something with it? Something positive and productive to try and change the world and perhaps make it a better place? That would be the real long-term challenge. Only time would tell whether any of us, alone or together, could accomplish that, but many of us were determined to try…

I'm on the plane again – this time to Singapore, for work for a couple of days….

At the airport, I picked up the latest issue of Yoga Journal and there is a great article in there this month about finding the calm within….

The article explains that upeksha stresses the importance of balance – a balanced heart is not an unfeeling heart; a balanced heart feels pleasure without grasping or clinging at it and it feels pain without condemning or hating it. It stays open to neutral experiences with presence.

Beyond being with the pain of seeing and witnessing suffering (both in Nepal and now everywhere I go), I realize that I held a lot of judgment towards many of the other participants of YFF, and I had struggled with acknowledging that feeling. I felt disappointed and sad because I had expectations and projected them. With this concept of upeksha, I finally feel at peace with all of the drama that took place in Nepal. I had wondered whether I would be able to stay friends with those people, how can I be real and authentic with them if I always held a sword over them, feeling justified? And, I also didn't like being fake either, just to please people – it was a bit tormenting. But now, I do feel freedom. It is neither an indifference to the suffering of others nor a bland state of neutrality, but rather it is a deeply rooted compassion and care for everything and everyone!

...With this trip to Nepal, I am a firm believer that the best way to go through life is to relinquish fear and control and to just live! I will never know which way my life's path will turn or what the ultimate consequences will be. Upeksha and equanimity allows for the mystery of this unknown space to be a beautiful space to be standing in.

Tingting Peng

For me, the first few weeks back in Ohio I felt like I was in two places at once. My body was in Cleveland, but half the time, sometimes without even realizing it, my mind was in Nepal. What brought me back to the present was a bug bite. I woke up early on the morning of July 6th and walked to the front door, staring out into the dawn of a beautiful summer morning. That was when I noticed a small bump on the back of my left thigh. I thought nothing of it then, and went back to bed. But the next day, the tiny bump had grown into a bigger one, from the size of a pin-head to the size of a dime or nickel. And it was sore. Strange I thought. Wonder what that could be? Did a mosquito or something bite me while I was out in the yard working the day before?

I went about my daily routine, worked on the early stages of compiling everyone's journals from the trip. I got an email from someone, Eve or Terri, saying that there would be a get together on the following Friday evening at Terri's apartment. A small wine and cheese gathering of all those who were feeling Nepal withdrawal pains. I was down for that. I hate goodbyes, and I have an almost pathological need to stay connected to people, especially those I've shared amazing experiences with. I was looking forward to seeing everyone.

The evening turned out to be a lot of fun. Terri, Eve, Marc, Joyce, Minling, Rachel, Jennette and Christina all showed up. We had a blast reminiscing, but it was clear too, that some of the issues from the trip had yet to be resolved…

Last night a bunch of us got together. It was nice to see the gang. We got to laugh and relive a lot of the special moments. But some people went back to some of the low points and playing the blame game. I did not have the patience to go over the same negative stuff again. That was the only negative.

_____**Marc Nathanson**

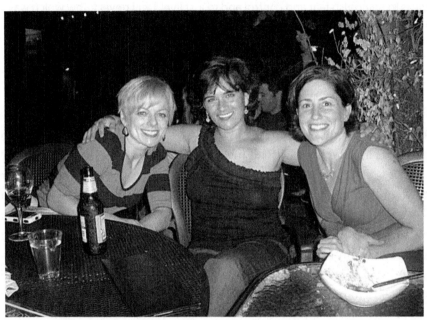

A night on the town, Cleveland style. Photo courtesy of Joyce Fijalkovich.

I wasn't all that interested in rehashing some of the more negative events. I had other problems. That little bump on the back of my left thigh had grown to the size of a tomato, and was just as red, and more importantly quite painful. It was hard to sit on that cheek. I shared my concern with the folks who had gathered. They all laughed at my predicament. They wondered if I'd gotten bit in Nepal. There were spiders everywhere…. Oh joy, I thought. And then they all wanted to see it. I was not prepared to show anyone my ass, at least not until I'd had a couple glasses of wine. But there was plenty of wine flowing that night, I had even brought a bottle myself, and so eventually my friends were checking out the back of my upper left thigh.

"Ohhhh…," said Terri. "You better go have that looked at. It might be infected."

Perfect. Here I am in Ohio, my health insurance and doctor are in LA, and I may have an infected bug bite on my ass. What a nice way to come home. By now I was running a low grade fever, so I called Kaiser and they told me to go to the nearest urgent care clinic. Their diagnosis: bug bite. The doctor there put me on antibiotics right away. Two days later I went back. It had gotten worse, not better. Time for a shot. And more antibiotics. And the recommendation to see an infectious disease surgeon. Happy happy joy joy, to quote Ren & Stimpy. Two more shots, and two more sets of antibiotics.

While I was dealing with the physical challenges presented by trying to sit on my infected bug bite, the others were dealing with more emotional and psychological issues...

July 17, 2010 _____

It has been almost two weeks since we came home from our adventure. It's funny, because in some ways it feels like yesterday. And in other ways, I feel like my whole life and me are now different. I continue to get less involved with the small stuff of life. I continue to think about those kids every day, and given the support & unity, share their way of being. In this world, my wish for all of us and our children is to possess their spirit of community and love for each other. I continue to share my experience with anyone who is interested and even those who aren't. I continue to think about my life and how I want to be. I seem more determined to serve than ever before. I cannot wait.

I will forever be grateful for the trip, and how it touched my view of the world, and how it is shaping my heart.

_____*Marc Nathanson*

At this point, it had been a couple weeks since I'd first realized I had a problem, and the pain had become excruciating, and the wound disgusting. Finally, after more than three weeks of treatment with four different antibiotics, I went to the surgeon, who cleaned out the last of the infection, and told me definitively it had been a spider bite. She pointed out the three punctures, one big one, and two smaller ones, just for good measure I suppose. She surmised that I'd been bitten in Ohio and not Nepal, though she couldn't say with 100% certainty. Maybe I had brought the little bugger home with me, and sat on him while unpacking. For a moment I thought of that first huge spider I'd seen at Norling, the one with the five-foot diameter web, and the way it had come to symbolize the fear that had followed us on our journey. Was there some deeper meaning to this spider bite, I wondered? What was I afraid of now? Coming home to Cleveland? Leaving again for LA? After three long, painful weeks of constantly looking for a gentle way to assume and maintain a seated position, finding the answer to that riddle didn't seem all that important; the doctor had pronounced me cured, and my ass felt great. That was good enough for me.

I was now sitting pain free, and just in time to attend another gathering of some of our group, this time at Eve's house, for a summer luau. The luau was a blast, and people were in good spirits. All this time, we'd been working on getting journals turned in by everyone. I emailed, texted, and otherwise cajoled everyone to turn them in. We were hoping to have them all in by the end of July.

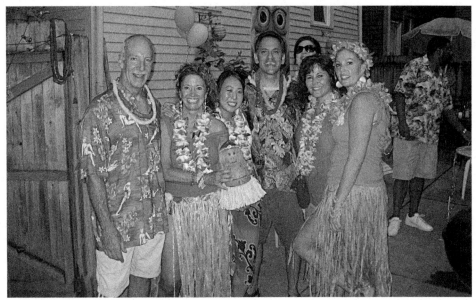

Luau party at Eve's house. Photo courtesy of Minling Chuang.

After a little added friendly persuasion from Minling, Journals began coming in rapidly, and from all directions. In fact, most people were very obliging. Some even typed up their own journals, which turned out to be a huge time and work saving thing for me. Once I started receiving the journals, I immediately began reading them. My thought was to go through each one in its entirety first, without taking any notes or marking it up, to get a visceral feel for the writing. Then I would go through them a second time to consider what parts to use for the book we wanted to put together. As I read through each journal, I was immediately sucked back to Nepal, into that time and place, into all the emotions, all the excitement, anticipation, the fear and drama of our trip.

July 26, 2010 _____

This is my last entry. The journal goes on to Minling and John. Saturday night I got together with a group of my fellow travelers from the trip. It's great seeing everyone, catching up, and hearing about their lives and those around them. We are all inter-connected…

What does a trip like this do to our beings? And why? Why does that kind of experience change our way of being in the world? Why and where does this sense of freedom materialize? Is it meeting Michael and witnessing the importance of one human being? Is it the impact of one human being on a cause, or others? Is it the freedom we felt from the kids? Was it the freedom we felt on the trip away from all the day to day responsibilities we create for ourselves? Not sure if all or more of these reasons are inspiring us and me, but I have felt a shift.

I feel like I am more honest with myself and others. If I want to try something, I am trying it. If I want to meet someone, I am meeting them. If I want to be busy for busy's sake, I am not. I feel more alive. I want to be more engaged in life. I am more excited to wake up and be more engaged. The trip touched my already open heart and soul.

_____ _Marc Nathanson_

July 28, 2010 _____

Cleveland Heights

I haven't written since returning home. I suppose the settling process was a whirlwind… a reflection.

In the time between returning and now, my dreams have been vivid…many of Nepal. One was wonderful: We were at a pool, the kids were swimming and I was continuously going off of the diving board and striking random yoga poses…the kids watched, laughing, loving life. I awoke with such a feeling of happiness; very similar to how I felt the day Jaime, Jesse and I spent at Papa's house Saturday before all of the traveling began. The joy I felt walking from front yard to backyard, inside and out…every inch with children playing, learning, laughing…free everywhere. It was so wonderful spending time with them. My cheeks literally hurt from smiling that day. The perfect day spent with the kids…the reason I went was to capture a day just like that Saturday….I will hold it so close in my heart, my memory for life.

_____ _**Rachel Vincent**_

So I am sitting here on the 28th of July, having procrastinated until 2 days before deadline in my classic style. I could use the excuse that I am a mother of 6 children, a yoga instructor, a photographer.... or I could speak the truth. The truth being that I am petrified to dig it up. Dig up the way that I felt in Nepal....

Kathmandu isn't a place to run away from the darkness. You have to be willing to take it all in for the bittersweet experience that IS life. You can't dig up the darkness without making space for the light, and the light shines brightly in Kathmandu. The light burns brightly in the children, in the power of hope, in the survivors. The seekers, the monks, the fallen alike. You will find the light in Kathmandu if you seek it, and you will realize that it's not coming for you after all, it's coming from you.

I believe in the good of man.

I believe equally in the darkness and the work to be done.

I believe in magic bracelets, and old new friends.

I believe in love, without judgment or fear.

I believe in the resilience of a child.

I believe in Michael Hess and every little soul at NOH.

I believe in the people who went on this journey called yoga for freedom, and the freedom we received on the journey.

I believe in my unbreakable soul.

Jennette Zimmerman

People had really taken the whole journaling thing to heart. They had opened themselves up quite a bit, revealing their innermost intimate thoughts and feelings about the events that had transpired over the last six months. And they had done so in clear, lucid, sometimes even poetic prose. I was impressed. And humbled.

Not everyone was as timely in turning in their journals as I'd have wished, though. Even I was procrastinating in finishing up. I guess maybe I wasn't really ready to let go of Nepal, or it wasn't ready to let go of me. I was getting moody, cranky from dealing with that bug bite, and in general struggling to summarize my thoughts about the trip into one last journal entry…

It's been 3+ weeks since we got back from Nepal. I'm beginning to feel like the bliss from that trip is wearing off. This is probably inevitable. Life goes on. The question remains, how much has this experience actually changed me, and how much of the experience will fold in on my old self (as Jennette, one of my fellow travelers, said just after we got back), leaving me unchanged.

Before I left on this trip, I was impatient, tense, frustrated, feeling caged in by the circumstances of my life, a cage I helped create myself. I don't want that feeling to come back. I think that's why I've been so unwilling to go back to LA right away. I don't want to pollute my newly cleansed soul with those emotions again. Not now. Not yet.

But I know myself, and I know what drives me, and I know that even if I never go back to LA, those emotions will return. Because I am not yet content to be like Siddhartha and row a boat back and forth across a river ferrying people from one side to the other, content in being only of service to others. Don't get me wrong, I think being of service is a blessing and a gift. I want to incorporate as much of that as possible in my life. I enjoy it immensely. But I have things I want to accomplish for myself as well. And they are not easy things. They require hard work, painful rejection, unending perseverance, discipline. And they also require patience, joy and even a realization that the outcome I seek is something I will never be entirely able to control on my own. The outcome is in the hands of God, of the Universe. And I learned on this trip to be at peace with that. Thank you, Nepal.

_____ **John Vourlis**

This first attempt to summarize my thoughts about the trip just got me more frustrated. Was I afraid to go back to LA? Or afraid to leave it, to come back to Cleveland, to come back home? I read over what I wrote, and it felt entirely inadequate, too selfish, like I'd missed the whole point of the trip somehow. So I took another crack at it...

Here's a few more things I learned from my trip to Nepal... a totally random list, from the silly to the profound:

Nepal has the best potatoes I've ever tasted—fried, mashed, mixed with vegetables, or with eggs, they are amazing.

20 people traveling halfway around the world can get along remarkably well almost all of the time. But they aren't going to always agree on everything,

especially regarding camping in a poor rural village way out in the countryside of a third world country. And there are times when the divisions will be so deep and so wide, that no amount of talking, sharing, powwowing, will close that gap. At this point, somebody's got to take charge, and that person is not going to get any love for doing so. But it has to be done. If you want to lead, you have to take the bad and deal with it. The good takes care of itself.

Poverty is the root of all evil. Give a poor person some money, and they can eat. Give them an education and a job, and they can, with a little luck, pull themselves out of poverty. Leave them with no education, no job, and no money for food, and they will resort to whatever they have to do to survive, including selling their own children.

There are a lot of people trying to do good in the world, and I was lucky enough to meet and travel with a bunch of them on this trip. They're not saints; they're not perfect, noble creatures. They have issues, battle their own demons, wrestle with their own fears, struggle to throw off the shackles of their own upbringing, their own cultural conditioning. They can be selfish, petty and even do wrong on occasion, but something about all of them makes them want to make the world a better place. Some of them are changing the world, slowly but surely. All of them in their own unique ways are making a difference for the better.

Children are the real superheroes, especially the ones growing up in poverty. The children of Nepal Orphans Home and Lawajuni are some of the finest kids I've ever met anywhere, more resilient than Superman, more adaptable than Spiderman, and nowhere near as dark and brooding as Batman. I was blessed to have had the opportunity to meet them. They helped me put a lot of things in my own life into perspective. They are remarkable.

In many ways, I am the same person I was before I left. In a few, I know I am not. And both of those are good things.

Namaste.

_____ *John Vourlis*

My second attempt made me no happier than my first. Too disjointed, too unfocused. It was even less satisfying, with respect to my overall thoughts and feelings about the trip, and to how I felt now that I was back, than my first feeble attempt had been. There was only very minor comfort in knowing that I wasn't the only one struggling to wrap up my thoughts in a neat little package…

I Officially Suck at Journals.

Hi again! It's been a while (for me, at least). I'd have written sooner, but my most wonderful factory job (I put stickers on football helmets for ten hours a day, six days a week) kept me from having much free time.

Anyway, I feel as though going to Nepal, however briefly, has really done wonders for me. Back at work in Elyria, some of my co-workers even noticed a difference, calling me more of a "free spirit" (as if I weren't one already). I most definitely agree with them. That trip opened my eyes to what's really happening on the other side of the Earth, and even what I did see was only a small fragment of the whole. After going, I feel as though I need to make a habit of traveling to places like that, as meeting those children especially brought about the most amazing feeling in the world. It kind of reminds me of the last stanza of a poem I wrote once about standing next to moving trains (odd, I know):

> *"I stand there—*
> *eyes closed*
> *arms outstretched*
> *hair blown back—*
> *facing the sun*
> *and*
> *feeling infinite"*

Infinite. That's exactly how Nepal, the kids, everything made me feel. I love it.

_____ *Jaime Furda*

I began to think there was no way to really summarize in a paragraph or three what this trip had been all about to any of us, what it had done to us, brought up in us, forced us to examine and deal with. Not in the few short weeks since we got back. That kind of introspection, I began to suspect, was going to take some time. Then I read Candy's last journal entry, and it all made sense why...

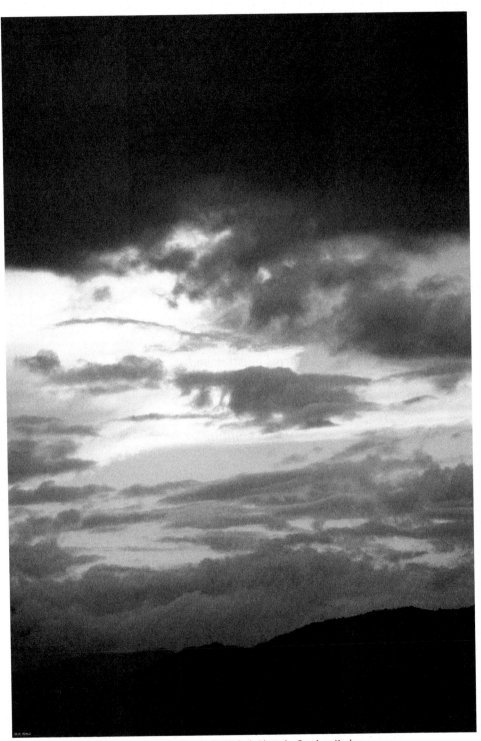

A picture is worth a thousand words. The Nepali sky at dusk. Photo by Candace Koslen.

When Words Fail Me

When words fail me...
I take it in.

When words fail me...
I stand in awe.

When words fail me...
her eyes show me the
depths of the oceans.

When words fail me...
his smile melts all
sadness from my heart.

When words fail me...
there is a peaceful warrior.

When words fail me...
love is abundant.

When words fail me...
God takes up space.

When words fail me...
I am free.

Candy Koslen

Right now, words were too inadequate a medium for expressing the feelings and emotions that were still roiling around in our heads and hearts. Now we just needed some time to process the whole experience… Words on paper, at this point, were not going to be enough.

The end of July arrived, and it was clear that we weren't going to have all the journals turned in on time. People asked, begged, pleaded, for more time to finish writing, to type up their own handwritten entries. I completely sympathized with their struggles. I also thought it was best if we could get as many, if not all, of the remaining journals turned in before I started writing. The more voices, the more perspectives, the better the book would be, I felt. So we extended the deadline to the end of August. A few more people turned in their journals.

August 6, 2010 _____

After the trip

I didn't know – couldn't know what would happen to me. I had no expectations for the ways I would be moved. But I will never forget the moment and the blanket of emotion that swept over me the first time we met the girls at the Imagine house. The herd of happy girls and boys came running up to us. They were open and eager. They were bright as the sun. They were amazing. I realized that the true hero is Michael Hess – a soul of greatness that I hadn't even met. But this man transformed the lives of all these children that were pouring out to meet us. And who were we? Were we a group going to Nepal to change lives, or were we a group of people whose lives would be forever changed?

I needed that moment at the Imagine house to feel. It was a gush. I felt my body and awareness more with the understanding of what it means to support this cause. It's the difference between a beautiful 10-year-old child working 18 hours in the field, and dying in a few years in morbid decay…Or having a childhood with love and laughter, an education, the opportunity to learn and expand. A child allowed having choices, as well as health and happiness.

So what matters to me is not that I didn't have the opportunity to experience a personal rescue, or an opportunity for a pen-pal. What matters to me is I know that every time I talk of the N.O.H. or the Kamlari – I am giving another child a choice. It takes the spread of the word to ensure Michael Hess's work continues.

My inarticulate leader, Jesse Bach, was completely articulate when he said that we are here to witness. That was the vision. Now we are back. It is our duty and our mission to make sure those children have choices.

_____ *Eve Ennis*

But by extending the deadline, we were also allowing life to get in the way of completing this project, as it often does with any long-term plans, interrupting them with reality…

August 11, 2010 _____

I found out that Kathy is moving to Switzerland. She got a job at our corporate headquarters. I'm happy for her, but also super bummed for myself because she was someone I could turn to at work to talk about all my thoughts and feelings. We shared a bond, she was my roommate for the trip, we've been through so much and she is leaving. She leaves the end of the month...I am sad for me and happy for her. She always said that Nepal would be the catalyst that changes something in her life. Boy was she right.

_____ *Minling Chuang*

Before she left for Switzerland, Kathy finally turned her journal in to Minling. This was her last entry...

August 2010 _____

When I think of the children, I don't think much about the NOH experience as much as Narti and don't think of Narti as much as the day in Namo Buddha. In Namo Buddha I met local children -- 3 young boys. I heard their laughter as it climbed up from the hillside to the top of Namo Buddha -- where prayer flags fluttered like a thick forest of wildly colored leaves. The day spanned out before me...no itinerary...no touring...no talking!! I wandered about trying to weave my way through the maze-like terraces to the mountaintop -- the

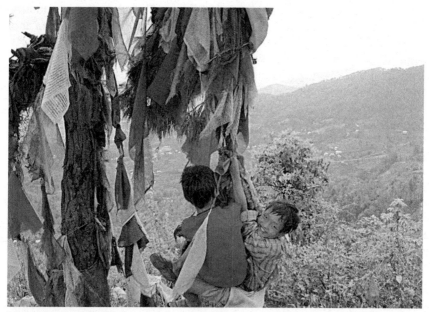

The local boys' makeshift swing made from prayer flags high atop Namo Buddha. Photo by Kathy Hayes.

energy radiated from that place -- it pulled you there but made you work to find it. After many dead ends, u turns, walking in places that seemed I was invading people's homes, finding monks' underwear hanging to dry…I found this special place. Perhaps it was so unique because we had been traveling, absorbing experiences for 2 weeks and now we had time to process, to settle, to be. So I stood there in the wind, delighted in my being. Spread my arms and breathed deeply. Feeling like my energy was pouring out into the wind. That skin and bones no longer confined me. I wasn't a tourist any longer, or a yogi or a friend…only breath and wind. Ahhhhhhaahhhhh. I watched a small boy instructed by his mother climb high into the pine trees. Far higher than would be seen safe by my standards. He tied the end of the prayer flags onto the trunk and scrambled down. Found another tree (after much pointing and instructing from mom) climbed it, again far too tall to be safe, tied the flags and found his way safely to the ground.

I couldn't help but wonder who hangs the flags when junior is too heavy for these thin pines? I guess they have to get their prayers in quickly!

So I'd reached my destination; the prayer flag covered peak and it's only noon -- what next? Then the laughter called me; a giggle of glee climbed up the hillside. I decided to check it out, after all I'd been at Narti playing patty cake, I can relate to kids, especially ones who are having fun. I found them swinging out from the edge of the hill beyond to the mountain side.

The swing isn't like ours, handmade by dad or bought from Home Depot, it was self-created from a tangle of prayer flags that had come loose from the tree tops. The boys seemed unfazed that I couldn't talk with them; they were curious, but cautious. I took out my camera, a modern day flute of the Pied Piper, and snapped a photo and showed it to them. They started posing for the camera eager to see themselves. Then I handed one of them the camera and showed him how to use it. From then on we were friends. They took many pics of me enjoying the prayer flag swing. At first I was a bit worried I might be too heavy for it and might go crashing down the mountain side. But after a few good tugs it seemed sturdy enough so off I swung out over the valley, using the tree trunk to push off, going higher and higher. The kids must not see adults play because they seemed very amused by my frolicking. I decided it was time to move along and let the boys play, but they adopted me and followed me back to the monastery, asking again and again for the camera, photographing themselves along the way. I went into the little store at the monastery and bought them penny candy. They sweetly took the candy and savored it, following me everywhere but inside the store. Tired, I headed back to the room, imagining the kids would depart when they saw the "private-guests only" sign but kids are kids and they ignore what doesn't suit them. Along they came following me to the rooftop delighted in this new venue and with their new subjects Joyce and Gabrielle to photograph.

My fondness of the trip is from the time I had with those boys; unplanned, unscripted, no expectations, just the sweetness of their spirits dancing with mine.

_____ *Kathy Hayes*

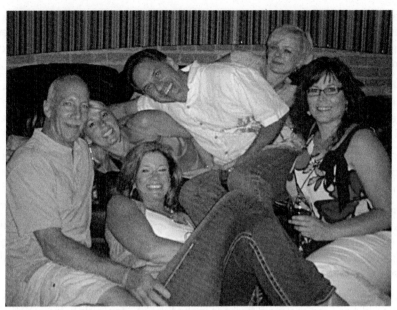

Group hug fun at Kathy's going away part. Photo by Joyce Fijalkovich.

On August 21st, a bunch of us attended the going away party for Kathy. We had a blast. Eve, Terri, Joyce, Gabby, Christina, Marc and I partied late into the night. But it was a bittersweet evening. Kathy would be going away, far away, for 3 years. Minling especially was really going to miss her. They had worked together for several years and were very close, and Minling couldn't be at the party because of a previous obligation.

Now that Kathy was leaving, and with Tingting already off in Hong Kong, the group was growing smaller. We might have Facebook and email to keep in touch, but it would be a long time, if ever, that we'd have the whole group together again.

The August deadline for turning the journals in stretched into September. For some of us, the trip had been a catalyst for positive change and personal growth. People ended bad relationships, started new, happier ones, and got on with the business of living...

September 8, 2010 _____

I am amazed at how this journey has inspired me. What has happened has been surprising. I feel like somehow I have been able to really reclaim "me". The past few years have been a slow reveal of who I truly am. Leaving a bad marriage and acknowledging who I am under all the weight of a 12 year I-don't-know-what-to-call-it relationship? A stifling/demeaning time in my life. It seems like I have always known "what's what", but my opinion has never been counted or acknowledged, so I buried what I felt to be "true" as wrong, or incorrect, or somehow "off."

With this trip, I have been able to really claim and own what's mine without shame or explanation. Maybe that's called confidence? I don't know, but when I see younger people, who have done so much less in their lives, exude this, I feel I'm finally ready to claim what is already mine; I can, and should, and it's ok.

Something else that's dawned on me is that I see cycles more clearly. Types of stages of life are crystal clear. I can identify them easily in other people and try to help where I can.

I have seen poverty and filth on a large scale and know there is suffering in this world on a massive scale. It is daunting and overwhelming if you really think about it. The best thing to do with that feeling of thinking "anything one person can do is just a drop in the bucket," is to acknowledge that's probably true and just try to impact 1 or 2 people directly.

I have a few causes I support—PETA, Sea Shepherd, and now NOH. I can't save the world, but I can make a difference in the lives of a few girls halfway around the world, and that's good enough for me.

I want to go back. I'm not "done" yet with my connection to Nepal. I'd like my daughter to go too. She's 12. I think it would be too much for my son, though, he's 10. I am eternally grateful for my spontaneity, for it led me to join this trip at the 11th hour, and it truly changed my life. Thank you!

_____ *Gabrielle Stickley*

September 9, 2010 _____

I know that we walked away spiritually, mentally, and emotionally transformed and much more awareness and gratitude, and we bonded with each other in ways that we never would have back home. For all this, and for all the things I learned and felt and saw, I am grateful. The only thing I wish were different was I wish we could have spent much much more time with the kids, the reason why we came. I feel like we hardly got to see them. I would love to go back someday and do more of a volunteer trip, so let's see how that manifestation comes together ;) It's hard to articulate the feelings and experiences of this trip, one of those times when words fall short of properly explaining the subtleties of emotion, and for much of us the trip was very personal and experiential…

I will always send my love to Nepal and I will never forget the new friends I met and cherish the bonds that were made with new and old friends. And I send the best wishes always to the kids we met and prayers for the kids who have yet to be saved.

_____ *Deanna Lee*

Fall 2010

Dashain

We weren't completely floundering. We had made efforts at growth as a group since our return. Shortly after our return from Nepal, Terri Bahr decided to put on a small fundraising event for the girls of NOH. It would center on the Nepali holiday of Dashain. Dashain is sort of the Nepali equivalent of Easter here in the West, a holiday of sacrifice, death, and re-birth that commemorates the victory of the goddess Durga over the demon Mahishasura. Just like at Easter, people in Nepal, especially women, put on their finest new clothes for the celebration. It was Terri's idea to help all the girls of NOH get new dresses for Dashain, which this year was going to be celebrated in September. She asked me to write up a little flyer for the event, and I gladly did:

SHOW A LITTLE LOVE

TO THE CHILDREN OF NEPAL ORPHANS HOME

This past June, 20 Yoga teachers and students from across Cleveland traveled on the inaugural Yoga For Freedom trip to Nepal. The purpose of the trip was to raise awareness and funds for the children at the Nepal Orphans Home, many of whom have been rescued from the Kamlari system of child slavery/ indentured servitude. In this illegal practice of indentured child labor, young girls, called Kamlaris, are sold by their impoverished parents to local landlords or urban households as domestic laborers. Some of the girls tragically end up in the sex trade. This band of Yoga brothers and sisters who traveled to Nepal not only were able to meet and work with the great kids of NOH, but in the process they became a part of the NOH family. And part of the cost of the trip went to sponsor a child at NOH for a whole year! It was an amazing, deeply moving experience for everyone involved.

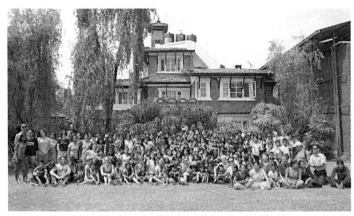

A Small Donation For A Big Festival

Once a year, in late September, the people of Nepal get ready to enjoy Dashain, the biggest festival on the Nepali calendar. Virtually every person in Nepal, regardless of their social caste, celebrates. The entire festival lasts fifteen days and is a riot of color, festivity and religious rites. Every home is cleansed and beautifully decorated, painted as an invitation to the mother goddess, so that she may visit and bless the house with good fortune. During this time the reunion of distant and nearby relatives occurs in every household. Many of the girls from the Nepal Orphans Home will return to their native homes to visit any remaining family; others will stay at NOH and celebrate. In either case, the girls need new dresses. A small minimum donation of $10 USD (750 Nepali Rupees) will help get a girl a new dress for Dashain. These girls have been through so much... Wouldn't it be great to show them some love?

Let's help make this year's Dashain festival one that they will remember forever!

The event was to be held at the TavCo Bar & Restaurant in Cleveland Heights. There would be food, and some music, and we'd invite all our friends. I had no idea what to expect or how many people would show up. Minling went all out and put together a video of our trip made from photos she'd taken for people to watch on the TV's over the bar. The event turned out to be quite a little success. We raised almost $2000, enough money to get a new dress for Dashain for every girl at NOH. When the kids in Nepal found out, they were overjoyed. We got all kinds of posts from them on Facebook, thanking us, including pictures of the girls in their newest finery.

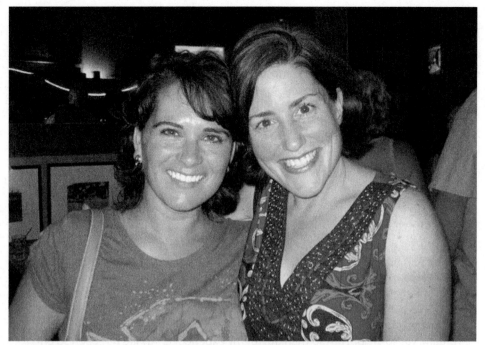

Gabby and Kathy at the Dashain fundraiser at TavCo. Photo courtesy of Kathy Hayes.

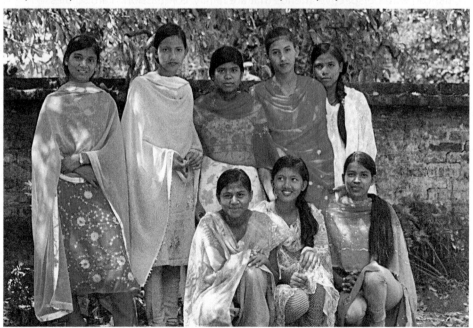

The NOH girls in the new kirtas they got for Dashain with our help. Photo courtesy of Carola Drosdeck.

Afterwards, we were all justifiably proud of the success of the event. If we could pull that off, we thought, we could aim higher. So we turned our focus to something bigger, the annual Imagine Foundation benefit fundraiser for Nepal Oprhans Home, set for the end of November. I wanted the book to be a part of that event, and pushed hard to get the last of the journals, which were emailed or delivered to me personally by Jaime, Rachel, and Deanna. Several people even volunteered to type up the handwritten ones. It had taken some serious cajoling, but we had done it. I was impressed with the level of commitment everyone had given to the effort. In my mind, having all these participants' voices heard could only make the book better in the long run. Rachel's turned out be the last journal that was turned in and typed up… Here's her final entry:

September 23, 2010 _____

There's an absolute chemistry about Nepal. There is an overwhelming feeling that takes over my body, mind, being when I take a moment to recall Nepal. Chills, welled tears, warm heart…a longing. I am convinced there is a magic about Nepal. It definitely cast its spell on me. I become drawn right back to the moments, the emotions…it's all so clear. It has a strange ability to feel like a dream, yet so vivid. I am so thankful for my experience. My life has been so enhanced with perspective, friends that are family, compassion. I am so blessed to have met the tiny bodies that house the largest of spirits…the children of Nepal.

My dreams, all of them, of Nepal and not of Nepal are more intense. I am stronger, more independent, more aware of my strength and independence. I am more willing and able to express, to share, to be open. Nepal lives within a part of me that will be forever reserved for Nepal.

_____ *Rachel Vincent*

Now it was time for me to really get to work. I actually thought I might possibly have a draft of the book done by the time of the Imagine Benefit in November, if I put my mind to it. I re-read all the journals, and then began selecting what I thought were the highlights of each one. Gabby and I began scanning pages from the handwritten ones into the computer so I could share them with Minling and Lauren Yanks, our friend and a New York-based editor who had been to Nepal and had kindly agreed to help us get started with the project. We held half a dozen meetings and phone discussions on how to make sense of all these journals, how to turn the multitude of voices into one coherent narrative. It was becoming clear to me that this was going to be no small task. Lauren pushed me to take on the role of narrator for the book. Minling had many excellent suggestions, including how best to integrate the volunteers' story into the overall structure.

Time passed. Summer turned to fall. As the seasons changed, so did my thoughts about returning to LA. I wasn't going to do it. I was loving every minute I was spending back in Cleveland with friends and family, and I wasn't missing the stress, the daily, soul numbing grind of living and working in Los Angeles. I made a quick trip back to grab some winter clothes, and the few short days I spent there convinced me that I was on the right track. I would miss my LA friends, no doubt, if I moved permanently back to Cleveland, but I realized I had to get out of there, get back to my roots, my old friends, my family, my home — that was what my heart had been telling me. Return home, it had whispered. This is where you belong now. And thanks to the Nepal trip, I was finally listening.

In August, Jesse returned from Nepal, having accomplished his own personal goal of building a playground for the kids there. When he got back, the group had a get together at a local restaurant in Beachwood. We were going to discuss the Imagine fundrasier and the necessary logistics. We set a date for the event— November 21st. It was only three months away, but we thought that would be enough time to organize everything. We held several meetings at Carola's house, and they included Jesse as well as some of his harshest critics. To everyone's credit, we all gave our best effort to make the benefit a reality, but in the end the planning fell apart before it had barely begun. Bickering about venues led to more bickering about finances, which ultimately led to a return to the negativity that had erupted in Narti. At that point, Carola, who'd been working diligently to help organize the benefit, stepped in, at the strong urging of several group members, and postponed the November benefit indefinitely.

We were all disappointed. It seemed like the YFF crew had reached the end of our journey, and we'd have to be satisfied with the modest success of the Dashian event. I became frustrated by the inability of the group to find common ground for selfless cooperation again. And that made me question my involvement with the book project, which I knew was going to be a massive undertaking. What should I do, I wondered? Should I stay the course, stay committed, or let myself drift away, quietly. Maybe I should just bail on the whole business, I thought, and get on with my life.

Then something happened that began to change my mind...

Spring 2011

Celebrate the Possibilities

The Cleveland winter was in full swing now. There was more than a little snow on the ground and a serious chill in the air. Totally not LA, and I was loving it. 2011 had arrived, and Carola invited the YFF crew to a dinner party to celebrate the New Year. I decided to go. Not just because I liked and respected Carola, but also because of the free food. And to my pleasant surprise, almost all of us attended. Candy, Christina, David, Deanna, Eve, Gabby, Jennette, Marc, Minling, Rachel, Terri, myself, and Jesse, we were all there at Carola's behest. She made a remarkably delicious vegetarian chili, and we all brought a little something—wine, cheese, bread, fruit, dessert—to add to the feast. I hadn't seen some of the YFF people in months; a few I'd kept in touch with through Cleveland Yoga regularly, and it was a blast getting together again. We quickly realized that we missed hanging out with each other. We were a fun group when we all got together. And it seemed like time had healed most, if not all of the wounds from the trip we'd all taken six months earlier. I for one was very happy about that.

Then, after we'd eaten more than our fill and had a few drinks, Carola spoke up. She said she was preparing plans for a spring fundraiser for Nepal Orphans Home, and she had talked with Jesse and they'd decided it would be a benefit for and about NOH, and that Imagine would step aside and let NOH and our YFF group take the lead if we were so inclined. The idea appealed to everyone instantly. Committees were formed, individuals assigned to them, and tasks written down for us all to carry out. We decided on a date: May 1st, 2011. Everyone was suddenly, genuinely excited again. It all felt right. One more big bash for NOH!

At Terri's prompting, we decided to hold it at Michaelangelo's Restaurant in the Little Italy neighborhood of Cleveland. Rachel worked there, and her boss, John was friends with several of the group members. And more importantly, he was a big fan of what we were trying to do. He set aside that Sunday night in May to close the restaurant to regular business so that we'd have it exclusively for our fundraiser.

With Rachel's help, food and wine was donated by the restaurant's regular distributors. Eve and Terri, along with Carola, took over the bulk of the logistics. Jennette's husband Adam helped design flyers and postcard invitations, and along with Jennette designed posters of many of the kids of NOH, complete with text in the children's own words, that we would hang around the restaurant for the event. Everyone who attended that first meeting ended up putting in real time and effort to make the event as great as it could possibly be.

We had people from all kinds of businesses donate goods and services for a silent auction. A massage therapist donated massages for people the night of the event. Toni Thomson, who had made the short documentary trailer on Michael Hess and NOH, agreed to come down from Canada to show the trailer and give a short talk, along with Carola, on NOH. Boo Hess, NOH's treasurer, would be there.

Join us for

Celebrate The Possibilities!

An Education Fundraiser for Nepal Orphans Home in Kathmandu, Nepal

Let's Celebrate The Possibilities of these children!

Sunday, May 1, 2011
Michaelangelo's Italian Food and Wine Bar
2198 Murray Hill Road - Little Italy
5-9 PM

Proceeds from the fundraiser will go toward paying the educational costs (tuition, uniforms, books, and supplies) of the over 100 children now living in the four homes of Nepal Orphans Home.

The only possibility of ending the cycle of extreme poverty in Nepal is through education.

To donate to the silent auction or for more information on sponsorship opportunities, contact

Eve Ennis
(216) 407-1203
elennis@aol.com

Tax-deductible donation levels:

$25 Individual
includes one drink ticket plus*

$50 Patron
includes three drink tickets plus*

$100 Sponsor
includes three drink tickets and a limited-edition gift from local jewelry artist extraordinaire, Gai Russo, plus*

*delicious hors d'oeurves provided by Michaelangelo's Italian Food and Wine Bar, an exciting silent auction, presentations by those who have witnessed the work of Nepal Orphans Home, and a preview of Canadian filmmaker Antonia Thomson's upcoming documentary on Nepal Orphans Home! With Tarot Card Readings, Henna Tattoos, Mini Massages and Magic Tricks!

Mission Statement:
Nepal Orphans Home is dedicated to helping children in need

Nepal Orphans Home (NOH) attends to the welfare of children in Nepal who are orphaned, abandoned, or not supported by their parents. NOH provides for the children's basic needs of food, shelter, and clothing, as well as schooling and health care.

NOH also administers to their emotional needs with love and compassion allowing the children to grow up in a nurturing environment. The mission of NOH is not just to rescue children from poverty, but to enable the children to develop and realize their potential.

Nepal Orphans Home, a 501(c)3 public charity incorporated in Davidson, North Carolina, was founded in 2005 by Michael Hess. As a volunteer in Nepal, Michael was moved by the plight of the children he witnessed living in poverty, often exploited, and vulnerable to the political turmoil and social upheaval in contemporary Nepal.

nepal orphans home
www.nepalorphanshome.org

We'd sell 50/50 raffle tickets. We'd sell drink tickets. We'd sell T-shirts, and other handcrafts. We set up an app on one of our iPhones to handle credit card purchases. We mailed out or dropped off hundreds of invitations, posted dozens and dozens of flyers in local businesses, and several local papers ran notices about the event. We made decorations for the restaurant, and got Deanna and Rachel to be volunteer bartenders for the evening. We did all of that and more, and we did it not for ourselves, but to raise money for those amazing kids we had met almost one year before at NOH. And then we held our breath and waited to see if anyone would actually attend…

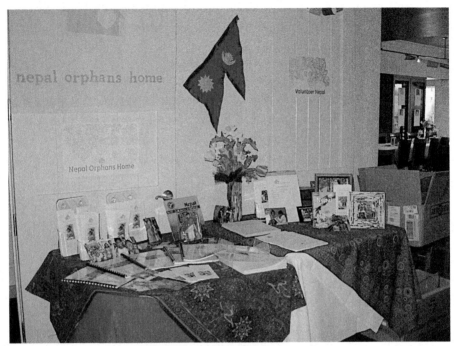

The information table at the Michaelangelo's fundraiser. Photo by Carola Drosdeck.

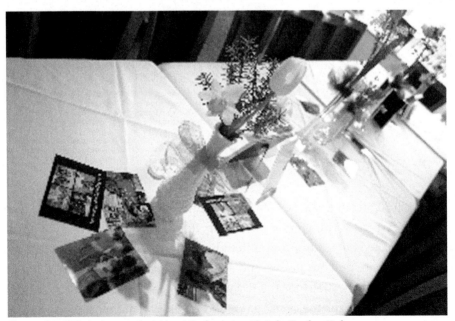

Photos of our YFF trip decorate the tables at the fundraiser. Photo by Candace Koslen.

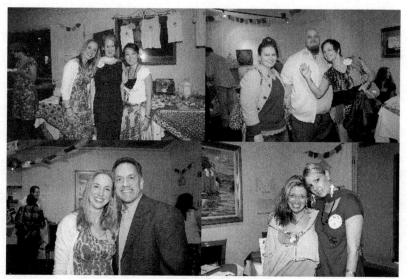

Canadian documentary filmmaker Toni Thomson (top left, center) and Jesse's sister Marina Bach (top right, left) join us for the celebration. Photos by Carola Drosdeck.

That first Sunday in May dawned cool and overcast. It had been a very wet spring in Cleveland, and there was a threat of rain this day as well. Terri had to run a workshop that afternoon, so Eve took over the day's logistics. Several people, including Minling and a few others, came early to help set things up, then went home to get dressed up for the event, which was scheduled to run from 5 p.m. until 9 p.m. I arrived a little before 4:00 and helped with the final preparations. Marc and I set up a table outside the front door of the restaurant to be used to greet arrivals and sell admissions tickets. Eve set up a table inside to sell drink tickets. Carola handed out large buttons to pin to our lapels that read "I've been to Nepal/Ask Me", and we all proudly pinned them on our shirts, jackets and dresses. When everything was finally ready, we all took a deep breath, hoped the rain would hold off, and prayed that at least some of the folks we'd invited would show up.

And boy, were we surprised. The turnout was huge. Eve, Marc, and John from Michaelangelo's estimated at least 300 people in attendance that night. Over 200 admission tickets were purchased. Drink tickets sold briskly. Rachel and Deanna were slammed with drink orders at the bar all night. Christina and Eve worked the crowd selling raffle tickets. Auction items were browsed over and quickly bid upward. Michaelangelo's was hopping. People indulged in all kinds of food to go along with their drinks. They also took the time to check out all the posters about the children of Nepal Orphans Home. Nearly everyone who'd been on the trip showed up, except for Kathy and Tingting, who were at that time out of the country. Our friends showed up, our families showed up, our brothers and sisters and husbands and wives and children, boyfriends and girlfriends showed up. Total strangers we had never met before joined in the fun.

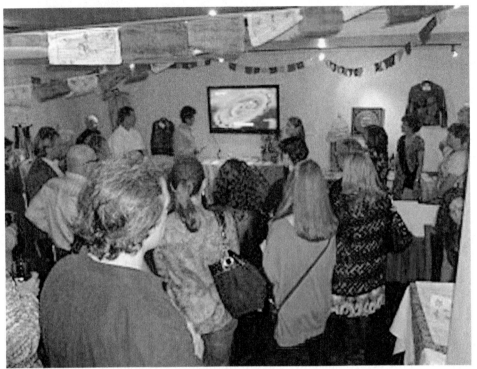

The crowd at the Michaelangelo's Fundraiser. Photo by Marni Task.

Around 7 p.m., Toni Thomson showed the trailer for her film about Michael and NOH. Carola followed up with a short, powerful speech about NOH, and the great reception and support they had received over the last few years from the Cleveland community. She concluded by reading a letter from Michael, thanking everyone for their interest in NOH. The response to the film and to Carola's talk was enthusiastic. People opened up their wallets, their checkbooks, and their piggy banks and bought up the auction items and raffle tickets.

By the end of the night, we were pleasantly exhausted. The last remaining stragglers hung around until 10:30 p.m. Most of us stayed on to help clean up the restaurant, reset the tables and chairs, and then finally headed home ourselves around 11:30, wiped out, but very very happy.

A week or so later, Carola reported the results. We had raised over $12,000, after expenses, for the Nepal Orphans Home. We were all blown away. The event had been a tremendous success! People reported that they had a wonderful time, and looked forward to coming back again the next year. Not only had the fundraiser been a great accomplishment, but the whole Yoga For Freedom idea had been a total success. Combined with the $12,500 we had raised for NOH as part of our Yoga For Freedom trip costs, and with the nearly $2,000 we raised the previous October for new dresses for Dashain for the girls at NOH, our little band of Yoga For Freedom brothers and sisters had raised nearly $27,000 for Nepal Orphans Home.

Our trip had finally come full circle. The journey we started back around Christmas of 2008 was now complete. And we could all be justifiably proud. Despite the hardships, the drama, the acrimony and the clashes of personalities, the 20 individuals who had originally come together for a cause, had managed to successfully complete our journey from 'me to we'. As a group, we had done far more than any one of us alone could have achieved to help make the world, in some small way, a better place. Whether we would ever be together again as a group, stay in touch, remain friends or not, or would eventually move on with our own lives, no one could take away what we had now accomplished. It wasn't always easy, but in the end, it had been, to my mind, unquestionably worth the effort.

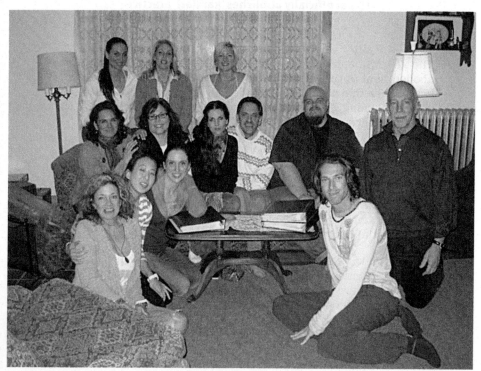

The New Year's dinner gathering at Carola's where we planned the big fundraiser. Photo by Carola Drosdeck.

It was that realization that convinced me to put aside all my concerns and doubts, and once again resume the task of writing this book. And this time complete it. In that way, I could make one final contribution to the group, and quite possibly, an enduring contribution to the children of Nepal Orphans Home. I would tell our story, the story of Yoga For Freedom, and through this book, perhaps pass on the inspiration to help that motivated all of us from day one of this incredible adventure, and beyond.

That journey to a finished book, has taken me three years, and a lot of hard work. Just as I was completing what seemed like this never-to-be-finished writing task, almost three years to the day that we had returned from our amazing Nepali adventure, I saw an article posted on Facebook from the Asia News Network that made me think that all my time and effort may have had some greater purpose. Maybe now was exactly when I was supposed to complete it…

ASIA NEWS NETWORK[16]

The Kathmandu Post— Friday, 19 July 2013

Nepal officially abolishes 'kamlari' practice

~ Weena Pun

The government of Nepal officially announced on July 18 the abolishment of the "kamlari" (bonded labour) practice, raising both hopes that legal action will finally be taken against those who hire young girls as kamlaris or bonded servants, as well as fears that those hopes will be dashed.

Even though the practice is already prohibited under Nepal's Human Trafficking Control Act, Child Labour (Prohibition and Regulation) Act, and the Kamaiya Labour (Prohibition) Act,

the laws have since failed to protect young girls from being hired as kamlaris, primarily in the western Tarai—Dang, Kailali, Kanchanpur, Banke, Bardiya and Surkhet districts.

According to the United Committee for the Elimination of Kamlari Practice (UCEKP), which led a 10-day protest in May this year, there were 12,776 kamlaris hired and working in Nepal, of which 642 are yet to be freed.

Former kamlaris believe that the announcement has finally brought their issues to the forefront. They feel that the issue

[16] http://www.asianewsnet.net/Nepal-officially-abolishes-kamlari-practice-49304.html

was often sidelined, because kamlaris were usually children and female.

"The government has admitted publicly, for the first time, its responsibility to protect children from the kamlari practice. Now, it must enforce the three laws," said Phakala Tharu, programme manager at the UCEKP.

The announcement is seen as the culmination of the "Save the Girl-Children" movement launched by former kamlaris on May 28 this year. Manjita Chaudhary, a 21-year-old former kamlari and central chairperson of the Freed Kamlari Development Forum, said the formal announcement was only one of the 10 agreements made between agitating anti-kamlari activists and the government on June 7.

She demanded that the distribution of identification cards to former kamlaris start right away. In the absence of ID cards, former kamlaris are unable to obtain scholarships provided by the government. As a result, they are unable to enroll themselves into colleges.

The other agreements included freeing the remaining kamlaris and rehabilitating them, investigating deaths, disappearance and pregnancies of kamlaris, and amending the Kamlari Education Guidelines to increase the amount of scholarships provided for former kamlaris.

At a meeting with the press on July 18, spokesperson for the Ministry of Women, Children and Social Welfare, Upendra Adhikary, said that the government was working on the agreements made. He said the ministry has allocated 3 million Nepali rupees (US$31,323) for the kamlaris this fiscal year.

Mina Chaudhary, a 15-year-old former kamlari from Kailali district hopes that the government would keep its end of the bargain. She had sustained injuries when the police attacked protesting kamlaris on June 3.

Revealing a bruise on her left leg, Chaudhary said, "If needed, I'll come back and fight."

It had finally happened. The Nepali government, the Nepali people, and the Kamlari girls themselves, had taken action to rid themselves of the scourge of child slavery. I re-read the article, amazed and overjoyed. Did I think our little 15-day Yoga For Freedom trip had anything to do with bringing about this change? Not really. Do I believe all the hard work put in by people like Michael Hess and the generous volunteers of the Nepal Orphans' Home had helped bring about this change? I couldn't say with any certainty, but definitely not alone. None of these people, organizations, or events, by themselves, led to this change. Together, though, I have no doubt that they did. It only takes a few small pebbles, rolling down the right mountainside, to start a landslide. And perhaps we, the Yoga For Freedom group, were one of the many small pebbles that had started rolling, most well before our naive group of yogis had even arrived in Nepal, and together, all those little pebbles, rolling down that enormous mountain, created something profound, something so much bigger than ourselves and our brief 15-day Nepali adventure. Whatever small part we may have played in that change, the change had come. And reading Mina Chaudhary's courageous words from that article, I know it's a change that's not going to be easily ignored or undone. Freedom for the Kamlari girls was and remains something worth fighting for.

I hope that you will take a moment now and think about all those courageous girls like Mina, and about all the children of NOH. Take the time to check out the Nepal Orphans Home website: www.nepalorphanshome.org. Open your hearts, to help out an incredibly worthy cause. If you've purchased this book, you already have, and I thank you. The majority of the profits from the book will be given

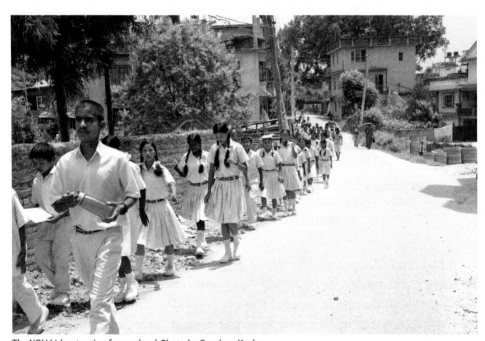

The NOH kids returning from school. Photo by Candace Koslen.

directly to NOH. If you are considering making a thoughtful donation directly to NOH, here is the link to the NOH website for you to do so: http://www.nepalor-phanshome.org/donate.

Kindly join me and all of us, the Yoga For Freedom crew, the volunteers and children of Nepal Orphans Home, to become a part of something greater than yourselves. Become a part of us; join the journey from me to we, the journey that the 20 of us along with our Nepali friends started back in 2010. Or start your own version of Yoga For Freedom. I promise you, you won't regret it. If you'd like to see for yourself, take a trip to Nepal and experience this breathtakingly beautiful country, and the mindful work being done by so many kind-hearted people. You'll never forget it, I promise you that, too…

Epilogue

The Nepali Perspective

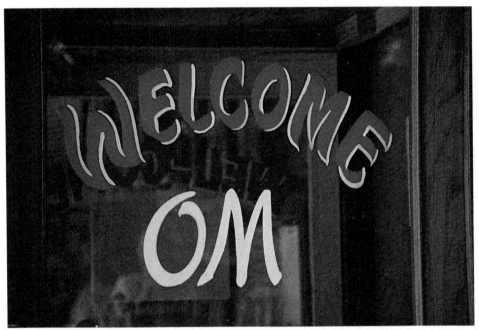

This hand-painted sign on the window of a shop door in Kathmandu says it all. Photo by Candace Koslen.

Fall 2010_____

Earlier this year, I was asked to consider teaching a yoga class for the Yoga For Freedom trip by Ram Barakoti and Basu Panday of Nepal Social Trek. I went along with Ram to meet Jesse Bach at Papa's House in Kathmandu. I was amazed to see all the great work being done by NOH. Jesse dai gave me a brief introduction to the trip and asked me about the type of yoga classes I conduct. The interview went well, and a few weeks later I was formally asked to join Yoga For Freedom. At that point in time I was excited and a bit afraid.

I had thought this was only a yoga trip for some foreigners, but upon joining Yoga For Freedom, I began to familiarize myself with the so-called Kamlari people. Up to that point, I had known about it only from the news. After that, I began thinking about our country, our political system, our laws, our social status—all of it filled my mind. Just making laws doesn't make any sense in the life of the under-privileged and Kamlari people because our government has already abolished the Kamlari system long ago. But the government hasn't given any assistance to the people to improve their livelihood. They have to depend on landlords, and thus are exploited by landlords.

NOH and Jesse had done a great job raising funds and organizing different activities for the kids and this was visible in the children's happiness, their natural smiles, and by the new life that they got at NOH. When these children grow up and are able to stand on their own feet they will bring awareness to and fight against the Kamlari system. Once that happens, there will be no more Kamlari system in our country. But right now they need assistance from organizations like NOH and people like Jesse dai.

Our trip started at the beautiful Norling Resort (heaven on earth). The stay at Kathmandu was fantabulous. We all enjoyed sightseeing, meeting the children, and doing yoga in the beautiful loving and pleasant surroundings of the resort.

Once we set off to Lumbini we had a bit of a tough time because the bus ride was long and adjusting to all the changes was difficult for some. Afterwards, we headed to Narti (home of Lawajuni Nepal Orphanage Home for Ex-Kamlari girls). The welcome we received from the girls and the traditional dance put on by the villagers all were unforgettable. They all performed beautifully and won our hearts. The stay at Narti was a little bit difficult too. It is said that "the past should be an experience, but not a burden." It was a great experience, despite facing some tough challenges, and we all were very positive and enjoyed each and every moment of the rest of the trip from Chitwan to Namo Buddha and back to Kathmandu. The silent meditation at Namo Buddha made us all more calm and quiet and helped us to understand the true value of our emotions.

The entire trip was awesome. Without yoga it wouldn't have been possible to bring [17] people together for 15 days. We all were here for the same objectives: travelling, helping, relaxing, and ultimately gaining peace of mind. One of the greatest things that yoga teaches is getting attached and detached at the same point in time. We all learned this during each and every day of this trip. For me it was not only a teaching experience, but it was also a learning experience. It was a give and take relationship wherein I not only taught but also learned.

For all this I want to sincerely thank Nepal Social Trek and Jesse dai for giving me such an amazing opportunity, and all the amazing and enthusiastic YFF participants. I tried to give my best the entire trip but if I did make any mistakes I apologize thoroughly from the bottom of my heart. I will be glad to stay in touch with this association and to help and be a part of this wonderful group.

Lastly I am sure that this book will turn out to be highly informative about the Nepal Orphans Home, the Kamlari system of trafficking girls, and in raising funds for rescuing and assisting more and more children.

Wishing a very happy and successful life ahead to all.

Love,

_____ **Subash Adhikari**

Fall 2010 _____

My name is Basu Panday and it is my pleasure to be able to express my feelings and share some of my experiences during the Yoga for Freedom trip. I helped organized "Yoga for Freedom" through Nepal Social Treks and Expeditions with the ultimate goal of raising money for Nepal Orphans Home. It was my great pleasure to get the chance to be part of the adventure as a tour guide and also as a participant in the Yoga for Freedom experience.

In December 2009 Michael Hess (the founder of NOH, also known as Papa) and Jesse Bach approached me with the idea for Yoga for Freedom. Since that day I had been working on making the trip a success. I was excited about the trip personally because yoga was a new experience for me and I was looking forward to being not only a guide but also a participant in the Yoga for Freedom trip.

When all the yogis arrived I met them in the airport and quickly realized what a great group of people they were. I found them all to be very friendly and easy to get to know. They were all kind people. At times during the trip some of the yogis became upset and afraid, I believe mostly because they were in a new place and were not mentally prepared for what they experienced. Once the people who were upset reflected and understood that they were here to help the victims of the Kamlari system, attitudes changed for the better.

During the Yoga for Freedom trip we all had the opportunity to visit many of the different places and people of Nepal. First the yogis arrived in Kathmandu, where we were all acquainted over sightseeing and other activities around the city. I was glad to show everyone around and spend time with them. After Kathmandu we traveled to Lumbini (the birth place of Buddha). This was an excellent place to practice yoga and meditation which was great experience for everyone.

From Lumbini we traveled to Narti. The visit to Narti was the main goal of the trip. In Narti we visited the Lawajuni girls' orphanage where we were able to meet and play with the girls that the money raised was helping to save. Playing with the girls was a great experience; they are all so happy and full of life. However when playing with the girls you are always thinking about how they are former Kamlari, which makes you think about all the other girls still out there who have not been saved. I had a lot of time to reflect on this point and it is upsetting now thinking about the failed system and how there is no one stopping these girls from becoming Kamlaris. Even with all the NGO's and all the foreigners giving money, until the attitudes of people change and the government actually steps in nothing will be solved and young girls will continue to be bought and sold. It's important to remember that it is not the girls' families fault that this system exists; they are just trying to survive whichever way they can. The poor people of Nepal will continue to be poor and it makes me think what can I do? When will the Kamlari system end? I learnt a lot myself about the Kamlari system when I was in Narti. Meeting the girls was a great experience, something I will never forget.

After that we continued to Chitwan, but in my heart I felt like I was still in Narti. Chitwan was a great place for the yogis to recharge and have some fun on the safari trip. Seeing everyone having a good time and smiling also made me happy again.

From Chitwan we traveled to Namo Buddha. When we travelled there it was late and getting dark on the way. This made some of the yogis very nervous and panic seemed to take over the bus. But after we arrived at the monastery the whole group had a day of silence (excluding phone calls I was required to take). This allowed the yogis to reflect. This is the place where people believe the previous Buddha sacrificed his body to the hungry tiger. This makes people think about why he did this. Namo Buddha helped me to reflect on who Buddha is and how people should live their life; giving not only taking. If more people reflected on this point then the whole world would be a better place.

Namo Buddha was our last destination before traveling back to Kathmandu. In Kathmandu we were able to spend some time at Papa's House with the children of Nepal Orphans Home. I have worked with NOH for a while, mostly helping the volunteers travel around Nepal, but this visit to Papa's house allowed me to spend more time with the kids. It made me feel great to meet again and play with the kids we were helping by being on this trip. Papa's House also made me feel hopeful because these children who are orphans and who have been rescued from the Kamlari system are now happy and well cared for, going to a great school and will have everything they need for a better life. I am so thankful to all the yoga for freedom participants for their help and love and for caring about Nepal and all of the kids.

The Yoga for Freedom trip was different from anything I have ever done before. The trip changed me in so many ways. It helped to open my eyes even more to some of the problems of Nepal. I think about all the great yogis who taught me about yoga and helped to love it. The money and awareness raised from this trip, and hopefully many more like it, will help save the life of many Kamlari girls and other orphan children, which is something I feel very proud to be a part of. Practicing yoga in Nepal is a great experience since yoga beliefs originated from the Himalayas. I believe the Yoga for Freedom trip really helps people to learn how they should live their lives and to help them see Nepal. The trip also allows people to understand the Kamlari system and inspires them to see the real Nepal, the mountains and the beautiful places and people but also the reality of the Kamlari system in Nepal. Overall it was the greatest experience of my life thus far.

Never ending Peace and Love – Kathmandu, Nepal

_____ *Basu Panday*

Spring 2014
WHERE ARE THEY NOW?

Three years later, we've all continued on with our own journeys through life. But that doesn't mean that any of us are less committed today to making the world a better place than we were when we all decided to go on this amazing journey. We all keep in touch with what's going on with Michael and the kids. Some of us have returned to see more of Nepal, and to do more volunteer work at NOH, and several of us have gone on to be involved in other worthy causes. Virtually all of us are keeping up with our yoga practice, and we stay in touch with each other whenever we can. Without further adieu, here's where we are, more than three years after the trip, in late Fall 2013…

Jesse Bach

If there was a hero of this trip, in my opinion it was Jesse Bach. Without him, without his initial drive, there would have been no Yoga For Freedom trip, and no $27,000 raised by the participants of that trip for the children of Nepal Orphans Home — and ultimately no Yoga For Freedom book. Some might see Jesse as a flawed hero, who like Icarus tried to fly a little too high, and who was sent by the gods tumbling back down to earth. I don't really see it that way at all, because really, who among us is without our faults?

While he no doubt took an emotional bruising during those two weeks we were in Nepal and for several months after our return, the fall, if there was one, was brief. Though he left the yoga world and has not returned to Nepal, like the Phoenix, Jesse has risen again to take on new challenges. Upon returning to Cleveland, he went back to school and is now working on his PhD in Urban Education at Cleveland State University. He was recently accepted to present a paper at Harvard University on 24-7 teaching: short, instructor made videos in the STEM fields which give at-risk & behind students full-time access to lessons so they have time to catch up to their peers.

Taking everyone to Nepal may have ended everything Jesse had hoped to achieve there, but he continues to work to end human trafficking in the world every day since then, through his Imagine Foundation. Though the YFF journey changed Jesse profoundly, perhaps more than anyone else who went on this amazing journey, he remains an inspiration to those of us who went, and who will never forget what we experienced there.

Terri Bahr (in her own words)

After almost 10 years of being a part of the Cleveland Yoga teaching team & calling Cleveland my home, it is with bittersweet emotion and also impending excitement that I am about to embark on a new journey, the next big chapter of my life. I re-located to New York City to live with my boyfriend, Robert and as serendipity would have it, I was recently invited to be a founding teacher with a brand new Baptiste Yoga studio in NYC called Lyons Den Power Yoga, opening in TriBeCa this November. I will be back to visit and teach classes & workshops in Cleveland! But, I am also extending an invitation to all of you to come to New York, show up and check out the new studio and share the love lighting up NYC!

I am also continuing my passion of community service that began in part with our trip to Nepal and Yoga For Freedom with my involvement with the Africa Yoga Project (http://www.africayogaproject.org/), a program that empowers young people in Nairobi's urban slums through yoga. I have been a mentor to Bernard Gitonga, an aspiring Baptiste yoga teacher there, for the last 2 years. Through mentoring Bernard, I have discovered a passion that runs deep within me. It is a realization that this is more than just making a difference in his life, but in every life he touches. I can see first-hand how this program has given Bernard strength to stand in his own power, to live his life with purpose and without fear. AYP is changing and saving lives!

I teach yoga because I want to make a positive difference in the world, and nowhere is that difference more evident than in the growth and learning I see in my students. Though I am very sad to leave Cleveland, yoga teaches us the only constant we have is change. And change is good.

Robb Blain (in his own words)

*Still living single in Broadview Heights, Ohio

*Working in sales at Levin's Furniture (Oakwood Village Store) and loving it.

*Teaching Yoga at the Spiritual Life Society in Hudson... Also have taken on private Yoga Students.

*Expanding my Yoga experiences to Kundalini Yoga, Mahamudra practices and Tantra as taught by Osho. I would like to expand these practices in the Cleveland area.

*April 2013 I traveled to Perth, Western Australia. Made contact and studied with Buddhist Society WA, Ven Ajahn Brahm. I also integrated with the Aborigines' cultures. As noted in my Nepal journaling I still have strong beliefs that the interference with what is natural is challenging nature and what is natural. My question is, "Is it better to be normal or natural?" Always keeping in mind who is determining what normal is????????

*My children are doing great: My daughter just received her BSN and is practicing and will be going back to school to become a Nurse Practitioner. My oldest son is a Chef in Maui and will be the executive chef shortly. My youngest son is in communications sales in Toledo. My 10 year old granddaughter is being a 10 year old. I'm loving every moment of it.

Minling Chuang (in her own words)

When I stepped foot on the plane to Nepal, I could not imagine how this one trip would shape my life. Since that day, my life has completely changed. In a way the trip was the catalyst for me to start a new chapter in my life as it had a profound effect on how I viewed life.

A year after I returned from Nepal, I found myself on the plane again headed to the unknown. I quit my job at Nestle and decided to return to California. I didn't know exactly what I would do yet, but I knew I had to do something that brought meaning to my life. The memories of the kids I met on our trip reminded me why I needed to leave and start something on my own.

So I started a website called {the JOY depot} (http://thejoydepot.com) to help people find their own passions and their own inner JOY. As I helped others find their path, I was also forging my own path, creating a business to help entrepreneurs with brand and social media consulting. I also found and fell in love with Kundalini Yoga and have been primarily practicing this beautiful style of yoga for the last 2 years. Now I also teach Kundalini Yoga at RA MA Institute for Applied Yogic Science and Technology in Venice, CA.

I fondly remember each day of the YFF trip like it was yesterday and hope to return to Nepal in the near future. I am forever grateful for all the lessons I learned there, and I have taken those lessons with me forward as I go on with my life. Thank you Michael and the entire NOH team for your tireless efforts in making a difference in people's lives. You have made a huge difference in mine.

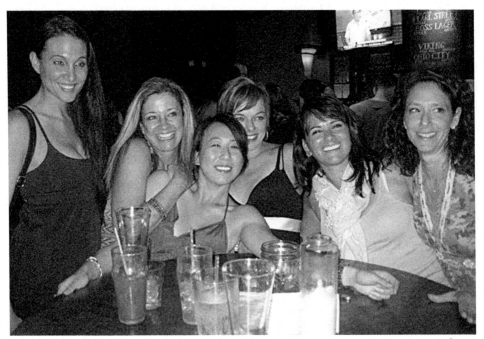

The YFF ladies decked out in their finest at Michaelangelo's for Minling's going away party. Photo courtesy of Minling Chuang.

Eve Ennis – married, now Eve Ennis-Kilbane (in her own words)

My husband and I are experiencing wedded bliss. After one year of marriage the honeymoon is still going strong. We are happily living in the historic Ohio City neighborhood of Cleveland. After 15 years of a difficult yet rewarding career in property management I resigned to pursue real estate sales full time. My career change has literally changed my life. I feel extremely fortunate as all my dreams have come true.

Reflecting back on Yoga For Freedom, the trip for me was twofold: first, an amazing opportunity to join my yoga comrades in the adventure of a lifetime.

Second, when I learned the story of Michael Hess, his undying devotion and dedication to the children in Nepal, to the orphans, I realized that real life heroes exist. His amazing work to help the forgotten children was the inspiration that took me to Nepal. I will always and forever be grateful to Jesse for making Yoga For Freedom happen.

Joyce Fijalkovich (in her own words)

I regret not sharing my journal, but I was going through a very difficult transition during the trip to Nepal in 2010. The events of the trip, our group and the children had a significant impact on my life, however. I came to feel like my simple, stupid, typical American girl problems that I let nearly end my life were so insignificant compared to what we were seeing. Initially I felt like a complete outsider in our group, but all the invitations I got to get together with everyone in those first few months after we got back home really moved me. I couldn't believe such amazing people wanted me around. That trip got me past some difficult stuff and helped me grow up.

I think about the children every day, especially [one] little girl who stole my heart. I still wonder what life would be like if I could have adopted her. I am

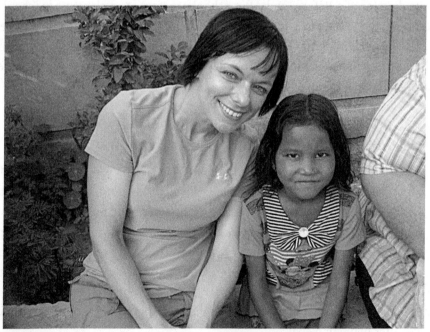

This is the little girl who stole Joyce's heart without saying much at all. Photo courtesy of Joyce Fijalkovich.

Facebook friends with Anita Mahato (the House Manager of Imagine House), and I ask her how [that little girl] is doing from time to time. I married a wonderful man in April of 2013. I have no children of my own, but am now a step-mother of a 14 year old girl.

I still feel a special bond to those of us who traveled together. I feel fortunate to have the close friends that I made during that trip. I do not look at life the same ever since my return. I appreciate what a wonderful country we live in and how easy it is to take that for granted. From having electricity 24 hours a day, to driving on paved roads, having clean water to drink and not being looked over simply because I am a woman, are some of the things that our trip gave me a deep appreciation for.

The resilience of the children we spent time with has also impacted my life. As bad as I may have thought my problems were, they paled in comparison to the untold stories of those young lives. Those kids taught me about the ability to heal, take care of each other, and move ahead. I am eternally grateful for their lessons.

Jaime Furda (in her own words)

I'm still living in the Cleveland area after graduating from Heidelberg University this past May (BA degrees in Psychology and Music). I'm currently working as the site director of a Before- and After-school program at an elementary school in Macedonia, OH. After the trip, I began attending Friday yoga sessions at the 'Berg and have been trying lately to get back into it at home. I wish more than anything to go back to Nepal, preferably as a volunteer at NOH (though I certainly have a few student loans begging me to stay).

Kathy Hayes (in her own words)

Here's what has happened in my life... after Nepal I moved to Switzerland for work for several years. I traveled to many third world countries during my stay there... connecting with people in a more compassionate and holistic way than ever before. One of my favorite projects was doing in home interviews with 'emerging' consumers - consumers who essentially earn just enough to get by - often without running water and often in a three room home with no doors or windows - just fabric hanging in the openings. I treasured getting the opportunity to understand these people, their wants, dreams, desires and challenges...and looked with different eyes after being in Nepal.

I came back to the USA recently and continue to be amazed with the freedoms and opportunities we have here. I deeply respect the opportunities and quality of life I have as a woman - I am educated, can vote, can own property, can live independently, feel safe and secure and can create the life I want... and I am glad that I can teach yoga. In Switzerland there was very little yoga. There is such peace and calm there, calming the mind any further may mean passing to the next world! But I met people interested in yoga so we began a yoga class in my living room, overlooking Lake Geneva and the French Alps... but soon the class size was larger than my space so another yogi offered up her space, and upon my departure from Switzerland my yogis made a nice donation to the Nepal Orphans Home.

I still have a photo on my desk from the trip. ☺

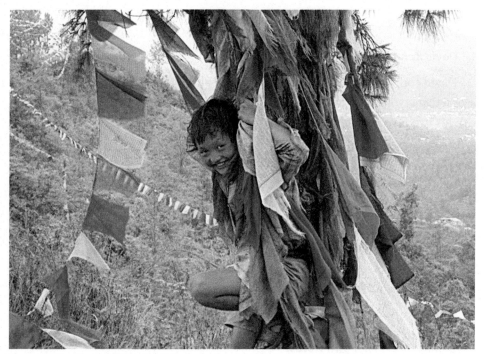

The photo, from Namo Buddha, that Kathy keeps on her desk at work. Photo by Kathy Hayes.

Christina Jankus (in her own words)

My life was forever changed by my experience in Nepal. I feel more loving kindness towards others as I don't know what they're dealing with. I no longer use the phrase, "I'm starving." My yoga and meditation practice is as strong as ever. I have also added journaling to really get to know myself. There's nothing like your honesty in black and white.

I love to bliss out to chanting and dancing to Kirtan - Om Namah Shivaya is my favorite! I traveled to Joshua Tree, CA For Bhakti Fest to camp, chant and dance with Minling. Camping?! I know! Right? I have also attended Bhakti Fest in the Midwest in Madison, WI. Bhakti meaning devotional worship.

I have had no changes in my job, location, or status. Cleveland remains my adopted home (I was born and raised in Queens, NY). I offer my time and assistance to local charities that ensure that all Clevelanders have enough to eat. I continue on my path of compassion by moving from vegetarianism to veganism.

I think about those children on a nearly daily basis. I enjoy receiving the updates from Nepal Orphans Home by email and Facebook posts. The smiles on the children's faces make me smile.

David Kampinsky

David continues to teach yoga in Chagrin Falls, Ohio. When he's not teaching or practicing yoga, you can find him hiking the trails of the Cleveland Metroparks with his two favorite people — his German Shepherds, Bella and Xento.

Candace Koslen (in her own words)

I am currently taking care of 1 husband, 2 children and have started rescuing animals... 12 right now of various sorts :-) 2 horses, 5 chickens, 3 dogs and 2 cats. I take pictures for local shelters and sanctuaries, and continue running a photography studio/business with my husband. I am only subbing yoga classes now because there is so much work to do at home!

Deanna Lee (in her own words)

I'm sure everyone who went will agree, our trip to Nepal was life changing.

Before the trip I was always working 7 days a week, every week. I was looking for a change of pace, burning the wick from both ends on high was leaving me feeling close to burnt out. I had this conflicting world of opposites - teaching yoga and working at the studio, and bar tending downtown at Lola. My days and nights were always filled and began coming and going much too quickly. I got to Nepal on what seemed to be pure luck, from raising money to borrowing money and taking time off all my jobs. While we were there, I encountered issues from both my past and (then) present situations and was able to release and finally move past old negativities, and, through retrospection after our travels, recognize new opportunities for growth. The people we met along the way and places we went all had an impact upon me on some level and upon returning home I was filled with humility, peace, a sense of connection and change in perspective, and gratitude. It felt less like luck and more like I'd needed to go. To be honest, the multitude of emotions are impossible to articulate, it was highly experiential!

Once back home, I felt a shift within myself, and had several "ah-ha" moments - from being ready to find life-work balance, to being more open to love. I felt cleansed, able to forgive and be forgiven, ready to begin again. I eventually phased out of bar tending and serving and began working at lululemon athletica, heading the community team, while still teaching and being involved in the yoga community. I was making less money but finding more satisfaction in how I earned it. Shortly after finding balance there, I met the love of my life, Vincent. A romantic, fairy tale love story ensued (and is still unfolding); I will keep that story short here since I could tell it in every amazing detail, but that would take quite awhile! I will say that he is beyond my wildest dreams of what I had ever hoped true love would be. We had a long distance relationship for a while, as he was from New York and I was still living in Cleveland. We were soon engaged and I moved to Manhattan with him. We were married on a beach and eventually decided to come back to Ohio, ready for more peace and quiet than the big city had to offer.

Not long after, we became pregnant with our first child. Olivia Maya was born in April of 2013. Her name was inspired from my time teaching yoga and our trip to Nepal. Her initials are OM, and Olivia means "symbol of peace" in reference to the extension of an olive branch. Her nickname will be "Liv", also "Live". Maya is the Buddha's mother's name, and the Nepali word for love. So her name has several meanings; live in peace, live, be peaceful, love, wisdom, kindness, OM, and more. And true to her name, she is the most peaceful, loving, attentive, sweet baby girl. Needless to say, we are planning to expand the family more! We've been bouncing around all over the place, and are settled currently in PA, for now. We are open to going wherever the flow takes us and when Olivia gets older plan to travel often with her.

I still do yoga, although I am currently not teaching. I was in yoga classes and doing yoga at home pretty much up until Olivia was born. Now, I like to do yoga while she's in the room so she begins to pick up the moves and the energy. My practice and my life are certainly not the same as they were before Nepal, as I'm sure everyone on the trip would echo.

Although I haven't made it back to Nepal, I stay in contact with several of the girls on Facebook, and would love to one day return for another visit. And that is the end of my story, for now. I wish I'd contributed more in my journal of the trip itself so I wanted to expand upon its impact here. Thanks for listening. Namaste, and we love you Nepal Orphans Home!

Marc Nathanson (in his own words)

Three years later:

1) Still doing yoga - Twice a week at Cleveland Yoga

2) Continue to do mission trips - I went to El Salvador a second time. I went with a group of high school seniors and the mission was to meet the families and high schoolers of a small village called Chiltupan. The teens compared life styles and we met with the El Salvadorian teens to discuss school, their lives, and their hopes and dreams.

3) Continue to work in the non-profit sector - For the past two years I have been the Senior Development Executive at Youth Opportunites Unlimited. We provide summer jobs for Cuyahoga County teens (3,000) and during the school year we teach employability skills and resiliency skills to at-risk Cleveland youth (500).

4) Personal life - My sons are doing well. My younger son is still looking for that perfect mate to raise a family with. My older son has blessed me with three wonderful grandchildren; two granddaughters, 11 and 5, and one grandson; 10.

5) More Personal life - I have not found Ms. Right and maybe that is because I am Mr. Wrong, not sure what the correct answer is.

6) More, More Personal life - I still feel totally blessed to have gone to Nepal; to meet Michael, the kids of NOH, and the privilege to meet my fellow Yogis. It was an experience that will forever be in my Heart!!

Tingting Peng (in her own words)

I can't believe it's been 3 years since our Nepal adventure - it doesn't sound like a long time but I feel like so much has happened since that summer.

Where am I now? I am still living in Hong Kong - but that's about the only thing that hasn't changed. I have switched jobs twice and am now working at a social venture think tank working on executive education programs. I am still practicing and teaching yoga and have taught around the world since 2010 including several retreats in Nepal. I led two Charity Yoga Adventure Treks - one to Everest Base Camp and one to Annapurna Circuit in 2011 and donated the proceeds to Papa's House. Besides these two trips, I have been back to Nepal on several other occasions to visit the kids. Unfortunately, I was not able to go back this year because I was pregnant for most of the year and just gave birth one month ago to an amazing little baby boy named Jack. My husband, Mark, and I got married last November and have been busy getting the hang of parenthood.

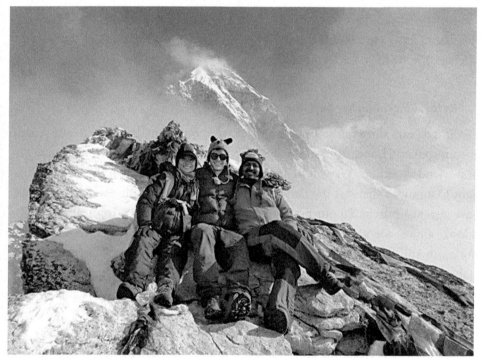

On the Everest Base Camp Trek, with the summit a mere 14,000 feet or so above them, are Tingting, left, and Basu, right, with a fellow trekker. Photo courtesy of Tingting Peng.

Gabrielle Stickley, married, now Gabrielle Goodman

Gabby continues living in Cleveland, Ohio. She recently began studying to become an art and antique appraiser. She also got married in January, 2013. Since Nepal, she's traveled to Mexico, Greece, Turkey, Istanbul & Israel.... She keeps in touch with the kids at Papa's House via Facebook, and "definitely will go back there – who knows when!" She continues to practice yoga twice a week.

Marni Task (in her own words)

Where I am now? I am still practicing and teaching yoga, leading teacher trainings, workshops and retreats. I have a team of amazing women assisting me with my Indu aromatherapy business mixing my lotion, soap and spray, and I am getting ready to create Indu bar soap and aromatherapy lotion candles (Marni created the scent of Indu in her tiny NYC apartment back in 1998). My husband Rick and I now have a daughter named Lila (leela)—which is a popular name in both India and Nepal and means to dance, act or play with the divine.

I haven't been back to Nepal, but I have stayed in touch with NOH through emails and letters to a few of the girls I made connections with, and of course with Michael. I hope to go back someday!

Rachel Vincent (in her own words)

Three years since our journey to Nepal... A monumental event of beauty, pain, encouragement, hope, faith, struggle, support. Three years later I am engaged to my best friend, Matthew. We will be married in September of 2014, shedding a little light to a month that has the dark memory of my dad passing away in 2005. We have also just purchased our first house, a Tudor built in 1935. Ironically enough, it looks almost identical to the house my parents bought as newlyweds and where my mom still lives. I am a recruiter for a local company that helps people find stable jobs, and clients find qualified employees. Nepal is often in my thoughts. I am extremely grateful for my experiences there, although they seem almost as if they weren't my own. As if I was dreaming... I try to vividly remember all, to relive the days, situations, feelings. I guess I was just in the moment and now that it's past, I will forever appreciate the glimpses into those memories. Thanks to Facebook, I get to see what many of our sisters in Nepal are up to. I would love to return, but for the time being am focused on building memories here and a family of our own.

John Vourlis

A lot has happened since I returned from Nepal, and almost all of it has been good. I moved back to Cleveland permanently in November of 2010. In 2011 I accepted a great job as an Adjunct Professor of Film & Digital Media (hopefully full-time one day soon!) at Cleveland State University, where I now teach some amazing kids of my own about one of the things I love most in life: the movies. I made a short film of my own shortly after taking the job, with many of my new friends at CSU, and that movie made it into a couple of great local film festivals, the Ohio Independent Film Festival and the Indie Gathering International Film Festival (where it won 2 awards!).

I am currently working on a couple of other really fun, creative projects, including a comic book/graphic novel and a documentary feature film about the game of bocce. And I have managed as I write this to finish my first non-fiction book, which you now hold in your hands. I see my family and friends nearly every day, and though I miss my friends in Los Angeles (who I stay in regular touch with via Facebook and email), I am happier now than I've ever been in my life. This newfound contentment, and long burst of productive creativity, I owe in no small part to the amazing Yoga For Freedom trip to Nepal I took with nineteen truly fine human beings in June of 2010. Namaste, Nepal. And thank you, Yoga For Freedom, for the time we spent together, and for being the catalyst for so much wonderful change.

Jennette Zimmerman (or Jothi as the kids at Papa's named me; in her own words)

3 years (since our trip), eh? Whoa… Things are great. Still in Cleveland. No new kids :-) Teaching yoga and meditation.

I went back to Papa's House September to December of 2011 where I volunteered at the KAT center (Kathmandu animal treatment center) for all the street pups. I also volunteered at a safe house for recently rescued girls ages 7 to 17. I went back again September/October of 2012. I mostly meditated on that trip and made friends with lots of the street kids in Thamel. I didn't stay in Dhapasi at Papa's that time though.

I heart Nepal :-)

Subash Adikhari (in his own words)

The Yoga For Freedom experience encouraged me to delve deeper into yoga, so I went to India in August 2010 to get my Bachelor of Science in Yoga at Swami Vivekananda Yoga University in Bangalore, where I graduated in June 2013. I then went to Singapore where I just completed 200 hours of hatha yoga teacher training certified by the Yoga Alliance. I was trying to find employment in Singapore, but the work permits are tight here, so I decided to go to Vietnam to work there as a yoga instructor at the California Fitness and Yoga center. I am currently single. With love and regards — Subash.

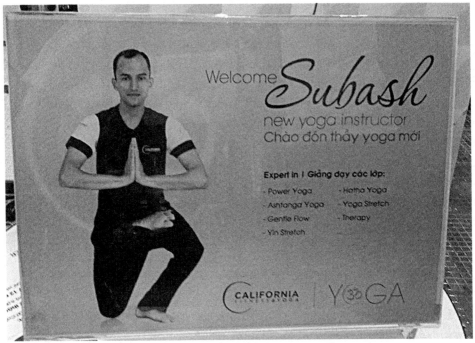

Placard announcing Subash's new job in Vietnam. Photo courtesy of Subash Adikhari.

Basu Panday (in his own words)

As the years have passed by, it has become clear to me that the Yoga for Freedom trek that helped to rescue Kamlari girls and helped raise funds for the Nepal Orphans Home was the beginning of something bigger. What we started was very important I felt. The kind of work we do can have an extremely positive effect on the Nepalese as well as all the Yogis who came and experienced yoga from another side, within Nepali culture and in Himalayan nature, to feel part of it all and inspire change in the community.

To be a part of that change, I focused on developing my company, Nepal Social Treks, and on trying to make the company grow and become the best it could, by creating a good team upon whom I could rely. The entire purpose is to create a local company in synergy with the culture and the tradition of the people of Nepal, and through our work to help the country to develop by helping and embracing all Nepalese. Hence, these last three years have been all about that, about traveling around Asia and Europe as well as making contacts in America, meeting people from all over the world who in one way or another helped or contributed to this change. Nepal Social Treks has kept our focus on Charity Yoga Treks, on Yoga and Meditation retreats, on climbing and trekking the Himalayas, and on helping our people and the foreigners who come to visit to create a synergy with each other.

From the first YFF group, Tingting was the one who helped me most to make this happen. She was our yoga teacher on several of the treks, but not only that,

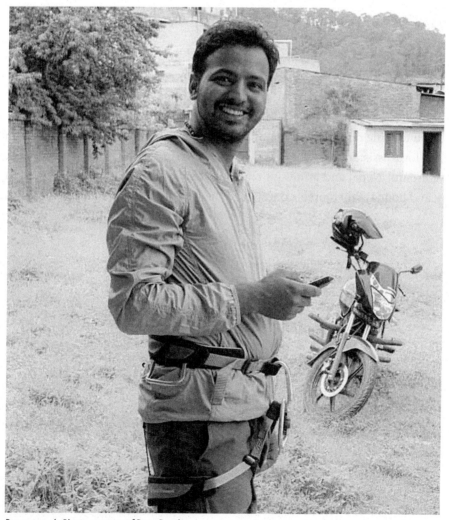

Basu at work. Photo courtesy of Basu Panday.

when she wasn't able to come she spread the word to her friends, and to other yoga teachers, and they have come full of energy and now are also a part of our project. The ultimate goal of all this work will be the Nepal Social Foundation which we hope will help to make possible all projects focused on the children in Nepal.

Personally, I know this is a lot of work. It isn't easy to combine family life and friendships with taking care of this project, but with enthusiasm and confidence I know it is possible to pursue our goals. Step by step, one thing at a time, I manage to have time for work, for this project, for my family and for those of you who may come to visit us here.

Namaste,

Basu Panday, Nepal Social Treks and Expedition,

Kathmandu, Nepal, www.nepalsocialtreks.com.

Buddha Saktia & Sun Tze

Basu told me recently that Buddha Saktia, our magnificent bus driver, and Sun Tze, his loyal assistant, and our porter on the YFF trip, are still helping travel groups move around Nepal and as always enjoying their work making others' vacations, trips, and holidays memorable ones. And they are still driving the very same bus!

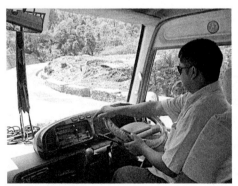
Buddha driving his bus.

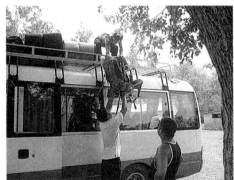
Sun Tze atop the bus, lending a hand.

Acknowledgements

Special thanks to the following people for their help in assembling this book: Minling Chuang and Jesse Bach for coming up with the original idea, and then coaxing me into getting involved with the project; Minling again for doing such a great job in her journal of recounting each day's activities (I relied heavily on her accounts to jog my own memory at times); Gabrielle Goodman for providing the scanner to upload all the handwritten journals; Cal Trause, Rachel Vincent and Jaime Furda for their diligent work transcribing the handwritten journals; Lauren Yanks for her initial, exceptional editorial insights; Minling for her assistance with the initial editing and structuring of the book; early readers Chris Lambert, Beth Wilson-Fish, Barbara Lewis, Nancy Wingenbach and Anup Kumar for their feedback and encouragement; Kitty Werner and Lawrence Meyers for their kind help with navigating the self-publishing world; Candace Koslen for her invaluable help in selecting and laying out the photographs; Candy again, as well as all the others who snapped the images we used in this book, for their brilliant photographs; Diana LeBlanc, for her mindful, thorough and professional final editing of the entire manuscript; and Jaime Lombardo for his exceptional skill and talent in designing the cover and layout of the book... Without all their help, this book would not have been possible.

A note about the journals: Joyce and David chose not to have their journals be a part of this book, a decision which I respected. All the others presented their journals with the clear understanding that they would be used in this book. I read the journals first, to get a general sense and feel for the material. It was a very humbling experience having been given the trust of so many people, with some of their most intimate thoughts from the trip. I went through the journals a second time, along with Minling and Lauren Yanks, to cull out the parts we thought were the most useful for the book. The criteria were simple: 1) Was it well written? 2) Did it provide insight into the person? 3) Did it provide valuable commentary on the trip? Once that was done, I turned the handwritten parts over to the various transcribers we recruited, who did the difficult, invaluable work of transcribing. I strung these pieces together in a rough outline of how I thought the book should be constructed. Minling and Lauren then gave me helpful feedback. Finally, nearly a year after the trip, I began writing the narrative portion of the book.

A note about the photos: All photos in the book are credited to the person who took the photograph and accompanied with a "Photo by…" credit, except the ones I took (no need to keep repeating my name). Where it wasn't clear who took them or impossible to find out, the photos are listed as "Photo Courtesy of [the source of the picture]".

Appendix 1

A Few Words from Michael Hess
Founder and Director of Operations of Nepal Orphans Home

May 1, 2009 (updated October 2013)

On behalf of Nepal Orphans Home, thank you for your interest in our work in Western Nepal. Publicity has in the past helped to give freedom and life to a child.

I would like to introduce you to one of those children, Sabbu, who was rescued this fall from indentured servitude. Her father died many years ago, her mother remarried and sold Sabbu to be done with her. Sabbu is 7 years old and has never hurt a soul; she is quiet, smiles a lot, and very helpful. Seven years old, she was a slave deprived of education, freedom, friends, a healthy environment, adequate clothing, nutrition, rest, warmth in the winter; and if that wasn't enough, abused. In seven short years to have lived a life worse than a Dickens tale you would think she would be sullen, withdrawn, and wracked with emotions. But she isn't.

Sabbu didn't know what life was supposed to be like; she simply accepted it as it unfolded, and did her best. She works really hard in school now, always helps our didi with her work without being asked to, and is respectful and sweet. In 2008, Nepal Orphans Home while working with SWAN, a local Tharu community group, took in 54 girls like Sabbu rescued by SWAN. When we are able to take a new girl, SWAN will rescue one more. Sadly there are hundreds of Sabbu's still living the nightmare of indentured servitude.

The Dang district in Western Nepal is one of about five that have traditionally sold their daughters to others. Brokers come each January and visit village after village and make arrangements for the girls' purchase. Parents are given on average 5000rs, or with the current exchange $62.50. In a part of Nepal that is one of the poorest, where most are unemployed and depend on very small plots of land for subsistence, where the average income is still less than $1.00 per day, this represents a great windfall, and they have one less mouth to feed. It is important to understand this aspect of the Nepalese culture to help understand how this practice could exist. Girls are reason for a parent's depression, or even worse a wife being ostracized by her in laws and husband should she not bear them a son. Girls grow up to be married, often very young, and will then leave her parents' house and live with and work for her in laws. Girls are deprived of an education most of the time so that they can help in the field; while boys are the little princes that receive the lion's share of food, have the warm clothes, go to school, and are spared the labor.

When a restaurant owner, an industry owner, or a wealthier family buys a girl, they put her to work. She is not paid, nor allowed to go to school. They are seldom allowed out of the establishment. If they live with the family that has bought them, they will be subject to the whims of all the family members who do not recognize the human in the little girl. The Kamlari girls are not able to have friends or make a society for themselves.

Interestingly these girls upon being freed have no anger with their parents, and though they have been mistreated, they will harbor no resentment or anger with the family that has bought her. Like Sabbu, they simply know this as life and can't contrast it with being a loved and cared for daughter. Laws have been passed and are on the books outlawing the Kamlari practice; but this hasn't had much effect on the practice. It is an economically and culturally fueled way of life.

As of May 1st, 2009 we have 92 ex-Kamlari girls in our homes, out of a total of 151 children that we care for.[1] As we are able to afford the cost to take care of another child and have room for her, we then authorize SWAN to rescue her. SWAN has a complete list of all the girls who have been sold in the Dang district, and most of those in neighboring districts. They will send a team of men and woman, all Tharu, to the establishment where the girl is working and talk to the owner of the girl. In almost every case the girls end up in a district far removed from their homes. By applying social pressure and reason the rescue team will usually persuade the owner to release the girl to them. Typically money isn't required in the exchange. The girl is asked if she wants to be freed and live in Lawajuni, which means New Beginnings, our Narti Home.[2] They have all said yes. The girls are then placed in Lawajuni and begin school. Those who have no parents are first on the list to be placed in one of our Dhapasi homes where the education is top notch in an English medium school. We receive papers from the VDC (village development committee) handing over the guardianship of the girls to Nepal Orphans Home. NOH has had a total of 101 girls brought to Lawajuni, nine of these have been repatriated with their families and remain under the monitor of SWAN to ensure they are cared for and not sold again. These girls returned to their families when an illness of, or the loss of a parent compelled them to return to care for the family. They all have gone willingly and without complaint; it is an admirable quality of these girls but one in which I regret they have had to learn.

NOH will raise all these girls, like all our children, in a manner no different than good parents raise their children. We guide them to either academic or vocational education, and we allow them to be children, to be cared for instead of being the care givers. We will ensure that they are strong and independent, with a clear vision of their future, prior to allowing them to venture out on their own. We are a family at NOH, a somewhat large one, but that only provides for a greater amount of love in our homes.

Please take time to read the updates section of www.nepalorphanshome.org to be absorbed by the life and times of these marvelous children. And for further information about NOH and the Kamlari system from a technical standpoint, or to review our standing as a 501(c)3 nonprofit organization, please contact the President of NOH Peter Hess at pehess@davidson.edu. Thank you very much.

Sincerely,

Michael Hess

Dhapasi, Nepal

---

[1] Currently (November 9, 2013), NOH operates five homes (known locally as Papa's Houses) in Dhapasi, all within a short walking distance of each other. Over half of the more than 140 children provided for in Papa's Houses are rescued Kamlari girls. Nepal Orphans Home and SWAN have been working separately, by mutual decision, since 2011.

[2] As of April 2010, Lawajuni House is no longer operated by NOH.

Appendix 2

Nepal Orphans Home Report of Interviews with Rescued Kamlari Girls

Peter Hess

President of Nepal Orphans Home

November 13, 2008 (updated October 2013)

"Child labor is a reality for one in every three Nepalese children, with each child laborer a tangible living symbol of a vulnerable and marginalized family; a reminder of an inadequate education system, a government's inability to act, and above all, a society's acceptance of a social wrong. Child labor destroys children's potential, robbing them of opportunities and perpetuating a cycle of poverty and marginalization." [1]

As affirmed in the United Nations Universal Declaration of Human Rights (Articles 1 and 4): "All human beings are born free and equal in dignity and rights," and "No one shall be held in slavery or servitude." Moreover, as stated in the United Nations Convention on the Rights of the Child (Article 2): "All appropriate measures [should be taken] to ensure that the child is protected against all forms of discrimination or punishment on the basis of the status, activities, expressed opinions, or beliefs of the child's parents, legal guardians or family members."

The Kamlari system in rural Nepal, whereby poor families are pressured by hardship to sell their daughters as indentured laborers, is an affront to humanity. Nepal Orphans Home, together with Society Welfare Action Nepal, is committed to rescuing and providing for Kamlari girls and ultimately ending this tragic practice.

Between October 17 and 19, Nepal Orphans Home (NOH) conducted interviews with ten of the rescued Kamlari girls at the Lawajuni hostel in Narti, near Lamahi in the Dang district of western Nepal. In addition, on October 31, six rescued Kamlari girls now residing at Papa's House in Dhapasi in the Kathmandu valley were interviewed. Before summarizing these interviews, a brief background to the system of Kamlari will be given.

Child Labor in Nepal

In 2001 the International Labor Organization (ILO) estimated there were over 17,000 Kamaiya children employed outside their homes, most under some form of bonded labor. At the time, the ILO estimated that 75% of these children were working more than 12 hours per day, 43% were working without pay, 15% were below the age of 10, and 95% did not attend school.[2]

Kamaiyas, under a system existing in Nepal for decades, refer to agricultural laborers forced to work for landowners to repay debts incurred earlier, sometimes by their parents or grandparents. The overwhelming majority of Kamaiyas are Tharu, an ethnic group indigenous to the terai, a fertile region of Nepal along the border of India which includes the five western districts of Dang, Banke, Bardiya, Kailali, and Kanchanpur. Until the 1960s, the Tharu were the primary inhabitants of the terai, in large part due to their natural immunity to malaria. Then malaria eradication along with land reform, intended by the powers in Kathmandu to help integrate the nation, led to hill people moving into the lowlands of the terai. Many Tharus did not have legal title to their land and were soon displaced, becoming sharecroppers. Meager wages and the exorbitant interest rates charged by the landowners on the small loans taken by the Tharu, whether to buy seed or to pay for medical emergencies, funerals, or weddings, resulted in unsustainable debts, eventually binding the Tharu families to the same landowners. Often to have any access to land, the Kamaiyas would have to pledge children, usually daughters, as working collateral. The bonded children would also be forced to labor for the landowners.[3]

In July 2000, the Nepali parliament declared the practice of Kamaiya and the associated debts of the bonded laborer illegal.[4] There were existing laws in Nepal intended to protect children. For example, the 1990 Constitution of Nepal protected the interests of children by conferring on them certain fundamental rights. The 1992 Children's Act ensured their 'physical, mental, and intellectual development' ... [and] ...'contained a number of provisions on child labor.'[5]

Moreover, Nepal has ratified ILO Convention 182 (Outlawing the Worst Forms of Child Labor) and Convention 138 (Restricting work carried out by children below a minimum age) and the UN Convention on the Rights of the Child. 6 Nepal was even chosen by ILO and IPEC (International Program on the Elimination of Child Labor) as one of the first three countries in which to implement a large-scale Time Bound Program to eliminate the worst forms of child labor, including bonded child labor.[7]

Nepal is one of the poorest countries in the world, however, ranking 142nd out of 177 countries in the United Nations Development Program's Human Development Index.[8] The combination of political instability, corruption, the lack of a coherent development strategy, and the Maoist insurgency have all contributed to the lack of enforcement of this legislation. Moreover, Nepal's Child Labor Act of 2000 does not cover family-based work, work in private homes, or work in agriculture--which account for the overwhelming majority of Nepalese child workers. [9]

Ironically there is evidence that the legislation that freed the Kamaiyas has actually increased the practice of Kamlari, as destitute parents remain unable to provide for their children. That is ex-Kamaiyas are still being pressured by land-owners to sell their children to the landowners as laborers as a condition for leasing land. Or, poor families without land may contract their daughters for employment outside their villages.[10]

To wit, as reported by the Nepali non-governmental organization, Friends of Needy Children...

"In five districts (Dang, Banke, Bardiya, Kailali, and Kanchanpur) of western Nepal, families 'sell" their daughters as bonded laborers in nearby landlord's houses or in faraway cities for an average of Rs 3,500 ($50) a year, paid to the family. These girls are called "Kamlaris" (Indentured Daughters). An estimated 25,000 girls have been indentured from this area. These girls, as young as 7 years, have never been away from home, and do not speak the language of the families for whom they work. No one checks on their welfare; the parents often do not know where their daughters live. The situation is tailor-made for abuse. Some of the girls never return. They do not go to school, and they work from early morning to late at night." [11]

Results of Interviews

The mission of Nepal Orphans Home (NOH) is attending to the total welfare of children in Nepal who are orphaned, abandoned, or not supported by their parents. Currently for nearly seventy children, our Papa's Houses in Dhapasi provide for the basic needs of food, shelter, and clothing, as well as schooling and health care, and administer to emotional needs with love and compassion. Nepal Orphans Home seeks not just to rescue these children from abject poverty, but to enable them to grow up in a nurturing environment where they can develop and realize their potentials.

Thus, it was a natural extension of our mission to collaborate with the nongovernmental organization, Society Welfare Action Nepal (SWAN) to provide for rescued Kamlari girls in the Dang district. The Lawajuni (New Life) hostel was founded at Narti in early 2008. Since then, over fifty girls rescued by SWAN are being provided for by Nepal Orphans Home...either at Lawajuni or at the Papa's House for girls in Dhapasi. The purpose of the interviews in October was to understand better the conditions of the Kamlaris so that we can mobilize the resources to provide for more girls rescued from lives of exploitation.

In the interviews of the sixteen former Kamlaris, we asked for their current age, the age they began work as a Kamlari, the number of employers, their job(s) as a Kamlari, if they liked working as a Kamlari (and why); whether they lived with their employer, whether they attended school after becoming a Kamlari, their current class or grade in school, their favorite subject, the number of brothers and sisters they had, whether they were happy not to be a Kamlari (and why), what they would like to be or do when they were older.

We would ask the questions. Sushmita, an impressive young Nepali woman recently hired by Nepal Orphans Home, would sit next to the girls and translate. The girls would then reply to Sushmita, who would translate (and paraphrase) back to us. Although a standard set of questions was asked, the interviews were fairly free-flowing. We heard sometimes about the girl's family histories. We always prefaced the interviews with how we were interested in their stories and ended with our appreciation for their talking with us. We tried to make the girls as comfortable as possible; and occasionally by the end of the interviews we were even able to have them smiling.

No pretense is made that the interviews were conducted in a rigorous academic manner or that the sample of girls was random. Of the forty-two girls then living at Lawajuni, thirteen were interviewed--and ten of these girls are former Kamlaris. Of the forty-five girls then living at Papa's House in Dhapasi, the nine who had earlier been at Lawajuni were interviewed, including the six former Kamlaris.[12] While each girl and her story are unique, we found some common themes.

To begin with a summary of the descriptive statistics, the current ages of the 16 rescued Kamlaris interviewed ranged from 11 to 16 years old. The ages the girls reported beginning work as Kamlaris ranged from 3 to 12 years old. Some of the girls had worked as a Kamlari for as little as one year; others had worked nine or ten years before being rescued. The number of employers the girls had ranged from one to six. All of the rescued Kamlaris interviewed had lived with their employers. Most did not attend school while working as a Kamlari. Consequently, most are behind in school and are now attending classes well below the representative ages. When asked their favorite subject in school, math was mentioned by nearly half, with Nepali a close second. Four of the fifteen girls expressing an aspiration, wanted to become teachers, three aspired to becoming doctors, and three to becoming nurses. Vocations also expressed by the girls were: pilot, singer, social worker, cricket player, and working in water supply.

When asked what type of work they did, or to describe a typical day as a Kamlari, all noted they worked in the households of their employers. Often the Kamlari would rise before dawn and begin a day that included fetching water, cleaning the house, washing dishes, doing laundry, and frequently cooking. Sometimes the tasks might include feeding cows and cleaning the shed, collecting wood from the forest, and caring for children of the employer. Their days usually ended well after sunset.

Not surprisingly, none of the girls liked being a Kamlari, although most seemed to accept their fates, recognizing the poverty of their parents or guardians. Many of the Kamlaris had lost one or both parents. Others were from broken families. Almost all had brothers and sisters. If their parents had remarried, then the girls often experienced harsh treatment from step-parents before their sale.[13] The most frequent reason given by the girls for disliking their positions as Kamlaris was not being able to go to school. Also mentioned all too frequently was the ill-treatment suffered, including being scolded and beaten by the employers, insufficient food to eat, and having to sleep on the floor. Most received no money for their work, although their parents or guardians might have received payment for their sale. Some, however, did report earning a pittance.

When asked if they were happy not to be Kamlari, there was universal agreement. Just as they all would emphatically shake their heads no when asked earlier if they liked working as a Kamlari, the girls would clearly affirm their happiness with no longer being Kamlari. Here too, the most prevalent reason was the opportunity to attend school. Also mentioned was no longer being required to work, no longer being subject to scolding and beating by employers, and now having friends, freedom and enough to eat. In sum, the results from this small survey correspond to the literature on Kamlaris.[14]

Society Welfare Action Nepal

While in Lamahi, we also talked with the leaders of Society Welfare Action Nepal (SWAN). Founded in 1994, SWAN's stated mission is to eliminate poverty through the mobilization of the community. In particular, SWAN is dedicated to the eradication of the Kamlari system and works to rescue and rehabilitate girls sold into indentured servitude.[15] SWAN's efforts are supported by Friends of Needy Children and Plan Nepal, among other organizations. As noted, Nepal Orphans Home (NOH) has collaborated with SWAN to provide for those girls rescued by SWAN who are unable to return to their parents or guardians. NOH has restored two buildings on the public school grounds in Narti, near Lamahi in the Dang district of western Nepal and provides shelter, food, clothing, and schooling for the rescued Kamlaris.

In addition to actually rescuing Kamlaris from their servitude, SWAN seeks to raise awareness of this terrible practice. SWAN recognizes, however, that underlying the problem of indentured child labor is profound poverty. Thus, SWAN is working to restore land rights to the poor and has a program to train farmers on improved technologies. SWAN also has programs for remedial education, vocational training, microcredit, and family planning.[16]

Endnotes

1. This quotation is from "An Analysis of the Determinants of Child Labor in Nepal, the Policy Environment and Response," by B. Gilligan, Country Report (January 2003), Understanding Children's Work Project, page 13.

2. See "Understanding Children's Work in Nepal," Country Report, July 2003, Understanding Children's Work Project, University of Rome, page 27.

3. See United Nations Commission on Human Rights (Geneva, June 2000) at http://www.anti-slavery.org/archive/submission/submission2000-Nepal.htm and "Nepal: Land Reforms, Key to Social Harmony," by Suman Pradhan (Sept. 15, 2008) at http://www.ipsnews.net/news.asp?idnews=34736.

4. As noted on the Government of Nepal's Ministry of Land Reforms and Management web site, the eradication of the Kamaiya system meant that "... no landlord can employ anybody as Kamaiya, and the debt or sauki has been declared null and void. If anybody wishes to engage an agricultural and household laborer, s/he should be paid to minimum wage and the working hours as laid down by labor law should be maintained." See: http://www.molrm.gov.np/programs.php.

5. See International Labor Organization, "National Legislation and Policies Against Child Labor in Nepal," http://www.ilo.org .

6. ILO Convention No. 182 stipulates that any person under 18 is to be protected from employment in the worst forms of child labor, including slavery, debt bondage, forced recruitment in armed conflicts, prostitution, pornography, illicit activities, and work that has adverse effects on the child's safety, health (physical or mental), and moral development. See "Bonded Labor Among Child Workers of the Kamaiya System: A Rapid Assessment," by Shiva Sharma, Bijendra Basnyat, and Ganesh GC, International Labor Organization, International Program on the Elimination of Child Labor, Nov. 2001, Geneva, pages 9-11.

It should also be noted that bonded child labor in Nepal exists outside of Kamaiya system... with children found working in hotels, restaurants, brick kilns, stone quarries, and the carpet industry, among other areas. ILO-IPEC (International Labor Organization-International Program on the Elimination of Child Labor) estimates 12,000 Nepalese girls are trafficked each year with most ending up in brothels in India...with nearly 40% trafficked before the age of 14... See "Understanding Children's Work in Nepal," pages 27-28.

7. See Sharma et al, page 9.

8. The Human Development Index is a weighted average of life expectancy at birth, school enrollment rates, adult literacy rates, and per capita income (adjusted for differences in purchasing power). See Human Development Report 2007/2008, United Nations Development Program (Palgrave Macmillan, 2007).

9. See "Understanding Children's Work in Nepal," page 34. It should be noted that even in the United States child labor laws are not comprehensively enforced. In particular, child labor is not well protected in the agricultural sector.

10. As noted by Sharma et al, under the Kamaiya system there are two basically types of child laborers: those who work in or around the village of origin usually as domestic servants and agricultural laborers, and those who migrate to urban areas and work as domestic servants or in the informal service sector (page 13). Often middlemen arrange the contracts for child laborers during the Maghi holiday in January of each year.

11. From Friends of Needy Children (FNC), "Indentured Daughters Program" brochure.

12. That is, in addition to the sixteen former Kamlari girls, six girls who were not former Kamlaris were interviewed. These six (three still at Lawajuni in Narti and three now at Papa's House in Dhapasi), initially brought to Lawajuni by SWAN because of their desperate circumstances, have also been rescued from hardship.

13. As described by Gilligan (page 65), "Widespread legal and illegal discrimination against women and girls in issues such as property, inheritance, access to justice, education, and health care, all conspire to increase the levels and types of vulnerabilities which create the supply of girls for child labor. It also permits child marriage, limited mobility and control over income, a lack of access to resources, an unequal distribution of household work, drudgery, celebrates boy children at the expense of girls, and offers limited protection from domestic violence. "

14. See Sharma et al.

15. There are other NGOs involved in the Kamlari abolition movement, including Friends of Needy Children (FNC) and Nepalese Youth Opportunity Foundation (NYOF).

16. Sharma et al. (page 37) attribute the child labor problem among children of the Kamaiyas mainly to their large family sizes and landlessness. Sadly, Sharma et al. (page 40) also observe, "Although the government has promised to redistribute land to ex-Kamaiya laborers, very few Kamaiyas have been issued with the necessary certification to claim the land." And, as Gilligan (page 52) notes, "Without the capacity to absorb existing child laborers into rehabilitation programs and alternatives, 'rescued' child laborers will find themselves, as did the Kamaiyas, vulnerable to further and perhaps worse exploitation."